The
Pregnancy
QUESTION
&ANSWER
Book

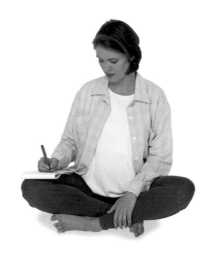

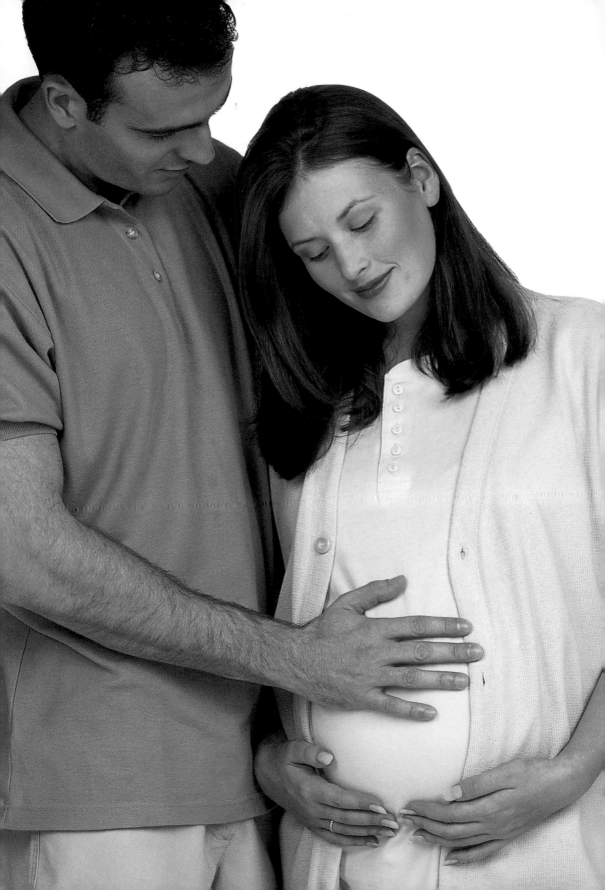

The Pregnancy QUESTION & ANSWER *Book*

Dr Christoph Lees MD, MRCOG, BSc

Dr Karina Reynolds MD, FRCSEd, MRCOG

Grainne McCartan RGN, RM, BScHons, MA

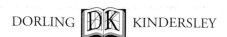

DORLING **DK** KINDERSLEY

LONDON, NEW YORK, MUNICH, MELBOURNE, DELHI

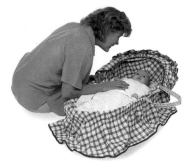

REVISED EDITION
PROJECT EDITOR Julie Whitaker
DESIGNER Edward Kinsey
EDITOR Claire Cross
ART EDITOR Glenda Fisher
MANAGING ART EDITOR Tracey Ward

ORIGINAL EDITION
MANAGING EDITOR Jemima Dunne
PROJECT EDITOR Jacqueline Jackson
EDITOR Claire Cross
MANAGING ART EDITOR Philip Gilderdale
SENIOR ART EDITOR Karen Ward
ART EDITOR Glenda Fisher
DESIGNER Chloë Steers
PHOTOGRAPHY Steve Gorton and Andy Crawford
PRODUCTION Antony Heller

First published in Great Britain in 1997 by Dorling Kindersley Limited
80 Strand, London WC2R 0RL

A Penguin Company

4 6 8 10 9 7 5 3

Reprinted 2000
This edition 2002

A CIP catalogue record for this book is available from the British Library

ISBN 0 7513 3975 X

Colour reproduced by Colourscan, Singapore
Printed and bound in Singapore by Star Standard

See our complete catalogue at
www.dk.com

FOREWORD

During the past five to ten years, a bewildering number of new techniques have been introduced into the field of obstetrics and midwifery, all aimed at improving your prospects of having a normal, healthy baby. For example, ultrasound scanning, assisted conception techniques such as IVF, and major advances in the early diagnosis of genetic and chromosomal defects, are just a few of the discoveries that have revolutionized pregnancy care. At the same time, there has been a movement towards making pregnancy and childbirth a more natural and fulfilling experience for both mother and partner. Women are being offered different choices about the type of antenatal care they receive and where they should give birth.

All these issues and many more are explored in a simple question-and-answer format in this book. The authors are known to me personally to be a highly experienced team of two obstetricians and a midwife whose advice is both practical and professional. They have managed to communicate the more complex medical advances, and advice on more practical matters such as the preparations you need to make for birth whether in hospital or home, or choices for pain relief in labour, in a brilliantly clear and down-to-earth way.

I believe that this book will help you to make informed choices in your pregnancy in partnership with those looking after you and that this information will make your pregnancy a more enjoyable and rewarding experience.

Professor Stuart Campbell DSc FRCOG FRCPEd
DEPARTMENT OF OBSTETRICS AND GYNAECOLOGY
St George's Hospital
Tooting
London UK

CONTENTS

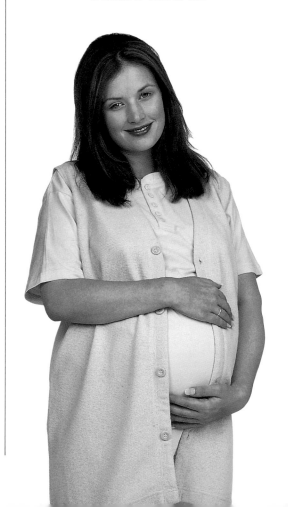

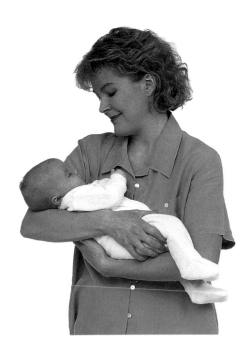

INTRODUCTION

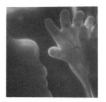 Without a doubt, having a baby is one of the most exciting, challenging, and life-changing experiences that life offers women. Having a healthy, happy baby is all-important, and you want the best advice and care for you and your baby. However, pregnancy and childbirth are uncharted territory for new mothers-to-be and their partners, who suddenly find that they need to understand and decide on vital issues such as antenatal care, what types of pain relief to use in labour, and where and how to have the new baby.

Changing attitudes to childbirth

The medical approach to childbirth has changed dramatically during the last few years, particularly in the developed world. Traditionally, until the 1950s, most births took place in the home, but with the advent of state medical health services and structured antenatal care for all, by the 1960s most births were taking place in hospital. With the current swing away from the medicalization of childbirth and towards the use of natural methods, antenatal care is moving away from direct (and often impersonal) hospital supervision and towards the midwife, and there is an increase in the number of women wanting, and having, a home birth. Understandably, with such major changes in approach, women today may be uncertain as to what is best in pregnancy and childbirth.

What this book aims to provide

One thing is certain: women are now playing a much greater part in making choices about many aspects of their pregnancies and labours. Doctors and midwives are increasingly giving women the chance to decide what they want. And to make an informed decision, whether it is about invasive tests, pain relief, or induction of labour, women need to be aware of all the facts.

In the past, women have been confronted by a barrage of conflicting and, at times, unreliable information from different sources. This book aims, in a simple question-and-answer format, to provide a source of detailed, balanced, and up-to-date information so that, armed with knowledge and confidence, women can assess, decide, and take a more active part in planning their pregnancies and labours – working with (not against) their professional carers.

Easily accessible information

The book is divided into chapters, beginning with pre-conception advice on preparation for pregnancy, fertility problems, and early pregnancy. Chapter 2 describes your choices in antenatal care. In Chapter 3, we explain in detail how your baby develops. Chapter 4 outlines what happens to your body during pregnancy, and also gives an indication of some of the emotional changes that you may experience. Advice on diet and keeping fit during your pregnancy is covered in Chapter 5. Chapter 6 outlines potential problems that may arise during pregnancy. Labour and birth are discussed in Chapter 7. The final chapter offers practical advice on coping during the first six weeks of your baby's life.

Throughout the book, each question is answered with equal seriousness; on some issues, however, there are discussion point boxes where controversial or difficult ideas or approaches are outlined further. Wherever possible, the advice given is explanatory, rather than dictatorial, and the reader is provided with cross-references to further sources of information, in order to allow informed choices.

Who are the authors?

This book is written from the collective professional and personal knowledge of two specialist doctors and one midwife, and we are well aware that each pregnancy is a unique and special experience. We also recognize that there are many ways of doing things – even in medical procedures. The book's questions and answers reflect some of the many queries (from the highly technical to the emotional) that we are frequently asked on a daily basis by pregnant women and by women in labour.

We hope that all mothers-to-be and their partners who read this book will find the guidance they need to help them towards a happier, healthier pregnancy and labour.

Dr Christoph Lees
Dr Karina Reynolds
Grainne McCartan

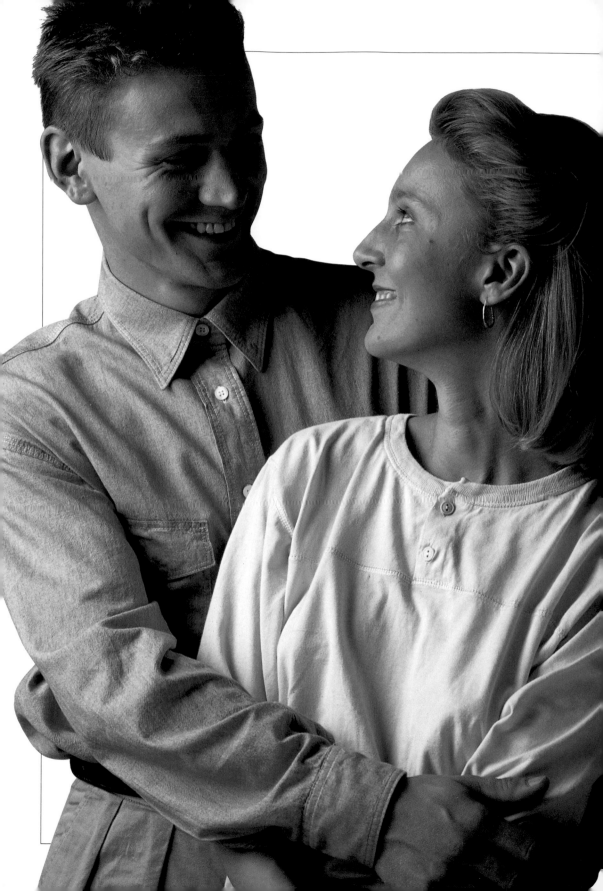

PREPARING FOR PREGNANCY

Deciding to have a baby is one of the most momentous decisions you can ever make. The impact that it will have on your body and daily life will be huge and possibly unsettling, but for most people the prospect of having a son or a daughter far outweighs any physical problems or lifestyle changes. Being fully prepared for pregnancy in both mind and body is extremely important; this chapter explains why you and your partner should attempt to improve your general health before trying to conceive as well as discussing fertility problems. As you begin your preparation, your questions and concerns as prospective parents are answered.

PREPARING YOURSELF

Q DO I NEED A MEDICAL CHECK-UP BEFORE TRYING TO CONCEIVE?

A Although no specific check-up is necessary, it is a good idea to check with your doctor to make sure that your cervical smear tests are up to date and normal – any treatment for abnormal smears should be carried out before pregnancy. Your doctor will also establish whether you are immune to rubella (German measles); if not, you can be protected by an injection before conception (see opposite). More thorough medical investigations are usually not necessary unless you have had problems with previous pregnancies or have a long-standing or serious medical condition.

Q WHAT CAN I DO TO IMPROVE MY CHANCES OF CONCEIVING?

A You can ensure that you and your partner are in the best of health by improving your diet and your lifestyle. Ideally, you should both cut out (or at least cut down on) cigarettes, alcohol, and illicit drugs six months before conception and reduce your stress levels at home and at work. You should also try to make love around the time that you ovulate (see below) when you are most fertile. Doctors recommend that you take folic acid supplements for three months before conceiving and during your pregnancy because this can reduce the risk of neural tube defects such as spina bifida.

WHEN AM I MOST LIKELY TO CONCEIVE?

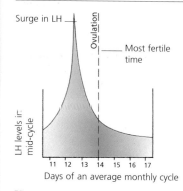

HORMONAL SURGE
The diagram (above) shows the LH surge indicating that an egg is about to be released.

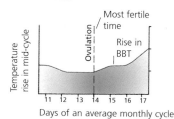

TEMPERATURE RISE
The diagram (above) shows the small rise in temperature that occurs around the time of ovulation.

The two or three days around ovulation (the time that an egg is produced from your ovary) is when you are most likely to become pregnant. This is normally in the middle of your monthly cycle. You can work out your most fertile period by these methods· by using an ovulation predictor kit or by the Basal Body Temperature method (BBT) (see below).

Using an ovulation kit
The kit tests urine for an LH (luteinizing hormone) surge. This hormone is produced by the brain and causes the release of eggs from the ovaries each month. Begin testing a few days before the middle of your cycle.

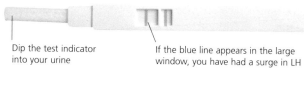

Dip the test indicator into your urine

If the blue line appears in the large window, you have had a surge in LH

Using the BBT method
Take your temperature every day. At ovulation there is a rise of about ½° above 37°C after which your temperature stays constant until menstruation.

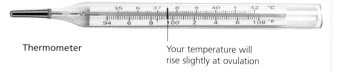

Thermometer

Your temperature will rise slightly at ovulation

Q WHY SHOULD WE GIVE UP SMOKING, ILLICIT DRUGS, AND ALCOHOL?

A Healthy parents usually have healthier babies, so if you both smoke (even as few as five to ten cigarettes daily), regularly drink alcohol, or take illicit drugs, you may reduce your chances of conception. Once pregnant, you also risk having a smaller and possibly an unhealthy baby who will need specialist care at birth (see p. 228).

Q I TAKE DRUGS FOR A MEDICAL CONDITION, SHOULD I STOP?

A No, do not stop taking your medication unless advised by your doctor. If you have epilepsy, high blood pressure, diabetes or other conditions that need long-term medication, your medication may need to be adapted once you are pregnant. Do not take any drugs you can buy over the counter unless you have consulted a doctor or pharmacist (see p. 107).

Q SHOULD I TAKE VITAMINS TO ENSURE A HEALTHIER BABY?

A If you eat a balanced diet, you are probably getting adequate vitamins – with the possible exception of folic acid. Doctors used to prescribe iron tablets routinely for all pregnant women but it is now only thought to be necessary if you are anaemic. Women on restricted diets, such as vegetarians and especially vegans, may need to take iron and vitamin B12 supplements if their diet provides insufficient amounts. Ask your doctor or midwife about this.

Q ARE THERE ANY RISKS INVOLVED IN TAKING FOLIC ACID SUPPLEMENTS?

A No there are not, but if you don't want to take supplements, you should make sure that your diet includes certain foods, such as dark green, leafy vegetables, that are high in folic acid (see p. 105). It is always a good idea to discuss issues like this with your doctor.

Q HOW SOON AFTER STOPPING CONTRACEPTION CAN I CONCEIVE?

A Ideally, you should stop taking the Pill a few months before you consider pregnancy. This allows time for your normal period cycle to become re-established and for your pregnancy to be accurately dated. If you have a coil, it is quite safe to conceive as soon as it is removed. If you have progesterone injections, you should wait at least three months before trying to conceive.

WHEN IS THE BEST TIME TO GET PREGNANT?

The ideal age
There is no ideal time to get pregnant; the advantages and disadvantages at any age will depend on your state of health, work situation, and relationship. Young women may not be as psychologically and emotionally prepared for pregnancy and the demands of childcare, while more mature women, that is, mothers over 35, are at greater risk of developing complications such as high blood pressure; and there is a higher risk of their children having chromosomal abnormalities, such as Down's syndrome (see p. 145).

After a miscarriage
Although it is possible for you to conceive as soon as you have your next period, sometimes it takes a little longer to be ready emotionally. If you have had several miscarriages, specific tests may be carried out to determine the cause and it is probably best to wait for the results of these before trying again.

After a rubella (German measles) injection
The injection contains a small amount of inactivated live virus that your body recognizes as foreign and to which it builds up an immunity. It takes three months to build up this immunity and during this time it is unwise to risk exposing a developing baby to the rubella virus.

Spacing between pregnancies
This depends on various issues such as personal relationships and work commitments, but from a medical viewpoint, a year between pregnancies is recommended to ensure your recovery. If you become pregnant while you are looking after and possibly breastfeeding a very young baby, this may take a toll on your physical and mental reserves and your health could suffer as your body tries to cope with these demands.

After a Caesarean
A Caesarean involves abdominal surgery that can take many weeks to heal, so you will probably need longer to recover than if you have had a normal delivery.

FERTILITY AND CONCEPTION

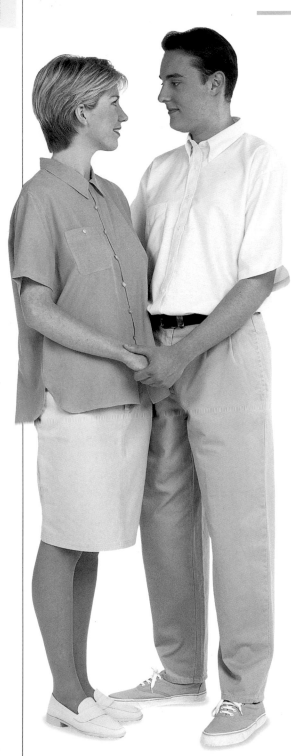

COMMON QUESTIONS ABOUT FERTILITY

QUESTIONS	ANSWERS
Will conception be difficult ...	
because I have painful or heavy periods?	Probably not, but if you have severe symptoms see your doctor to rule out an underlying cause such as fibroids, endometriosis or a pelvic infection.
because my periods are infrequent or irregular?	Possibly. Irregularity makes it harder to plan a pregnancy. You may need medical advice to work out when you ovulate (see p. 12).
because both my partner and I are over 30?	Male fertility is not greatly affected by age, but the fertility of women over 35 does gradually decline.
because we both lead very busy, stressful lives, and hardly ever feel like making love?	Too much stress can put you off sex, and may also make your periods irregular. Regular exercise such as yoga and swimming, can help to relieve stress. If regular sex is unlikely, find out when you ovulate (see p. 12) and try to make love then.
because my partner had a sperm test and was told he had a low sperm count?	A low sperm count reduces a man's fertility and usually means that your partner needs special tests, and maybe treatment. There are several causes; simple treatment includes wearing looser underwear and reducing cigarettes and alcohol.
because I recently had a pelvic infection?	Severe or recurrent pelvic infections may lead to blocked or damaged Fallopian tubes (see opposite).

Q WHAT CAN REDUCE MY CHANCES OF CONCEPTION?

A Even if you are having sexual intercourse regularly, three main factors can reduce your chances of becoming pregnant: irregular or non-existent ovulation; damage to the Fallopian tubes; and reduced numbers of, or poor quality sperm. (See the panel, left, for other factors.)

Q WHEN SHOULD WE CONSULT A DOCTOR?

A Don't worry if you do not become pregnant at once. You have a 90 per cent chance of becoming pregnant within one year and a 95 per cent chance within two years. However, you should probably consult your doctor after trying for one year. If either of you suffers from a medical condition or if you are over 35 years old, ask for specialist advice earlier.

Q WHAT IS MY CHANCE OF CONCEIVING EVERY TIME I HAVE INTERCOURSE?

A If you have intercourse at the most opportune period of your menstrual cycle, around the time of ovulation (when the egg is released from the ovary), and neither you nor your partner have any fertility problems, then you have a roughly 25 per cent chance of conceiving. At other times of your menstrual cycle, because sperm survives for only three days and there may be no egg available to be fertilized, the chances of conceiving are much less. An egg may be released from the ovary at times other than mid-cycle, however.

Q I'M 45. CAN I GET PREGNANT NORMALLY?

A If you are still having regular periods, then you are theoretically fertile. However, the egg quality is not as good as it was previously, and in some cycles your ovaries may not release eggs. So, it would be advisable to seek medical advice if you want to get pregnant.

Q MY PARTNER IS GOING TO HAVE A SPERM TEST – WHAT IS THIS?

A If you have had problems conceiving, a sperm test will determine your partner's fertility. The sperm will be examined to see how well they move and how many abnormal sperm there are. The lower the proportion of healthy sperm, the more difficult it is for you to get pregnant, and the longer it may take.

Q MY FALLOPIAN TUBES ARE BLOCKED – DOES THIS MEAN I'M INFERTILE?

A The egg travels from the ovary to the womb through a Fallopian tube. This can be blocked or damaged by pelvic or abdominal infections, or an ectopic pregnancy (see p. 18), which reduce your chances of pregnancy.

Q WHEN ARE FERTILITY DRUGS USED?

A Fertility drugs are used when hormonal problems prevent ovulation (the release of eggs from the ovaries).

Q IF I TAKE FERTILITY DRUGS, WILL I HAVE TWINS OR MORE?

A Not necessarily, although the odds do increase; your chance of having twins is one in ten, compared to one in 90 for women who do not take fertility drugs.

Q AM I LESS FERTILE IF I'VE BEEN TAKING THE CONTRACEPTIVE PILL?

A There is no evidence that using the combined oral contraceptive pill (COCP), even for prolonged periods, reduces your fertility. Although some people notice that their periods are less regular when they stop taking the pill, this is because the pill makes periods regular, so after stopping it, your periods may return to a more irregular cycle.

Q MY PERIODS ARE VERY IRREGULAR. WILL I HAVE LESS CHANCE OF CONCEIVING?

A This depends on why your periods are irregular. Irregular periods make timing intercourse to achieve conception much more difficult. They can also be a sign of you being underweight, having a thyroid problem, or a condition called polycystic ovary syndrome (PCOS). A blood test and ultrasound scan can usually help determine what is the cause of your irregular periods and whether you need any medical treatment.

Q WHAT OTHER OPTIONS ARE THERE TO HELP ME CONCEIVE?

A If simple treatments fail, options include surgery to unblock your Fallopian tubes, stronger fertility drugs, or your partner having treatment to improve his sperm count. If these fail, you may be offered assisted conception (see p. 16).

ASSISTED CONCEPTION

Q HOW IS CONCEPTION ASSISTED?

A There are several ways of bringing together the sperm and egg to achieve fertilization. The most commonly performed procedures are IVF (In Vitro Fertilization) and ICSI (Intra Cytoplasmic Sperm Injection). IVF is now a relatively common procedure, and is becoming cheaper as more people are trained in it. IVF has also become more successful in recent years. GIFT (Gamete Intra-Fallopian Transfer) and IUI (Intra Uterine Insemination) are still performed in some clinics, but less commonly now.

Q WHAT ARE IVF AND ICSI?

A IVF is fertilization of the sperm and egg "in the test tube" (more commonly a sterile plastic dish). It involves mixing sperm and eggs (typically 100,000 sperm to one egg) to allow one or more embryos to form. In certain conditions – where the sperm count is low or if sperm are unable to fertilize eggs – one sperm may be injected directly into the centre (nucleus) of one egg using a very fine needle; this procedure is called ICSI. In some circumstances, if sperm cannot be obtained from semen, they can be taken straight out of the testicles under an anaesthetic; this procedures is known as TESA (Testicular Sperm Aspiration).

Q WHAT ARE THE SUCCESS RATES OF THE DIFFERENT METHODS?

A There are two elements to consider here. The IVF procedure has a 30 per cent success rate for conception, while that for ICSI is slightly higher, at 40 per cent. However, as in the case of natural conception, becoming pregnant does not guarantee a healthy pregnancy and baby, as any pregnancy may miscarry early on (up to 12 weeks is considered the "risk" time). IVF has a successful pregnancy rate of 25 per cent, and ICSI has a successful pregnancy rate of 30 per cent.

Q HOW MANY CYCLES OF IVF CAN I HAVE?

A It is generally agreed that the chances of attaining a successful pregnancy with IVF tend to diminish after the fourth cycle, but couples have made up to 10 attempts before achieving pregnancy.

Q WHAT ARE THE RISKS OF TAKING DRUGS TO HELP ME OVULATE?

A Fertility drugs such as clomiphene citrate tablets (clomid) and hCG injections work by increasing your chances of ovulating (releasing eggs from your ovary). The number of eggs that you release cannot be controlled precisely, so if you were having IUI, there would be a chance that several eggs could be released at once, thereby increasing your risk of multiple pregnancy (twins, triplets, or more). In addition, there is a risk, particularly with injections, of "ovarian hyperstimulation", a condition in which the ovaries grow very large, with cysts in them. You can become dangerously sick, with abdominal pain and dehydration, and may sometimes need hospital admission and expert treatment. On another note, however, there is no current firm evidence of a link between IVF treatment and cancer of the ovary.

Q WILL MY PREGNANCY BE DIFFERENT FROM ONE THAT OCCURS NORMALLY?

A Medically, your pregnancy is unlikely to be any different from anyone else's, unless you have a chronic condition for which you are having treatment and needed IVF or ICSI. If you have twins or triplets, the situation is different from that of expecting a "singleton", and you will need much closer medical care. In any event, the emotional investment by you and your partner may well be higher, as you may have been trying to get pregnant for some time. This may modify your thoughts on prenatal diagnosis and the kind of delivery that you would like.

Q I'M HAVING IVF. CAN I DONATE MY EGGS (OOCYTES) TO SOMEONE ELSE?

A This will depend on the laws of the particular country in which you are receiving your fertility treatment. Sometimes, if many eggs have been collected from you and not all of them are needed in your treatment, you may agree to donate some of them to a couple if the prospective mother, for whatever reason, has few or no eggs of her own. This may reduce the cost of your IVF treatment under what are known as "egg sharing" schemes. However, the practice of selling unwanted eggs to strangers has now become illegal in some countries, including the UK.

WHAT HAPPENS IN ICSI?

If the sperm are too few, or not the right quality, to fertilize the egg, IVF won't work. This is because when sperm and egg are mixed, the sperm are unable to penetrate the egg. With ICSI, an embryologist will select a healthy sperm, remove its tail, and introduce the sperm's head directly into the egg using a long, fine needle.

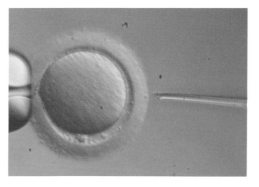
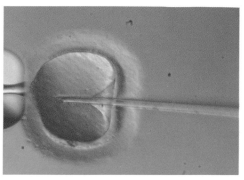

THE MOMENT OF FERTILIZATION

These images have been taken using an electron microscope; the egg is actually only 0.1 mm wide, the diameter of a human hair. The first image shows an egg (oocyte) being held in place, and a fine needle containing one sperm approaching it from the right. In the second image, the needle has pierced the egg and the single sperm is about to be injected. This will, hopefully, allow the sperm and egg to fertilize.

Q WHAT IS PREIMPLANTATION GENETIC DIAGNOSIS (PGD)?

A PGD is a method of identifying genetic abnormalities in an embryo before it is transferred into the mother's womb. It allows parents who are at high risk of transmitting an inherited (genetic) condition to their children to check whether an embryo carries that condition. The diagnostic method is rapid, and results can be ready within 24 hours. The healthy embryo(s) may then be transferred into the mother's womb, as happens in normal IVF, and will not carry the genetic condition in question.

Q WHAT DISEASES CAN PREIMPLANTATION GENETIC DIAGNOSIS (PGD) DETECT?

A This procedure can detect single gene defects such as sickle cell disease, cystic fibrosis, haemophilia, Tay-Sachs disease, Duchene muscular dystrophy, and others. It can also determine the sex of the embryo. This has special relevance for couples who are at risk of transmitting X-linked chromosome disorders such as Duchene muscular dystrophy and haemophilia, both of which affect males only.

Q DOES PREIMPLANTATION DIAGNOSIS AFFECT MY BABY?

A The most common method used is the removal of a single cell from a six to eight cell embryo for analysis of the DNA. This procedure does not affect the development of the embryo, nor its potential to implant and lead to pregnancy.

Q CAN I CLONE MY PARTNER AND HAVE AN IDENTICAL VERSION OF HIM AS A BABY?

A Cloning would involve taking DNA (genetic material) from one of your partner's blood cells or other body cells, introducing it to an empty egg, and allowing the egg to divide into cells to form an embryo, as if it were a normal fertilized egg. While cloning in humans is theoretically (and even practically) possible, there are far too many unanswered questions about the safety and long-term effects of the technique. For example, it is possible that cloned cells will age far more quickly than those derived from a more conventional mating process. So, at present, the answer is that the technique is not legal for use in humans in most countries, and no-one is quite sure about its long-term safety.

IF YOU LOSE YOUR PREGNANCY

Q WHAT IS A MISCARRIAGE?

A A miscarriage occurs if you lose your baby before it is capable of sustaining life – normally considered to be before about 24 weeks. Most miscarriages happen in the first ten weeks of pregnancy; in fact, at least 30 per cent of all conceptions end this way.

Q WHY DO MISCARRIAGES HAPPEN?

A There are several reasons why a pregnancy does not lead to a successful birth. It may be because your pregnancy was ectopic (see below); because the fetus did not develop normally; or because the placenta, the egg, or the sperm was defective, or there may be a chromosomal problem.

Q ARE ALL MISCARRIAGES THE SAME?

A Not all miscarriages happen in the same way – there are several terms to define what takes place: "threatened", "missed", and "inevitable". In the first trimester, if there is bleeding but no pain, and the fetus stays alive and healthy so that the pregnancy continues to term, this is called a threatened miscarriage. You may have what is called a missed miscarriage if the fetus dies, but stays in the womb and is either expelled later or is removed by an operation. An inevitable miscarriage is the term used when there is bleeding and pain, the cervix opens, and the fetus is expelled from the womb. If the miscarriage leaves small fragments of the placenta or blood clots in your womb, this is known as an "incomplete" miscarriage (see opposite).

WHAT IS AN ECTOPIC PREGNANCY?

When a fertilized egg develops and implants outside the womb, either in a Fallopian tube or, more rarely, in the abdominal cavity, the developing egg outgrows its blood supply and dies, causing severe bleeding. This condition is rare.

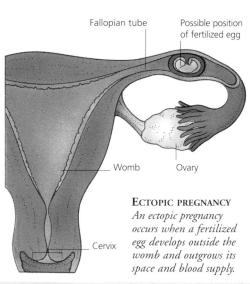

Fallopian tube

Possible position of fertilized egg

Womb

Ovary

Cervix

ECTOPIC PREGNANCY
An ectopic pregnancy occurs when a fertilized egg develops outside the womb and outgrows its space and blood supply.

Symptoms and treatment
If you are experiencing severe pain in your abdomen (usually on one side), heavy vaginal bleeding, and you feel faint (particularly if you have already had a positive pregnancy test), go to a hospital at once. If it is discovered to be an ectopic pregnancy, it can't be saved. The situation may be life-threatening because it can cause severe internal bleeding and will need prompt surgery. In serious cases, the affected Fallopian tube may need to be removed. Sometimes, an early ectopic pregnancy can "miscarry" itself, known as a tubal abortion, without your knowledge.

How likely is an ectopic pregnancy?
You are at risk if you have previously had an infection in your Fallopian tubes or a pelvic inflammatory disease, or your Fallopian tubes have been otherwise damaged. The chances also increase if you become pregnant while wearing a coil (IUD) or while taking the Mini-pill.

Can I still have a normal pregnancy?
You can still have a healthy pregnancy after having had an ectopic pregnancy, although your chances of conception are slightly reduced.

Q HOW DO I KNOW IF I AM HAVING A MISCARRIAGE?

A Vaginal bleeding with period-like cramps are frequently a sign that you are about to have a miscarriage. Bleeding at any stage of pregnancy, with or without pain, should always be taken seriously; seek medical advice immediately.

Q WILL I NEED TREATMENT AFTER A MISCARRIAGE?

A Yes, you will probably have an ultrasound scan to see what has happened. You will not need treatment if the scan shows that your womb is clear. If the womb is not entirely empty, known as an incomplete miscarriage, you may need a procedure called an ERPC (evacuation of retained products of conception) to clear your womb. If your womb is not treated in this way, an infection could develop which may affect your chances of a future pregnancy. You will have a general anaesthetic and a short stay in hospital for this procedure.

Q I HAVE HAD SEVERAL MISCARRIAGES, DO I NEED SPECIALIST TREATMENT?

A One or two miscarriages are unlikely to have a long-term effect on your ability to carry a baby to term. Early miscarriages are very common, and investigations are unlikely to help unless you have had more than three in succession. Even then, only if you have a treatable condition will further investigations prove useful.

Q CAN ANYTHING BE DONE TO PREVENT A LATE MISCARRIAGE?

A When a threatened miscarriage occurs in the second trimester and the cause is identified – if, for example, there is a weakness in the neck of the womb or an infection – this can be treated and miscarriage can often be avoided. If, however, no cause is found, nothing can be done to prevent it.

Q WILL I SEE AND HOLD MY BABY AFTER HAVING A MISCARRIAGE?

A If you miscarry in the second trimester, you can see your baby if you wish. However, not everyone wants to do this, and you should not feel you have to. Most hospitals have a trained professional, usually a doctor or midwife, to guide you and your partner through this time. If your baby is born and dies after 24 weeks, this is legally not a miscarriage but a premature birth, and the birth and death have to be registered; if you want a funeral, arrangements need to be made (see p. 193).

DISCUSSION POINT

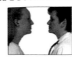

HOW WILL HAVING A MISCARRIAGE AFFECT ME?

Feelings of guilt and anger
You will almost certainly feel guilty and also possibly angry after a miscarriage, even though it is unlikely that you or your partner were in any way responsible for the miscarriage. These feelings are very understandable. Ask your professional carers to explain exactly what may have happened and to answer your questions.

The need to grieve
Whether you miscarried early in pregnancy, or very late, and particularly after you have felt your baby move, you may already think of your baby as a person and grieve for your loss. Grieving is important, just as it is when you lose any loved one, and it may take some time to come to terms with your loss.

Healing
If you lose your pregnancy early on, the chances are that you will not be able to see or hold your baby. But this doesn't mean that you do not imagine what might have been, and your mind may come back to this time and time again. It may be helpful to contact a support group, usually run by people who have experienced miscarriage themselves. They can help you come to terms with what has happened.

The future
You may want to see your family doctor, or specialist, to understand what happened and why, and to discuss future pregnancies. But remember that there is often no explanation, and cruel as it may seem, an early miscarriage is often nature's way of dealing with a pregnancy that, for whatever reason, is failing to develop. When you are both ready, the time will probably come to try again, but it is wise to wait until you are mentally and physically ready. Remember, most women who have had one or more miscarriages go on to have a healthy baby.

NOW THAT YOU'RE PREGNANT

Q I THINK I'M PREGNANT, HOW CAN I CONFIRM IT?

A There are three ways of confirming your pregnancy – by a urine test, a special blood test, or, occasionally, an ultrasound scan. A simple urine test is the most common method by far and can be done at home with a pregnancy-testing kit (with immediate results), or you can take a urine sample to your doctor or to a family planning clinic for testing. A doctor's or clinic's test is usually free, but it takes a few days to get the results. Your doctor can also do a blood test. Although not a routine procedure, ultrasound can also be used to confirm a pregnancy (particularly if you are not sure about your dates), but not for at least ten days after a missed period.

Q ARE HOME TEST KITS RELIABLE?

A If you follow the instructions carefully (see below), a home test kit is as accurate as a doctor's or family planning clinic's test. Its advantage is that it gives you an immediate answer; a sensitive testing kit can tell you that you are pregnant the day after your period is due

Q WHAT ARE THE FIRST SIGNS OF PREGNANCY?

A A missed period is the most common sign of pregnancy but sometimes a period may not happen for other reasons, such as illness, shock or even jet lag. However, if you are experiencing other symptoms (see below), you should consider having a pregnancy test. Although not everybody feels the full range of symptoms as soon as they become pregnant, you may experience some of the following, which are most characteristic:

Signs of pregnancy
- You have missed one or more periods.
- You need to urinate frequently.
- You may find that certain tastes and smells become unpleasant suddenly; or you may crave odd foods. Often there may be a strange metallic taste in the mouth.
- You feel nauseous and may vomit in the mornings (or at other times of the day).
- Your breasts are tingling, tender or more swollen than usual.
- You feel particularly tired.
- You feel emotional or tearful.
- You suddenly become constipated.

HOW DO PREGNANCY TEST KITS WORK?

Pregnancy test kits require you to test a sample of your urine. The absorbent wand (below) reacts if a hormone called hCG (human chorionic gonadotrophin), which is produced by the embryo, is present in your urine. As a back-up, many kits include a second test.

Results windows   Cartridge   Absorbent pad

HOW TO USE A TEST KIT
Remove the test wand from the cap or cartridge. Hold the absorbent sampler in your urine stream for a few seconds. Replace the wand into the cartridge. Wait as directed. If you are pregnant, both windows will show a colour. (Not all kits look the same as the one shown here, but they work in the same way.)

Results windows

Pregnant   Not pregnant

Q WHAT SHOULD I DO WHEN MY PREGNANCY HAS BEEN CONFIRMED?

A It is a good idea to discuss your pregnancy with your doctor at the earliest opportunity. At this early stage, you need to have a check-up to ensure that all is going well, and to discuss how you want to organize your pregnancy care (see p. 26). If you are not registered with a doctor, you do need to contact a professional as soon as possible, preferably a doctor and/or a midwife, or otherwise visit your local hospital's antenatal clinic. If you would like to contact a midwife for advice, ask at your doctor's surgery about community midwives and the midwife schemes available, or for names of local independent midwives (see p. 256).

Q WHY IS MY DOCTOR RECOMMENDING A SCAN TO CONFIRM MY DUE DATE?

A If your periods are irregular, you were on the Pill when you got pregnant, or you have a long cycle with infrequent periods, your doctor will find it more accurate to date your pregnancy by looking at the size of the baby on a scan.

Q I'VE MISSED MY PERIOD BUT THE TEST SHOWS NEGATIVE, WHAT DOES IT MEAN?

A The obvious answer is that your period may, for a variety of reasons, simply be late, or perhaps you haven't ovulated. Or you may be pregnant but your urine did not contain enough hCG (see box, opposite) to show on the test. Wait for a few days and try again.

WHEN IS MY BABY DUE?

If your periods are regular (about 28 days apart) and you have not been taking the Pill, your pregnancy is dated 40 weeks after the first day of your last menstrual period (LMP). There are several days around ovulation when fertilization could have taken place, so pregnancy is not dated from the time of fertility or sexual intercourse. You will be considered four weeks pregnant when you miss your first period.

HOW TO USE THE CHART

Look up the first day of your last period in the light-coloured line next to the months that are in heavy type. The figure below it will be the estimated date of your delivery (EDD). For example, if your last period began on April 15, you will see that your EDD is January 20. In a leap year add one day to any date after February 29.

JANUARY	1	2	3	4	5	6	7	8	9	10	11	12	13	14	15	16	17	18	19	20	21	22	23	24	25	26	27	28	29	30	31
Oct/Nov	8	9	10	11	12	13	14	15	16	17	18	19	20	21	22	23	24	25	26	27	28	29	30	31	1	2	3	4	5	6	7
FEBRUARY	1	2	3	4	5	6	7	8	9	10	11	12	13	14	15	16	17	18	19	20	21	22	23	24	25	26	27	28			
Nov/Dec	8	9	10	11	12	13	14	15	16	17	18	19	20	21	22	23	24	25	26	27	28	29	30	1	2	3	4	5			
MARCH	1	2	3	4	5	6	7	8	9	10	11	12	13	14	15	16	17	18	19	20	21	22	23	24	25	26	27	28	29	30	31
Dec/Jan	6	7	8	9	10	11	12	13	14	15	16	17	18	19	20	21	22	23	24	25	26	27	28	29	30	31	1	2	3	4	5
APRIL	1	2	3	4	5	6	7	8	9	10	11	12	13	14	15	16	17	18	19	20	21	22	23	24	25	26	27	28	29	30	
Jan/Feb	6	7	8	9	10	11	12	13	14	15	16	17	18	19	20	21	22	23	24	25	26	27	28	29	30	31	1	2	3	4	
MAY	1	2	3	4	5	6	7	8	9	10	11	12	13	14	15	16	17	18	19	20	21	22	23	24	25	26	27	28	29	30	31
Feb/March	5	6	7	8	9	10	11	12	13	14	15	16	17	18	19	20	21	22	23	24	25	26	27	28	1	2	3	4	5	6	7
JUNE	1	2	3	4	5	6	7	8	9	10	11	12	13	14	15	16	17	18	19	20	21	22	23	24	25	26	27	28	29	30	
March/April	8	9	10	11	12	13	14	15	16	17	18	19	20	21	22	23	24	25	26	27	28	29	30	31	1	2	3	4	5	6	
JULY	1	2	3	4	5	6	7	8	9	10	11	12	13	14	15	16	17	18	19	20	21	22	23	24	25	26	27	28	29	30	31
April/May	7	8	9	10	11	12	13	14	15	16	17	18	19	20	21	22	23	24	25	26	27	28	29	30	1	2	3	4	5	6	7
AUGUST	1	2	3	4	5	6	7	8	9	10	11	12	13	14	15	16	17	18	19	20	21	22	23	24	25	26	27	28	29	30	31
May/June	8	9	10	11	12	13	14	15	16	17	18	19	20	21	22	23	24	25	26	27	28	29	30	31	1	2	3	4	5	6	7
SEPTEMBER	1	2	3	4	5	6	7	8	9	10	11	12	13	14	15	16	17	18	19	20	21	22	23	24	25	26	27	28	29	30	
June/July	8	9	10	11	12	13	14	15	16	17	18	19	20	21	22	23	24	25	26	27	28	29	30	1	2	3	4	5	6	7	
OCTOBER	1	2	3	4	5	6	7	8	9	10	11	12	13	14	15	16	17	18	19	20	21	22	23	24	25	26	27	28	29	30	31
July/August	8	9	10	11	12	13	14	15	16	17	18	19	20	21	22	23	24	25	26	27	28	29	30	31	1	2	3	4	5	6	7
NOVEMBER	1	2	3	4	5	6	7	8	9	10	11	12	13	14	15	16	17	18	19	20	21	22	23	24	25	26	27	28	29	30	
August/Sept	8	9	10	11	12	13	14	15	16	17	18	19	20	21	22	23	24	25	26	27	28	29	30	31	1	2	3	4	5	6	
DECEMBER	1	2	3	4	5	6	7	8	9	10	11	12	13	14	15	16	17	18	19	20	21	22	23	24	25	26	27	28	29	30	31
Sept/Oct	7	8	9	10	11	12	13	14	15	16	17	18	19	20	21	22	23	24	25	26	27	28	29	30	1	2	3	4	5	6	7

CONCERNS IN EARLY PREGNANCY

Q WE'VE LONGED FOR THIS BABY, SO WHY AM I UPSET AND CONFUSED?

A Give yourself time to adjust to the idea of being pregnant. It is not unusual to feel confused, or to feel ecstatic one minute and scared the next when you first discover that you are pregnant. Once you accept that the coming baby is a reality, you should be able to enjoy your pregnancy to the full.

Q I DRANK ALCOHOL BEFORE I KNEW I WAS PREGNANT, IS THIS BAD FOR MY BABY?

A Although regular, excessive alcohol drinking during pregnancy is bad for your baby, the likelihood of your baby being affected by a little alcoholic over-indulgence during early pregnancy is very small. However, if you are planning to become pregnant or have recently discovered that you are expecting a baby, it is still best to avoid alcohol.

Q MY CERVICAL SMEAR TEST INDICATED AN ABNORMALITY, IS IT IMPORTANT?

A Smear abnormalities range from mild to severe. However, irrespective of the degree of abnormality, it is unlikely that you will need or be given treatment for this while you are pregnant. Nevertheless, you should not ignore any smear abnormality, and it is best to seek medical advice from your doctor.

Q I HAVE HAD TREATMENT TO MY CERVIX – WILL THIS AFFECT MY PREGNANCY?

A Modern treatments for an abnormal smear are very unlikely to affect your pregnancy but if you have had treatment to your cervix, you should mention this to your doctor at your first antenatal visit. Also, if you have had a cone biopsy (the removal of a cone-shaped area of cervical tissue), there is a slightly increased risk of having a late miscarriage or a premature labour. Most women have normal pregnancies after cone biopsies.

Q DO I NEED GENETIC COUNSELLING?

A You may need advice if you are over the age of 35; if you or your partner have or are carriers of a genetic or chromosomal disorder; if you have previously had a child with a chromosomal or genetic problem; or tests have shown problems in the baby you are carrying (see p. 33).

Q WILL MY SECOND PREGNANCY BE LIKE MY FIRST?

A In general, no two pregnancies are the same. Many women find that subsequent pregnancies are physically and psychologically easier than their first. To some extent this is because you are more aware of what to expect. Physical symptoms of early pregnancy, such as nausea and vomiting, are sometimes less severe.

I HAVE DISCOVERED THAT I AM PREGNANT ACCIDENTALLY…

… while taking the Pill. Will this have affected the baby?
The hormones in the Pill (both the combined oral contraceptive and the Mini-pill) are similar to the oestrogen and progesterone that occur naturally in your body. The amount of hormones in the Pill is very small and once you stop taking it the hormones will disappear very rapidly from your body, so it is very unlikely to cause any harm to the developing baby.

… while I have a coil in place. Should it be removed?
It is important to establish first that the pregnancy is in the womb rather than in a Fallopian tube; this can be established by an ultrasound scan. If the pregnancy is at an early stage, the coil is usually removed but there is a small risk of miscarriage. It is more difficult to remove the coil later on; it may be left where it is, with only a very minimal risk to the baby.

… while on tablets from my doctor. Could this have harmed my baby?
It depends entirely on what tablets you are taking. Most are relatively safe; these include many vitamin supplements (excluding those containing vitamin A, which should be avoided), anti-depressants, and antibiotics (except tetracyclines). Those that might cause a problem include anti-acne tablets and certain blood pressure tablets.

WHAT COULD HARM MY BABY?

	RISK TO BABY	ADVICE
Alcohol	Your baby's development can be harmed by alcohol because alcohol crosses the placenta and enters your baby's bloodstream.	It is probably best to avoid any alcohol in the first trimester. Binge drinking can be particularly harmful (see p. 107).
Animals and pet litter	Toxoplasma infection, which may cause blindness, mental retardation, and deafness (see p. 34).	Avoid direct skin contact with cat litter and use gloves while gardening.
Chemicals: hair dyes, permanents; chlorine in pools	There is no evidence of any harm.	There is no reason to avoid swimming pools. Follow the manufacturer's instructions when using dyes.
Cigarettes	Smoking more than ten cigarettes a day can reduce your baby's birth weight and cause problems during pregnancy, labour, and your baby's first weeks of life (see p. 106).	Smoking should be stopped completely during pregnancy – not only does it affect the blood and oxygen supply to the womb and baby, it also harms the mother's lungs and circulation.
Particular foods	Listeria bacteria found in some foods can cause miscarriage or stillbirth. Excess Vitamin A may cause birth defects. Salmonella can cause miscarriage.	Avoid pâtés and unpasteurized dairy products such as soft cheeses. Avoid all undercooked meats and offal, especially pork, as well as raw fish (sushi). Do not eat liver or liver pâté. Avoid raw or partially cooked eggs (see p. 106).
Infectious illnesses	Chickenpox, mumps, and measles are all potentially harmful to the developing baby (see p. 127). German measles (rubella) may cause severe abnormalities, but most women are vaccinated against this.	Avoid contact with young children who may have an infection. Contracting rubella may be a reason to consider termination. If you are worried, talk to your doctor.
	Genital herpes may cause severe infection in the baby after delivery.	Contact your doctor if you have herpes or develop genital blisters or ulcers (see p. 127).
Strenuous physical activity	Exercise in moderation will not harm you or your pregnancy.	It is sensible to avoid heavy lifting and any activity that involves the risk of injury. Don't take up any new strenuous physical activity.
Stress	There is no evidence of any harm.	Avoid becoming very stressed because it will add to your fatigue. It may also reduce your enjoyment of your pregnancy.
VDUs, microwaves, and photocopiers	There is no evidence of any harm.	Use them as you would normally.
X-rays	It is possible that X-rays during the first 13 weeks may harm the development of your baby's main organ systems.	X-rays (including dental ones) aren't usually done in the first 13 weeks. If an X-ray is necessary, make sure your doctor or X-ray technician knows you are pregnant.

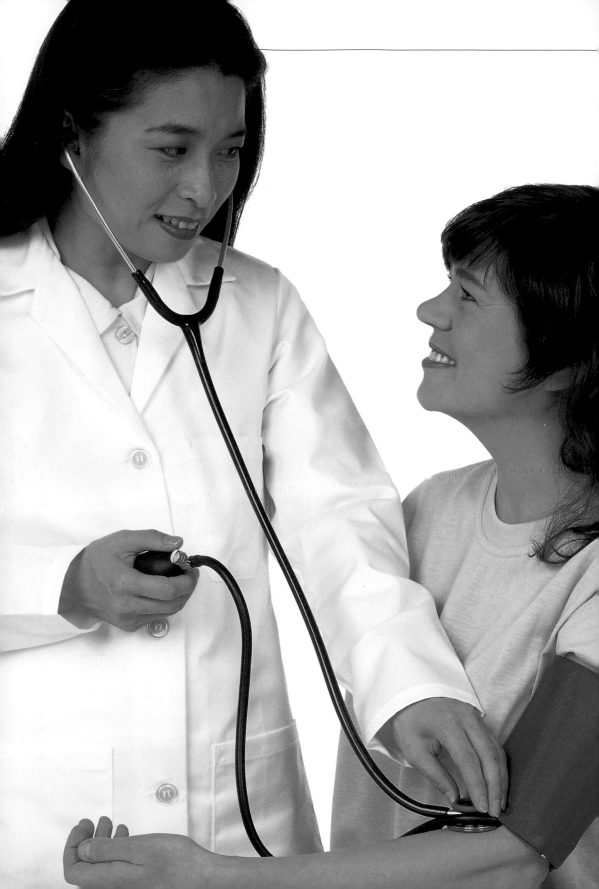

YOUR
ANTENATAL
CARE

Now that you know that you are pregnant, you
will want to find out as much as possible about
your physical condition, what to expect in the
coming months, and what plans you should be
making for your labour. This chapter provides
detailed information about the antenatal tests
you may have, as well as your choices in
antenatal care and labour so that you can decide
what would suit you and your partner. Whether
you would prefer a home birth or a hospital
birth, these options are discussed. It also
explains where you could have your antenatal
care, who your professional carers are likely to
be, and what happens at your first check-up.

CHOOSING ANTENATAL CARE

Q WHEN CHOOSING ANTENATAL CARE, WHAT SHOULD I THINK ABOUT FIRST?

A Before you choose a system of antenatal care, you should think about whether you would prefer a home or a hospital birth. This is an important decision and one that you and your partner should be happy with. Both locations have advantages and disadvantages (see opposite). If you are unsure now, you can make up your mind later. Also consider how long it takes to travel to the hospital or clinic for your check-ups and when labour begins.

Q I FEEL VERY WELL, DO I REALLY NEED ANTENATAL CARE?

A Even if you are feeling on top of the world, you should not miss your antenatal visits. The aim of antenatal care is to monitor your general well-being and identify potential problems for the mother and the baby before they become serious. This may involve simple interventions such as iron tablets for anaemia, or regular scans for twins; some women do, however, need help for a range of medical and psychological problems. Often, new mothers-to-be just need to hear that all is well.

Q WHERE DO I GET ANTENATAL CARE?

A You can discuss your antenatal care options with your doctor or a midwife (see opposite). If you are having your baby in hospital, a letter is sent to the hospital and you will receive an appointment letter or you can telephone and make this appointment. If you choose the Domino or Team systems (see opposite), a midwife will contact you and visit you at home for your first check-up.

Q I KNOW I WANT TO HAVE A HOME BIRTH, HOW DO I ARRANGE THIS?

A Discuss the options with your doctor or midwife as soon as you can. The possibility of a home birth will depend largely on whether your pregnancy is considered low-risk or high-risk (see p. 32). Women with high-risk pregnancies are usually advised to have a hospital birth. If you are told that you have a low-risk pregnancy, and no complications develop during your pregnancy, a home birth is an option to consider (see opposite).

Q CAN I ENSURE THAT I HAVE THE SAME MIDWIFE THROUGHOUT?

A In Team midwifery and midwifery group practices you have a high chance of being delivered by one of the same small group of midwives who have been involved in your antenatal check-ups. The only way to ensure that you see the same midwife throughout and have her attend your delivery is to pay for the care of an independent midwife.

Q WILL MY OWN DOCTOR BE ABLE TO ATTEND MY DELIVERY?

A Many general practitioners have had training in obstetrics and can therefore provide your antenatal care throughout your pregnancy, but few get involved in the delivery itself. Your own doctor may agree to attend you at home, but you need to discuss this with him or her before the labour.

Q I HAVE SPECIAL NEEDS, HOW DO I FIND OUT IF THERE ARE FACILITIES FOR ME?

A Many hospitals provide facilities and staff with extra training for those with special needs such as deafness and physical disabilities. Today, midwifery training usually includes instruction on helping women with special needs. Some hospitals also cater for particular diets including Halal or Kosher. Check with your chosen hospital.

QUESTIONS TO ASK

What is the reputation of the hospital according to parents, midwives, and doctors?

Is there any particular specialist knowledge or interest in the maternity department?

Are the midwives flexible about special requests and different types of delivery?

Is there a 24-hour anaesthetic service in case I want an epidural?

Will I meet the consultant?

How long do I have to stay in hospital after the birth?

Can I have a home delivery?

What is best for me?

In general, doctors recommend that first babies and high-risk pregnancies are delivered in hospital where equipment and expertise are on hand in case of complications. Where a pregnancy has gone smoothly, home birth is an option more women are choosing.

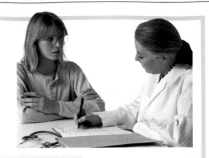

HOSPITAL BIRTH

Advantages
- Provides a good environment if your home is not suitable.
- Full medical back-up is available should a complication develop.
- You have contact with other mothers and babies.
- If you need help, 24-hour support is available.

Disadvantages
- There may be a lack of privacy and intimacy.
- Medical intervention is more likely.

How do I choose a hospital?
Often there is a choice of local hospitals and it is worth comparing their facilities and asking questions about their procedures (see below, opposite). Ask around; if you want your community midwife to deliver, she will usually be based at one hospital.

HOME BIRTH

Advantages
- Freedom from hospital rules and strict routines.
- A more private and intimate birth is possible.
- There is no need to travel or be moved about while in labour and afterwards.
- Your partner and family share more in the birth.

Disadvantages
- Should any complications develop, medical help involves transferral to a hospital.
- You may not get as much rest afterwards if you have to look after your family.

What should I consider?
- Is my home suitable (warm, comfortable, quiet, with adequate space and a telephone)?
- Will I worry that medical back-up is not on hand?
- Would I appreciate extra help with my baby?

ANTENATAL CARE

Where you decide to have your antenatal care will depend on what kind of birth you want and what is available in your area. Talk to your doctor or midwife about the local hospitals and care systems. Travel may also be a factor.

1 Shared care If you have decided on a hospital birth, check-ups are usually shared between the hospital and your doctor, most taking place at your doctor's surgery. Your doctor does not usually attend the delivery at the hospital.

2 Community midwife care Community midwives and group practices offer several pregnancy care options including the Domino system. This system, which means "in and out from home" usually involves a short stay in hospital for the birth (returning home about six hours later if all is well). The same midwives see

you for your antenatal check-ups, are with you at the hospital during labour, and visit you afterwards for about ten days. Community midwives will also look after you should you decide to have a home confinement.

3 GP units These small units are quite rare and are more commonly found in rural areas. You will be looked after by midwives who work with the GP. These units are designed to deal with normal deliveries; if there is the likelihood of a problem, you will be transferred to a larger hospital that offers more specialist expertise.

4 Hospital only After your initial visit to your doctor, all your check-ups and contacts are with the hospital antenatal clinic. This system is usually necessary for women with complicated pregnancies or medical problems. The birth is in hospital.

ANTENATAL VISITS

Q HOW OFTEN DO I HAVE CHECK-UPS?

A The first and longest check-up is the "booking" visit, between the eighth and twelfth week of your pregnancy. Routine check-ups are at monthly intervals thereafter until 28 weeks, then every other week until 36 weeks; finally, they are once a week until your delivery. You may need more check-ups if you are expecting twins or if a complication develops, and fewer if you are low-risk (see p. 32). If necessary, you can contact the clinic between visits.

Q DO I HAVE TO ATTEND EVERY APPOINTMENT?

A Antenatal care is a service that is offered to ensure the well-being of you and your baby. You may have to miss a visit for unavoidable reasons but this is unlikely to cause harm. It is, however, best to attend even if you feel well.

Q CAN MY PARTNER COME WITH ME?

A Yes, if he is able to, it is a good idea. During the first visit, he can answer questions about his medical history and that of his family; he can ask any questions, and see what happens when you have check-ups. Perhaps most importantly, your partner will feel more involved with his baby if he shares in the pregnancy process.

Q DO I NEED TO DO ANYTHING BEFORE MY FIRST VISIT?

A You may find it helpful to read any leaflets or information that the hospital has sent you. Check if there are any inherited abnormalities or diseases in either family. Make a note of the date of your last period, and the dates of any previous pregnancies and/or miscarriages. Think about and write down any questions you wish to ask.

WHAT DO THE NOTES ON MY ANTENATAL RECORD MEAN?

When you attend your first antenatal check up you will be given a wallet or a page of notes. Bring your notes to every appointment because they contain personal details such as your blood group. Your doctor or midwife will fill in information on your progress; certain abbreviations are always used by them (see below).

BP Your blood pressure.
NAD Nothing abnormal detected, usually in your urine.
Hb Haemoglobin levels that indicate anaemia if low.
Fe Iron tablets.
FHH/NH Fetal heart heard or not heard, usually from about 14 weeks. Also FHHR, which means fetal heart heard and regular.
FMF Fetal movements felt, usually from 16–20 weeks.
Ceph Cephalic, means baby is head down in the womb.
Vx Vertex, also means baby is head down.

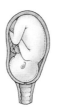

Cephalic or vertex   Breech

Br Breech. Your baby is bottom down in the womb.
Eng/E Engaged. The baby's head has dropped into the pelvic cavity ready for delivery.
NE Not engaged (see above).
SFH Symphysis fundal height is the measurement of the length of the womb (in centimetres) from the top of the pubic bone, and indicates the growth of the pregnancy.
PP Presenting part, which refers to that part of the baby that is lying lowest.
Primagravida A woman who is in her first pregnancy.
Multigravida A woman who has been pregnant before.
EDD Estimated date of delivery.
Oed Oedema, which means swelling of the hands, feet, and face.
CS/LSCS Caesarean section or lower segment Caesarean section.
TCA To come again.

Q WHO WILL I SEE AT MY FIRST ANTENATAL APPOINTMENT?

A At the hospital a midwife usually handles the history-taking and tests before passing you on to an obstetrician who will carry out a physical (and possibly an internal) examination. Should there be any complications, you may also have to see the consultant obstetrician. If you have opted for the Domino or Team system (see p. 27), this check-up is carried out by a midwife in your home, and lasts about 1½ hours.

Q WHAT HAPPENS AT LATER ANTENATAL APPOINTMENTS?

A The checks-ups at later appointments are less comprehensive and therefore shorter. There are several procedures that are routinely carried out at each check-up. Your weight is noted, your urine tested, and your blood pressure checked. Your baby's position and stage of growth are established and the heartbeat heard. You will be asked about your baby's movements. Blood tests are taken at intervals or if you are having special investigations.

WHO ARE THE PROFESSIONAL CARERS?

During your pregnancy, labour, and after the birth, you will meet a number of health professionals who will give the advice and care that you and your baby need. Your doctor or midwife will probably be the professionals you see most often; at most check-ups you may not necessarily see anyone other than a midwife. Usually you will need to speak to a consultant obstetrician only if you have a problem and, (apart from the first check-up) to a paediatrician only if your baby has one.

Doctor, general practitioner (GP)
Your doctor has a pivotal role during your pregnancy. He/she is also your first point of contact when you wish to find out about your pregnancy and your options. Usually, those looking after you and your baby will refer back to your doctor's initial contact and notes. Your doctor books the hospital or writes to the community midwife for you once you have decided where you wish to go to have your baby. Doctors sometimes have their own antenatal clinics or GP units. Some doctors are able to be involved with the delivery itself but if this is not feasible, he/she will visit you afterwards at home.

Midwife
A midwife is trained in the speciality of childbirth and is responsible for providing care in normal pregnancies. She (and it is usually but not always a woman) is recognized as an independent practitioner and may work within a hospital, in the community or both. Her role includes caring for you and your baby before, during and after the birth, either at home or in hospital, provided that all goes well. If there should be any complication, it is the midwife's role to work alongside the obstetricians to provide the appropriate care. A midwife is an excellent source of practical advice on pregnancy, birth, and baby care as well as of more technical medical information.

Obstetrician
This is a doctor who has trained as a specialist in the care of pregnant women and after many years and a wealth of experience will become a consultant obstetrician.

Consultant obstetrician
The most senior doctor in the obstetrics department, as head of the team of doctors looking after you, the consultant has the final say if there are any problems. His/her name will also appear on your personal notes. Consultants are experts in the complications of pregnancy, so you will probably have little contact with them if your pregnancy is problem-free. However, you have a right to speak with your consultant at any stage of your pregnancy should you wish.

Paediatrician
A doctor who specializes in the health of babies and children, a paediatrican attends all "abnormal" deliveries and multiple births, or when the baby is delivered with forceps, or by Caesarean section. All newborn babies are checked by a paediatrician before they go home.

Health visitor
A health visitor has had specialist training in family health and is often an ex-nurse or midwife. She will contact you before and after the delivery.

WHAT HAPPENS AT AN ANTENATAL VISIT?

Your first antenatal visit may seem a daunting prospect but in fact the procedures are not lengthy or arduous, although there may be some waiting time. The main purpose of these visits is to allow the midwives and doctors to gain a complete picture of your pregnancy, to troubleshoot for potential problems, and for you to get to know your midwife and to receive her support.

HISTORY TAKING

A midwife asks you about your partner and your families; your personal details, medical history, and the date of your last period are entered on your notes. You have to mention previous pregnancies, miscarriages or terminations but these do not have to appear on your notes.

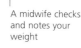

A midwife checks and notes your weight

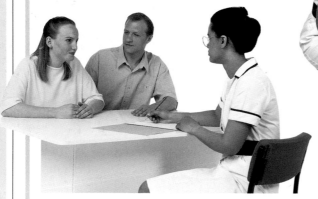

PERSONAL HISTORY
Your present weight and height are recorded. You will also be asked about smoking, drinking, and street drugs and given the chance to talk about any problems you have.

URINE TESTS

You will be asked to provide a urine specimen. This is tested on the spot by a midwife to confirm that there are no abnormalities.

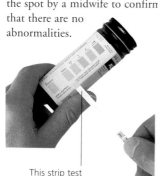

This strip test instantly shows any problems

Glucose (sugar)
More than a trace of glucose may be a sign of diabetes. You may need a blood test (see right).

Protein
When this is found in quantity in the urine it may indicate a kidney or bladder infection, or pre-eclampsia (see p. 138).

Ketones
These are substances that, if present, mean that the body's metabolic system is upset because you haven't eaten enough or you have vomited.

BLOOD TESTS

To establish your blood group and to ensure that you are not suffering from certain diseases and conditions, a series of routine blood tests is taken on the first antenatal visit (see p. 32). Blood is taken again at regular intervals thereafter to check on your haemoglobin (red cell) levels, which indicate whether you need iron supplements. Other routine blood tests include those that check your blood sugar level, and (if you are Rhesus negative) a blood test that detects the presence of antibodies.

PHYSICAL EXAMINATION

At the first check-up, the doctor will check that your heart, lungs, and general health are good, and that your baby is developing normally.

Checking your womb

At each visit your abdomen is measured to establish the height of the top of your womb (fundus); this indicates the baby's size. On some visits, you may have an internal examination (see right), which may be slightly uncomfortable. Your baby's heart is listened to; if an electronic sonicaid is used you can also hear it.

Checking your breasts

Your breasts are checked to make sure there are no lumps.

Smear test and cervical check

If your smear tests are not up to date, a smear may be taken. This is a routine test that involves a painless scraping of the cells of the cervix, which are then sent to be checked that they are healthy. Your cervix will also be examined visually.

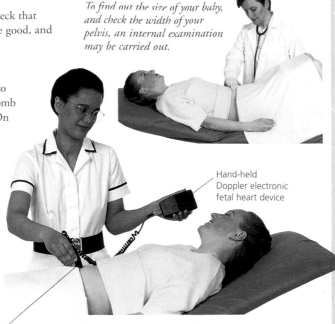

INTERNAL EXAMINATION

To find out the size of your baby, and check the width of your pelvis, an internal examination may be carried out.

Hand-held Doppler electronic fetal heart device

The baby's heart rate should be 110–150 beats per minute

LISTENING TO THE BABY'S HEART

Using a sonicaid, the midwife or obstetrician listens to the baby's heart, or after 24 weeks, a plastic or metal stethoscope that looks like a trumpet may be used.

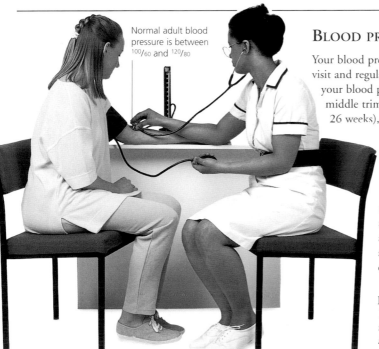

Normal adult blood pressure is between $^{100}/_{60}$ and $^{120}/_{80}$

BLOOD PRESSURE

Your blood pressure is recorded at your first visit and regularly thereafter. It is normal for your blood pressure to drop slightly in the middle trimester of pregnancy (13 to 26 weeks), and to rise slightly in the last trimester (27 to 40 weeks).

Any abnormal rise in blood pressure may be one of the first signs of pre-eclampsia (see p. 138) and will need close monitoring. The midwife also checks your legs and ankles for swelling which, if severe, can be a danger sign of pre-eclampsia.

BLOOD PRESSURE

Your blood pressure is a good way of assessing how your body is coping with pregnancy.

ANTENATAL MONITORING

Q HOW IS IT DECIDED WHETHER MY PREGNANCY IS LOW- OR HIGH-RISK?

A There are certain factors that constitute a risk to you and/or your baby. Some of these you can do something about, such as stopping smoking or not taking street drugs. Other factors, such as twins or a large baby, you can do nothing about. However, by careful antenatal monitoring the likelihood of unexpected complications is reduced; should something unforeseen happen, your professional carers will be prepared. In pregnancy care there is an adage that "the best predictor of the future is the past"; this means that if you had a problem in a previous pregnancy, the same problem may recur.

General risks that may affect your pregnancy
- Alcohol abuse.
- Smoking.
- You are very thin or very large.
- You have a restrictive diet or are malnourished.
- You take street drugs such as heroin or cocaine.
- You have a medical condition requiring drugs.

Risks that mean you need close antenatal care
- Previous pre-term delivery (before 37 weeks).
- Baby in previous pregnancy had an abnormality.
- You have diabetes and/or high blood pressure.
- Previous thrombosis (blood clot).

Risks that mean you need extra care in your delivery
- Very large baby (estimated weight over 4kg/8½lb).
- Very small baby (estimated weight less than 2.5kg/5½lb).
- Twins.
- Breech baby.
- A previous delivery by Caesarean section.
- Previous problems in delivery such as haemorrhage (excessive bleeding).
- High blood pressure in pregnancy (pre-eclampsia).
- Diabetes.

Low-risk pregnancies
If none of the risks listed above applies to you, and any previous pregnancy and delivery were normal and uneventful, it is unlikely that you will have a problem that needs special care. It is nevertheless essential to attend all your antenatal appointments so that your health and the health of your baby can be regularly monitored.

WHAT DO THE ROUTINE BLOOD TESTS SHOW?

Your blood group and Rhesus (Rh) status
It is important for your doctor to know which blood group you belong to in case you need a blood transfusion during the pregnancy or labour. The most common is group O; A, B, and AB are much less common. Your Rhesus status is either positive or negative, so that you may be O negative or A positive and so on. Rhesus positive simply means that there is a special identifying label on your blood cells, which is not there if you are Rhesus negative. If you are Rhesus negative, a further test will be done to check if any antibodies are present; the tests will be repeated at intervals during your pregnancy. If there are antibodies present, your partner will also need to give blood for testing.

Your haemoglobin (red blood cells) levels
Red cells contain iron and carry oxygen; if the test shows that the level of red cells is low, you are anaemic, and you will be advised to eat foods with a high iron content, or you may have to take iron tablets. Anaemia can cause you to feel very tired (see p. 128) and it will also be a problem if you bleed during your pregnancy or at delivery.

Rubella (German measles) A blood test shows whether you are immune to the disease. If you aren't, you could contract rubella in early pregnancy; this could cause blindness, deafness, and heart defects in your baby (see p. 127).

Syphilis Because it is now so easily cured, this sexually transmitted disease is rare these days. However, if the disease is present and untreated in pregnancy, it could cause the baby to have congenital and developmental problems.

Hepatitis B This liver disease, caused by a virus, can be passed to the baby and cause serious liver damage in the baby.

Other blood tests You may be offered other blood tests (see p. 34).

SPECIAL INVESTIGATIONS

Q WHY MIGHT I NEED SPECIAL INVESTIGATIONS?

A You will normally be offered further tests if there is a significant reason to suspect your baby might be suffering from a disease or an abnormality. The decision may be made on the basis of your age (over 35); if your routine scan (see p. 36) shows a problem; if you and/or your partner suffer from a hereditary disease; or if you have previously had a baby with an abnormality.

Q WHAT TESTS WILL I HAVE?

A There are several sorts of tests which detect or rule out problems. Initially, tests on your blood may detect problems in the baby such as Down's syndrome or spina bifida (see Triple Test, p. 34), or a problem you may have, such as diabetes. An ultrasound scan may reassure you that the baby seems to be normal and is growing well; it will also reveal any major defects. If the blood tests or scan do detect a problem, then further tests such as amniocentesis may be offered: this involves taking a sample of fluid from inside the womb (see p. 40).

Q WHAT ABNORMALITIES CAN BE DETECTED?

A There are three kinds of abnormalities that occur: congenital, chromosomal, and genetic. Congenital abnormalities can usually be detected on an ultrasound scan at 18 to 22 weeks (see p. 36). Chromosomal and genetic abnormalities are detected by invasive tests such as amniocentesis, cordocentesis, and CVS (see p. 40).

Q WHAT ARE CONGENITAL ABNORMALITIES?

A This term means that the baby has developed a physical abnormality, such as hare lip, heart and brain defects, spina bifida, absent limbs or extra digits, in the womb. There is no genetic or chromosomal reason for this and often no cause whatsoever is found; it happens rarely when, for instance, the mother contracts an infection such as rubella (German measles). Congenital abnormalities can also be the result of dietary imbalances (such as a lack of folic acid), or because a harmful drug was taken in early pregnancy.

Q WHAT HAPPENS IF A CONGENITAL ABNORMALITY IS DISCOVERED?

A The less severe abnormalities such as hare lip, club foot, and extra digits can usually be dealt with surgically after the baby is born; often the baby is otherwise completely normal. Severe abnormalities such as major heart and central nervous system (brain and spinal cord) malformations often result in miscarriage or death of the baby before 24 weeks. In either situation you will be referred to a consultant to discuss all the options.

DISCUSSION POINT

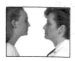

DO I HAVE TO HAVE SPECIAL TESTS?

The most difficult aspect of medical intervention is that it tells you facts about your pregnancy that you might have preferred not to know, and you may not wish to proceed with further tests.

Positive results
There is little point in having screening for any abnormality unless you have carefully thought through what you would do if the results were positive. Once you know there is a problem, and realize the severity of the condition, you will have to decide whether to continue with the pregnancy or not.

Difficult decisions
Whether to terminate the pregnancy on the basis of what tests show is a question about which medical and popular opinion is divided. Some couples want only a completely "normal" baby and so would wish to have a termination. Others are prepared to continue with the pregnancy and raise a child with special needs; some cannot consider a termination. Knowing how you feel about this issue will help you and your medical advisors should a difficult decision be necessary.

SPECIAL BLOOD TESTS

Q WHY MIGHT I NEED SPECIAL BLOOD TESTS?

A Special blood tests are the tools of diagnosis. There are three types of tests: the tests that detect existing diseases that might affect the pregnancy – these include diabetes and HIV; the tests that detect problem genes that you may be unaware of but could pass on to the baby – these include tests for thalassaemia and sickle cell anaemia (see below); tests that measure substances in your blood that indicate possible fetal abnormalities, and these include the Triple or Bart's test, which tests for Down's syndrome.

Q DOES THE TRIPLE BLOOD TEST GIVE A DEFINITE ANSWER?

A The Triple or Bart's test is a screening test, which means that the result of the test is not absolute, but an indication of the risk of your baby being affected. Carried out at 15 to 16 weeks, along with an ultrasound scan, this test is based on the level of hormones in your blood. Usually, if the test shows that the risk of your baby having Down's syndrome is greater than 1 in 270, you will be offered an invasive test, such as amniocentesis or cordocentesis, to confirm or deny that the baby is free of this condition (see p. 40).

WHAT ARE THE SPECIAL BLOOD TESTS?

TEST	WHO IS TESTED	WHAT IT TESTS FOR
Triple or Bart's test (for Down's syndrome, see above)	Depends on local policy but it is usually offered to women over the age of 35 or those with a higher risk of a Down's baby.	It shows the level of three substances that are found in the blood stream of the mother: alpha-fetoprotein (AFP), oestriol, and human chorionic gonadotrophin (hCG).
Glucose tolerance test (for diabetes)	Women at risk of diabetes include those who are known to have high blood sugar, sugar in the urine, diabetes in a previous pregnancy, or a large baby	After a sugary drink, four samples of blood are taken over the next two hours. If your blood sugar level remains high, this can indicate the presence of diabetes.
HIV test (for human immunodeficiency virus)	Anyone who is at risk may ask to be tested. This is done only with your consent.*	It detects the presence of antibodies for the HIV virus.
Sickle cell test (for sickle cell anaemia)	If you, or any of your ancestors, originate from an area where this trait is widespread, especially Africa and the West Indies.	It looks at the type of haemoglobin in your red blood cells and detects the sickle cells.
Haemoglobin electrophoresis test for thalassaemia	If you, or any of your ancestors, originate from an area where this trait is widespread, especially Asia and parts of Africa.	It identifies in red blood cells the different haemoglobins that denote thalassaemia disease.
Toxoplasmosis test	If you have had a recent flu-like illness, especially if you have been in contact with pets and farm animals.	It looks for antibodies to toxoplasma in your blood, which suggest that you have been infected.

*Anonymous HIV testing is carried out on blood samples in many hospitals. No samples are named and the result cannot be traced to you. If you want a "named" test, you will be offered counselling.

Q WHEN DO I NEED TO HAVE THE TEST FOR TOXOPLASMOSIS?

A Toxoplasmosis is a parasitic disease that is passed on to humans by domestic cats, and, more rarely, by sheep and pigs. If this disease is contracted during pregnancy, toxoplasma can cross the placenta and cause blindness, epilepsy, and learning difficulties in the baby. A blood test indicates whether or not you are immune to this disease. You will not usually be offered this test unless there is a high risk that you have been exposed to the illness. If the test shows you have contracted the disease, you may need an ultrasound scan to discover if the baby's growth has been affected. In the UK only about 20 per cent of women are immune to this disease.

WHAT HAPPENS IF A TEST IS POSITIVE

This test screens only. If it is positive you have an increased risk of having a Down's baby. To diagnose this absolutely, you need a further invasive test such as an amniocentesis or cordocentesis (see p. 40).

You are treated for diabetes, which means close control of your diet, possibly with insulin injections as well, and extra antenatal check-ups. You may also have to have more than the average two ultrasound scans.

Any infections that you develop must be carefully treated. The risk of transmitting HIV to the baby can be reduced by certain measures at delivery (see p. 130).

If sickle cell trait or disease is detected, your partner should be tested as well. If he is positive, the baby is at risk of being born with the disease. An amniocentesis or cordocentesis test will confirm this (see p. 40).

If this trait is detected, the baby may develop the disease. Also, you may become anaemic and require iron and folic acid supplements.

You may need to have antibiotics to treat the baby, and ultrasound scans to see if the baby's growth is being affected by the illness (see p. 36).

Q MY DOCTOR WANTS TO TEST ME FOR DIABETES, WHY?

A Your doctor is probably suggesting this because sugar has been found in your urine after several tests, your blood sugar level is high, or you are carrying a large baby – all may indicate diabetes.

Q WHY IS UNTREATED DIABETES A PROBLEM IN PREGNANCY?

A Diabetes occurs when your body is not producing sufficient insulin for its needs. When diabetes develops because of the demands of pregnancy on your body, it is called "gestational diabetes", which is not usually as serious as pre-existing diabetes (see p. 136). Insulin is essential for regulating sugar conversion and for the metabolism of fats and protein. If diabetes is not correctly treated by a carefully controlled diet or regular insulin, this condition can make you feel thirsty, weak, and very unwell, and may cause problems for the baby.

Q I HAD DIABETES IN MY LAST PREGNANCY, WILL I GET IT AGAIN?

A If you developed diabetes in a previous pregnancy, even if it subsequently got better after the delivery of your baby, you have a higher chance of developing it again. This means you will automatically be given an extra blood test for glucose between 20 to 26 weeks, or a "glucose tolerance test" (see chart, left).

Q WHEN SHOULD I HAVE AN HIV TEST?

A HIV stands for Human Immunodeficiency Virus. It is a "retrovirus", which means that it incorporates itself into the genetic material of the cells in your body, especially those white blood cells that are important for fighting infections. There is as yet no known cure. You should think about having a test if you or your partner are from an area such as Central Africa and parts of Asia where HIV is prevalent; if your partner past or present was a possible carrier of HIV; or if you have injected drugs and shared needles.

Q IF I AM HIV POSITIVE, WILL IT AFFECT MY BABY?

A If you are otherwise well, your pregnancy will not necessarily be affected. However, the disease can be transmitted to the baby but there are ways of reducing this risk at or after delivery. Some women opt for a termination.

ULTRASOUND SCANS

Q WHAT IS AN ULTRASOUND SCAN?

A A scanner probe is placed on your skin (see box, opposite) and very high frequency sound waves that are inaudible to the human ear are passed into your body. As the sound waves pass over objects in fluid, they produce a pattern of echoes. These echoes are converted into electrical signals, which are processed and displayed on a screen as a two-dimensional image.

Q DOES IT HURT?

A Not at all. As the scanner probe is guided over your abdomen, you will feel only the cold plastic. If the pregnancy is at a very early stage, you may need to have a full bladder for the scan to be effective; this may cause slight discomfort.

Q WHY DO I NEED A SCAN?

A There are several reasons why a scan is offered: to measure the baby and so give an accurate delivery date; to find out how many babies you are carrying; to check for any complications by looking at the baby's limbs, organs, brain, and spine; to check that the placenta is not lying over your cervix (see placenta praevia, p. 140); or to see the position of the baby.

Q CAN I SAY NO TO HAVING A SCAN?

A Yes, you can. You shouldn't feel forced into having a scan. Scans have been offered as routine for about 15 years, but if you feel that this is unnecessary interference and you don't need extra reassurance, you can decline (see panel, below).

Q WHEN WILL I HAVE A SCAN?

A This depends on your hospital, but an early scan may be offered 8 to 12 weeks after your last period, so as to date the pregnancy. You will be given a routine scan at about 18 to 22 weeks to check the development of your baby's organs.

Q WHY MIGHT I NEED MORE SCANS?

A Further scans may be recommended if it was not possible to see everything clearly because of the position of the baby; if the doctor suspects that there is a risk to the pregnancy; or if there is more than one baby. More detailed scans that investigate particular problems, such as slow growth or chromosomal abnormalities, may be required (see p. 38). You may also be offered a further scan within the last six weeks of your pregnancy to check on the position of the placenta, or to establish the baby's position.

DISCUSSION POINT

DECIDING ON AN ULTRASOUND SCAN

Although the safety of ultrasound scans has never been seriously cast into doubt, there are differing views about whether pregnant women should routinely accept having a scan.

Routine scanning

Most doctors support a routine early scan at 8 to 12 weeks to date a pregnancy, and another at 18 to 22 weeks to check the baby's organs and limbs. You will be offered "serial" scans every 2 to 3 weeks if doctors think there is a problem with the baby's growth or if other routine tests (see p. 30)

detect potential difficulties. Through close monitoring, a doctor can anticipate special circumstances, such as the need for an early delivery. Doctors feel that scans provide reassurance – whether you have a "normal" pregnancy or one that carries risks (see p. 32). Certainly, if there is any suspicion that you may have a baby with an abnormality that can be helped by intervention, then scanning is valuable.

Making an informed choice

Midwives agree that ultrasound scans should be available; however, you have a right to accept or decline them.

Q WILL AN ULTRASOUND SCAN HARM MY BABY?

A The most recent research indicates that ultrasound cannot harm your baby; nevertheless repeat scans are offered if your doctor feels they will enhance your antenatal care.

Q CAN I FIND OUT MY BABY'S SEX FROM AN ULTRASOUND SCAN?

A It is not always possible to detect a baby's sex accurately, as the cord, closed legs, or moving limbs can all contribute to a misreading. Many hospitals have a policy of not disclosing the sex of the baby in case they are not absolutely correct. However, doctors will try to establish the sex if there is a risk of an hereditary disorder affecting one or other of the sexes. If you are really keen to know the sex of your baby, you can always ask the ultrasound operator.

Q WHAT HAPPENS IF A DEFECT IS DISCOVERED?

A You will probably be referred for more conclusive tests (see p. 40) before any further discussions take place regarding the pregnancy. At every stage, make sure you understand the doctors' explanations. If you need to decide about continuing with the pregnancy, it can help to get in touch with a counselling service or support group (see p. 256).

QUESTIONS TO ASK

What does the scan show about my baby?

Does it confirm my expected delivery date?

Can I have a photograph of my baby?

What will you be looking for in further scans?

(see p. 40) ... (see p. 256).

YOUR ANTENATAL CARE

WHAT HAPPENS WHEN I GO FOR A SCAN?

If you have a scan in the early weeks of pregnancy, you may be asked to drink plenty of fluid, as an enlarged bladder will make it easier to scan the baby; this will not be necessary later on. You will lie on a bed beside the machine and lift up your clothes – so wear something loose. The procedure takes about 20 minutes.

THE SCREEN IMAGE
The image is not always clear. The scan operator will point out your baby's head, heart, and limbs. This scan shows an 18-week fetus.

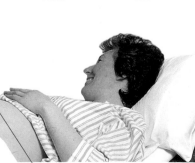

Head   Arm   Chest   Knee

THE MACHINE
The screen shows an image of the baby from which the necessary measurements are taken.

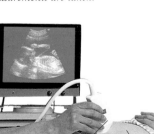

THE SCAN OPERATOR
An ultrasound scan may be done by a radiographer, an ultrasonographer, an obstetrician, or a midwife.

The probe is moved over the gel on your stomach to produce an image on the screen.

Gel is rubbed over your stomach to help conduct the sound waves. The gel is water-based and non-staining.

YOUR ANTENATAL CARE

DOPPLER AND NUCHAL SCANS

Q WHAT ARE THESE SCANS FOR?

A Doppler and Nuchal scans are both painless and non-invasive special ultrasound scans that are used to detect specific problems. Both types of scan are relatively new and they are available only at certain hospitals.

Q WHEN IS A DOPPLER SCAN OFFERED?

A A Doppler scan is used to examine the blood flow in the baby or in the placenta. It is used to check babies who are small in relation to their due date or not growing as fast as expected. The test may also identify women at risk of developing high blood pressure (pre-eclampsia), (see p. 138).

Q HOW DOES A DOPPLER SCAN WORK?

A It uses a different form of high-frequency sound waves, which are processed to show special wave forms. These sound waves reflect off moving objects, particularly red blood cells moving through arteries and veins. A Doppler scan shows the speed at which these cells are travelling; this tells doctors about the flow of blood through the blood vessels, indicates whether the placenta is working properly, or if the baby is short of oxygen.

Q IS A DOPPLER SCAN SAFE?

A The Doppler scan has been used in obstetrics, gynaecology, and many other areas of medicine for at least ten years and it has never caused any safety concerns. However, to be on the safe side, it is not used in very early pregnancy. It tends to be available only at larger hospitals with specialist units.

Q WHAT IS A NUCHAL SCAN AND IS IT SAFE?

A A Nuchal scan is an ultrasound scan in which the baby's neck is examined (see below). It is a fairly new but safe method of early antenatal screening for Down's syndrome. Although it does not give a definitive answer, it can show at a very early stage if there is a chance that your baby has Down's. It may be the best non-invasive test available at the moment. If it shows this risk is high, you can be offered amniocentesis or CVS (see p. 40).

WHAT DOES A NUCHAL SCAN SHOW?

"Nuchal" means neck; a Nuchal ultrasound scan, carried out at 11 to 14 weeks, is used to look at the thickness of the baby's neck. It is thought that babies with a particularly thick nuchal pad at the back of the neck are at higher risk of suffering from heart defects, Down's syndrome, or some other chromosomal or genetic disorder.

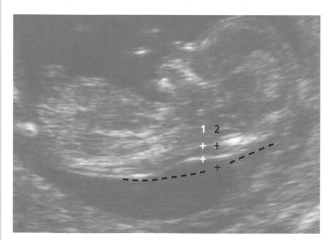

1 2

WHAT THE SCAN SHOWS
The picture (left) shows the scan of a normal baby (1). The dotted lines indicate where the nuchal pad would be thicker in a Down's syndrome baby (2). The baby's neck is measured between the points indicated as crosses; if the nuchal pad is larger than normal, chromosomal problems or heart defects are more likely.

1. Normal nuchal thickness measurement.

2. Increased nuchal thickness measurement.

CONFIRMING THE DIAGNOSIS

Q HOW IS A DIAGNOSIS CONFIRMED?

A If, as a result of what the special blood tests and/or the ultrasound scans show, there is reason to suspect that your baby may be suffering from a disease, or a genetic or chromosomal abnormality, further invasive tests will be suggested (see p. 40) to confirm, or rule out, these problems.

Q WHAT ARE GENETIC ABNORMALITIES?

A Genetic abnormalities are those diseases that occur usually because of a defective gene that you or your partner is carrying, but do not necessarily know that you possess.

Q WHAT ARE GENETIC DISEASES?

A Examples of these are: cystic fibrosis, a rare disease of the lungs and digestive systems that occurs in around 1 in 2,000 pregnancies; sickle cell anaemia and thalassaemia, which are common in certain ethnic groups. Babies suffering from these conditions are usually perfectly well in the womb and the illness only shows itself after birth. There are also some sex-linked conditions, such as muscular dystrophy and haemophilia, that are carried by the mother and passed to male children; you will almost certainly know if you have these genes in your family.

Q HOW MIGHT MY BABY HAVE A GENETIC DISEASE IF I DON'T HAVE ANY DISEASES?

A The genes for some diseases are recessive, or hidden. If both parents have the same gene, the two sets of genes may match up in your baby, which means that your baby will suffer from the full condition. Some genes are passed directly from one or other parent. Occasionally, diseases occur due to a spontaneous mutation of the genes.

Q WHAT ARE CHROMOSOMAL ABNORMALITIES?

A Chromosomal abnormalities include Down's syndrome and other, usually fatal but very rare, chromosomal syndromes. In Down's syndrome an extra chromosome 21 is present, which results in a child with physical abnormalities and learning difficulties (see p. 145). It occurs more frequently in babies of older mothers (see right).

HOW LIKELY IS IT THAT MY BABY WILL HAVE DOWN'S SYNDROME?

The risk of having a baby with Down's syndrome is related to your age, although parents of any age can have a Down's child; it is not related to how many children you have had, whether you have a new partner, nor to any drugs that you might have taken at or around conception.

YOUR RISK INCREASE

IN YOUR TWENTIES
You have a 1 in 1,000 chance.

IN YOUR THIRTIES
You have a 1 in 900 chance. At 35, this increases to 1 in 400. At 37, it becomes 1 in 250.

IN YOUR FORTIES
You begin with a 1 in 100 chance and by the time you are 45 it has increased to 1 in 25.

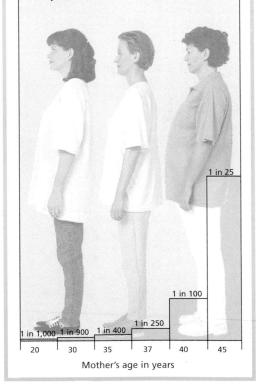

1 in 25

1 in 100

1 in 250

1 in 1,000   1 in 900   1 in 400

| 20 | 30 | 35 | 37 | 40 | 45 |

Mother's age in years

INVASIVE TESTS

Q WHAT ARE INVASIVE TESTS?

A These are special procedures where small samples are taken from the baby, placenta, or amniotic fluid inside your womb. They are called invasive because they involve piercing your skin and your womb with a fine needle.

Q WHAT EXACTLY ARE THESE TESTS FOR?

A These tests show the sex and genetic make-up of a baby. They will detect chromosomal problems such as Down's syndrome, or neural tube defects such as spina bifida, and genetic conditions such as cystic fibrosis, haemophilia, muscular dystrophy, or sickle cell anaemia. Cordocentesis can also show whether a baby is anaemic or suffering from an infection.

Q ARE THERE DIFFERENT KINDS OF INVASIVE TESTS?

A There are three kinds of test. When a sample of the placenta is taken it is called chorionic villus sampling (CVS). Taking a sample of the amniotic fluid is called amniocentesis. When some of the baby's blood is taken from the umbilical cord it is called cordocentesis.

Q WHO CARRIES OUT THESE TESTS?

A These tests are normally performed by a doctor who is experienced in ultrasound scanning. In some hospitals it may be an obstetrician or, more rarely, a radiologist. In specialist centres, difficult cases may be referred to an expert in fetal medicine, usually an obstetrician.

Q ARE THESE PROCEDURES SAFE?

A Any procedure that involves puncturing the womb carries a risk to the baby, albeit a small one, so do discuss this with your obstetrician. At present, one to two per cent of women have a miscarriage as a result of these techniques.

Q DOES IT HURT?

A It may feel a little uncomfortable as the needle enters the womb. You may be offered a local anaesthetic to numb the area around the needle.

Q WHY WOULD I BE OFFERED ONE TEST AND NOT ANOTHER?

A Whichever test you are offered will depend on the stage of your pregnancy. CVS can be performed after 11 weeks; amniocentesis is carried out between 14 and 26 weeks, and cordocentesis is performed from 20 weeks onwards.

Q HOW QUICKLY CAN I GET RESULTS FROM THE TESTS?

A The results take about two to three weeks after an amniocentesis, 7 to 10 days from CVS, and two to three days from cordocentesis. The amnio and CVS results take longer because cells need to be cultured in a special medium until they have grown mature enough for the chromosomes to be counted and analysed. You may be offered two new techniques: FISH (fluorescent in situ hybridisation) and PCR (polymerase chain reaction). These allow results within 2 days, but will only detect certain major chromosomal abnormalities.

Q CAN THE RESULTS EVER BE WRONG OR INCONCLUSIVE?

A In very rare cases, the cells that are obtained in the samples are found to be your own instead of your baby's; this is known as maternal contamination. Also, the cells can simply fail to grow in the laboratory and cannot be analysed. The procedure may then have to be repeated. These situations are very unusual but you should not worry if you are told that this has happened.

Q DO I NEED ANY SPECIAL CARE AFTER THESE PROCEDURES?

A You may be advised to avoid strenuous exercise for a day or two. You may feel drained, but unless you have a fever, do not worry. After a CVS, light vaginal bleeding is common. The blood should become dark brown and stop after a couple of days. If you bleed for longer than three days, or heavily with clots and pain, seek urgent medical attention.

QUESTIONS TO ASK

Will my care be affected by the test or result?

If I decide not to have the test, how would this affect my pregnancy?

How accurate are the tests?

What happens in an invasive test?

Invasive tests are not routine, because chromosomal and genetic problems affecting the baby are quite rare. You will only be offered such tests if there is a specific concern, perhaps because of your age, or if you or your partner suffer from a disease that can be passed on to your baby, or if an ultrasound scan warrants further investigation. These tests are commonly performed to rule out Down's syndrome.

AMNIOCENTESIS

This can be carried out from 14 to 26 weeks. A doctor inserts a fine needle into your womb and extracts 10 to 20 millilitres of amniotic fluid. The procedure takes 10 to 20 minutes. The cells are cultured in a laboratory, which takes up to three weeks, or sent for rapid PCR or FISH diagnosis.

GUIDING THE NEEDLE
First, to help the doctor be absolutely precise when inserting the needle, an ultrasound scanner is usually used to establish the baby's exact position in the womb. Second, a fine needle is inserted into the womb and into a pool of amniotic fluid

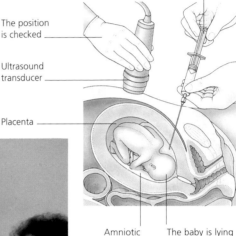

The needle is inserted

The position is checked

Ultrasound transducer

Placenta

Amniotic fluid

The baby is lying head down

HAVING AN AMNIOCENTESIS
You are made comfortable on a couch, then a doctor takes a sample of amniotic fluid from your womb. Your partner may be present during the procedure.

OTHER INVASIVE TESTS

Amniocentesis is the most common invasive test, but, depending on how advanced you are in your pregnancy and the specific circumstances, you may be offered a CVS or cordocentesis instead.

Chorionic Villus Sampling (CVS)
The advantage of CVS is that it can be carried out as early as 11 weeks. The basic procedure for this test is similar to amniocentesis (above), except that the doctor extracts a few fragments of the placenta through the needle. These cells are then sent off to a laboratory for detailed analysis, and the results are available a few days later.

Cordocentesis
This test can be carried out relatively late in pregnancy (from 20 weeks onwards) when the umbilical cord has developed. The doctor inserts a needle through your womb and into one of the blood vessels in the baby's umbilical cord. A tiny sample of blood is extracted and analysed.

REMEMBER
These procedures carry a small risk of miscarriage. You will be advised about your options and the possible outcome of your decision. You shouldn't feel hurried into an invasive test if you don't want one. Usually there is time to consider it and discuss it with your partner.

APPROACHING PARENTHOOD

Q WE WANT TO BE GOOD PARENTS, HOW DO WE BEGIN?

A There is no short answer to this question. But the fact that you want to do the best for your child is a good start. Most parents, if asked, would tell you that it takes a lifetime of learning to be a good parent. You will grow with your child. And no matter how much you read about childcare, you will always be learning something new. This is what makes parenting such a challenge.

Q WE'RE NO LONGER YOUNG, WILL WE BE UP TO SUCH A CHANGE IN OUR LIFE?

A Physically, things may well be harder for you in terms of sleepless nights and all the energy that having a new baby requires. Emotionally, older parents are often better prepared and more resilient than their younger counterparts. Having a child around will also broaden your horizons as you find yourself doing things you thought you had given up long ago. Don't worry about your age, the important thing is your willingness to give your child all the love and support that are needed.

Q HOW DO WE LEARN ABOUT THIS DEMANDING JOB?

A Very few people approach parenthood without some fears about their suitability and worry that they will be unable to cope with the extra pressures. This is natural, but there is no need to panic. There are several ways both of you can prepare yourselves for what will be a demanding and yet hugely rewarding part of your lives.

■ You could both attend antenatal classes, which will give you practical information about the birth itself and babycare (see p. 44), and meet other prospective parents with whom you can discuss and share ideas.

■ Discuss the coming change in your lives; think positively, and focus on the probable high points, but be realistic about coping with the low points.

■ If you can, talk to your parents and other parents with young babies and children; they may tell you about the difficulties of having children, but they will usually also admit that they could not imagine life without their child because of the richness the experience brings.

WHAT ABOUT SINGLE PARENTHOOD?

Will I have to go through labour alone?
Contemplating pregnancy without the father of your child does not mean that you have to go through the birth on your own. Family or friends are often only too pleased to get involved. You can choose an alternative partner such as a friend or sister who can be with you at the antenatal classes and during the delivery.

What practical support do I need?
If you are a single mother, it will help if you have good, reliable friends or family to assist you with baby-sitting, morale-boosting, and general all-round back-up. It is probably a good idea to establish a network of other single parents in your area with whom you can share your problems and solutions. There are several organizations and support groups for single parents, perhaps with a local group in your area (see p. 256). Make contact as soon as you can.

Will I be able to cope?
Remember that you are not the only one in your situation. Although being a single parent is not easy, more and more women are finding themselves in this situation, whether by choice, or because of the death or absence of a partner. Until it happens, you cannot predict how you will cope with the stresses and demands of single parenthood. Most single parents do cope, however. Few mothers ever regret having had their child, with or without a partner.

Are there any advantages?
If you are a single mother, your relationship with your child may be closer and you should be able to look after you baby in your own way. The relationship will also be more demanding because you will be the main focus for your child's love and for his or her needs.

YOUR FEARS ABOUT PARENTHOOD

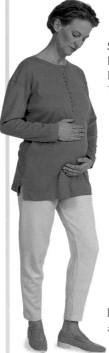

YOU

Since becoming pregnant I have changed; will I ever feel like "me" again?
You will probably not be quite your old self again because you are changing both physically and emotionally. Childbirth makes a woman mature very rapidly. Once you have been through the pregnancy and birth and have your own baby to care for, you will find that you have a different set of priorities. Try to look at it this way: having a baby is probably one of the most difficult and at the same time most rewarding experiences in life – go with it and enjoy your achievement!

I worry that I will become more and more like my mother, is this silly?
Many women experience this fear: you want to be a mother in your own unique way and not simply follow your mother's example. Of course, this also depends on the relationship you have or had with your mother. The relationship with your child, however, will be an entirely new one, although certain parallels may exist. You will find yourself taking pointers and examples from the good things you remember in your mother, and develop your own skills at the same time.

I find it hard to think of myself as a mother, when will this transformation take place?
This cannot be predicted. You may find the moment when you first hold your baby is so magical that it is no longer difficult to see yourself as a mother, but do not feel guilty if this is not the case, because it can take some time to bond. It should not be a question of transforming yourself, but rather of experiencing a natural feeling of love towards your baby. Being a good mother, however, takes time and practice, and is a learning process that takes a lifetime.

YOUR PARTNER

What can I contribute as a partner and father?
There is a great deal to learn about childbirth and your role as a supporter in labour. You can make time to attend antenatal visits and parent education sessions together. Often these classes offer a dads-only session, giving you a chance to have queries answered; you will also meet other fathers-to-be and perhaps in talking or listening to them you will realize more and more that this is just as much your baby as it is your partner's.

Will I be able to live up to my partner's expectations?
What are your partner's expectations? Find out what her needs are and then try to accommodate them. Certainly, the very least she will want is that you provide emotional support for her at antenatal visits, during the delivery, and after the birth; also that you provide practical help with the baby, especially in the first months after the baby is born. As long as you are willing and happy to do this, you are probably a fair way towards being the partner and father she wants.

I'm worried that I won't make a good father
The fact that you are worrying is probably a good sign that you want to do your best. No amount of books or classes can ever quite prepare you for this wonderful experience. You can learn how to change nappies and look after the baby, but this is merely the beginning. Remember that fathers are made, not born. You and your partner will both be learning how to be good parents. Talk to your partner about your worries. Realize too that instant perfection is impossible.

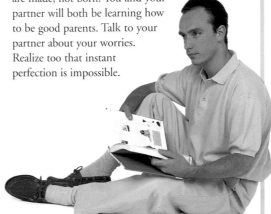

ANTENATAL CLASSES

Q WHAT ARE ANTENATAL CLASSES?

A Antenatal simply means before birth. These classes prepare you for childbirth. A better term might be parentcraft classes because, as well as covering all aspects of having a baby, from exercises before birth to the labour, these classes also advise on breastfeeding and babycare. Special classes may also be held for partners to encourage them to rehearse the role they will play during the labour, as well as show them how they can help to look after the new baby.

Q WHO RUNS ANTENATAL CLASSES?

A The classes are run by midwives and health visitors through your local health authority, doctor's surgery, or the hospital, and are usually free. There are also independent organizations that offer courses of classes (see p. 256). The teachers at these classes are trained to teach aspects of pregnancy and labour and will have had a child themselves, but they will not necessarily be trained midwives.

Q ARE ANTENATAL CLASSES USEFUL?

A Yes, they can be extremely useful because they provide a relaxed and informal setting in which to learn about and discuss the techniques of childbirth with other parents-to-be. If you are thoroughly prepared for your delivery, you will be less apprehensive and therefore less tense when you go into labour, which may result in a less painful and certainly less frightening experience. If the classes are held locally, they also offer an opportunity to meet other prospective parents.

Q WHEN SHOULD I START GOING TO ANTENATAL CLASSES?

A The classes are usually held once a week over a period of six to eight weeks. It is best to begin going to the classes around 31 or 32 weeks of your pregnancy. Classes that are run by your hospital or midwife usually take place during the day and there may be a large number of women attending. Other independent classes are held during the day or in the evening so that partners can be present. The number of women booked on a course may be limited.

Q DO I NEED TO BOOK CLASSES?

A Classes run by independent organizations tend to limit their numbers for a more intimate group, so it is best to book in advance. Hospital or local authority classes are usually larger but it is also advisable to book ahead.

Q HOW DO I FIND OUT WHERE MY NEAREST CLASSES ARE?

A Ask your doctor or midwife for information about the health authority classes at your hospital, or for contact numbers for the private classes in your area (see p. 256). You could attend both if you wish to have a broader perspective.

Q I WILL BE GOING ALONE – WILL I BE THE ONLY ONE WITHOUT A PARTNER?

A You will almost certainly not be the only lone expectant mother at the classes. There will be single mothers and women whose partners cannot attend because of work or because there are other children to look after. Some women have partners who just don't want to go to classes.

Q I HAVE HAD A BABY BEFORE – IS IT WORTH GOING TO CLASSES AGAIN?

A Yes, because there are special "refresher" classes. It will also be more than a year or so since your last baby, and you may find that the classes can update you on any changes that have occurred in certain procedures. Sometimes you can receive reassurance about a particular aspect of your previous labour that worried you. Equally important, you will also be able to meet other local mothers who are expecting around the same time, and they could be a great source of friendship and support.

QUESTIONS TO ASK

What is the emphasis of the classes?

Who normally takes the classes?

Is the teacher a professional childbirth educator or a lay person?

Can I contact anyone in your previous classes?

Do I have to pay for the course?

WHAT SUBJECTS ARE COVERED?

The exact content of the classes varies according to the individual taking the class. Before you sign up for a course, it is worth telephoning to establish if the approach is consistent with your ideas. Also, many teachers ask at the first class which topics you wish to discuss. In general, topics will include your health and any minor problems; exercises; labour (the mechanics, how to recognize its start, types of delivery); relaxation techniques; pain relief in labour; babycare, and so on. Classes held at your hospital will usually include a tour of the delivery rooms.

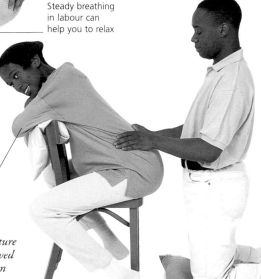

HOW TO LOOK AFTER YOUR NEW BABY
Nappy changing may seem a basic skill yet it often strikes panic into the minds of first-time parents. Practising on a model in antenatal classes will give you the know-how and the confidence to undertake this task for your new baby.

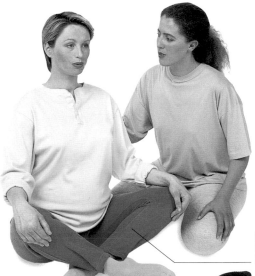

Steady breathing in labour can help you to relax

PAIN RELIEF IN LABOUR
Classes will discuss the merits of various methods of pain relief during labour, including relaxation techniques. These can be practised under the teacher's supervision in a calm atmosphere.

Leaning over a chair back can be a comfortable position in early labour

MASSAGE
Many women find that low backache is a feature of the early stage of labour and it can be relieved by massage. This is something your partner can learn and practise on you in the stress-free environment of parenting classes.

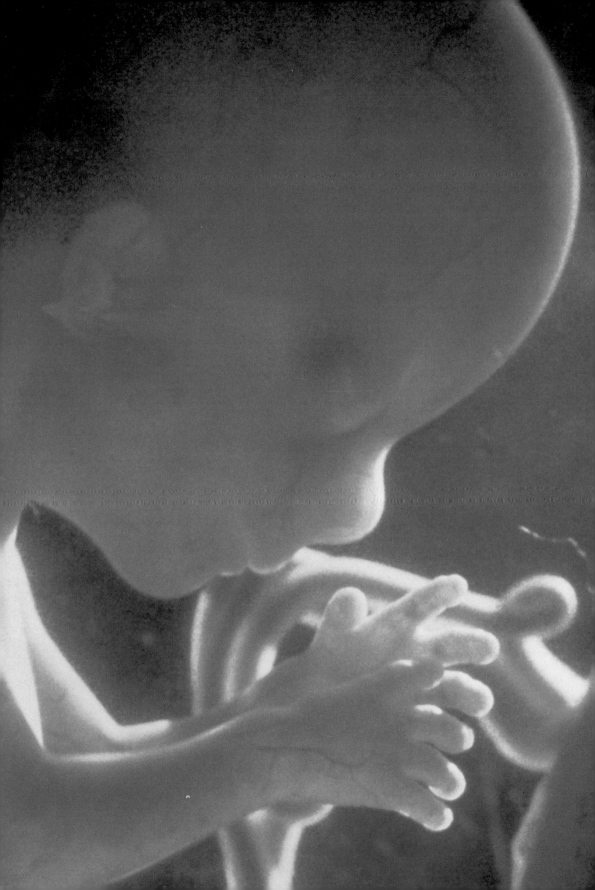

YOUR
DEVELOPING
BABY

Inside your expanding womb your baby is growing, taking from you all the nourishment he or she needs to become a unique human being. What started as a microscopic two-celled egg will, by only 12 weeks, have developed into a tiny but perfectly formed baby. Although, at this stage, you cannot detect any movements, as the weeks pass you will be able to feel his or her presence in your body. This chapter explores the miracle of this new life in detail, showing exactly how your baby develops from conception to term – month-by-month – and giving you a complete and fascinating picture of what is happening to you and your baby.

HOW YOUR BABY GROWS

AT THE MOMENT OF conception, when the sperm penetrates the egg, the genes from both parents join to make a new combination, and your child, a unique human being, is created. Below is a visual summary of this miraculous achievement. Your pregnancy is looked at in three stages. The first 12 weeks – the first trimester – are crucial for your baby's development. Although you may not be aware of it, the cluster of cells is multiplying into a fully formed (but immature) human being.

From 13 to 25 weeks – the second trimester – your baby grows rapidly, about 5cm (2in) a month, and can now make facial expressions, swallow, hear, and kick. By 26 weeks – the third trimester – your baby could survive if born. In the last three months, he or she should double in weight, weighing an average 3.4kg (7lb 7oz) at birth.

STAGES OF DEVELOPMENT

Fully formed but still thin

Fine hair (lanugo) grows over the body

The head grows faster than the rest of the body

The fetus begins to look human

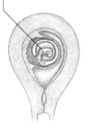
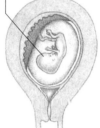
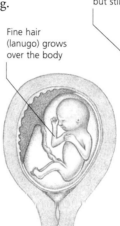
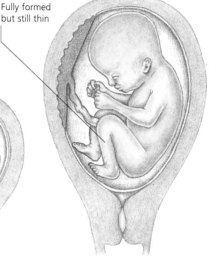

BABY AT 8 WEEKS
Your baby's limbs are developing and the major organs are forming.

BABY AT 12 WEEKS
The facial features are apparent. Your baby has no layer of fat yet and the skin is translucent.

BABY AT 16 WEEKS
Your baby now resembles a tiny human being; nails are starting to grow on the fingers and toes.

BABY AT 24 WEEKS
Your baby is much larger now and very active. All the major organs are working, but the lungs and digestive system need to mature.

HOW IS THE AGE OF MY BABY CALCULATED?

The length of your pregnancy is calculated by an old convention that began when it was thought that conception occurred during your menstrual period. Although we now know that conception usually occurs just after ovulation, which occurs between nine and 18 days after the start of your last period, the old system is still used when your date of delivery is calculated. Therefore, the number of weeks you are pregnant and the age of the baby will always be worked out from the first day of your last period (see p. 21). Throughout this book, when discussing the age of your baby, we give the gestational (development) age as dated from the first day of your last menstrual period (LMP) – not the age of the embryo. These dates will therefore correspond with the dates given to you by your doctor or midwife and so avoid any confusion.

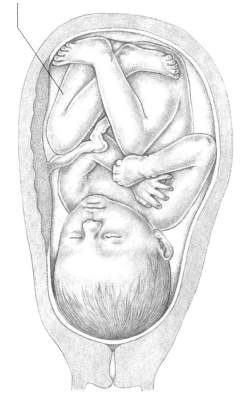

By this stage, most babies lie head down in the womb

There is not much space for movement in the womb

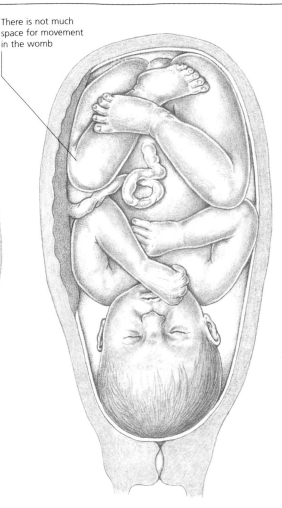

BABY AT 32 WEEKS
Your baby's head is now more in proportion to the body. Fat is accumulating under the skin. If born at this stage, your baby stands a very good chance of survival.

BABY AT 40 WEEKS
Now fully mature, much plumper and ready to emerge, your baby moves less and less as the surrounding fluid reduces and the womb is unable to expand further.

Are there different stages of development?
Pregnancy is divided into three-month stages called trimesters. Your pregnancy has three trimesters of 12 or 13 weeks, each trimester being distinctly different as regards the development of you and your baby.

PREGNANCY TIMELINE
To help you find information about the precise developmental stage of both you and your baby, this chapter and the next one feature a timeline running along the bottom of each page. It is shaded to indicate which trimester you are reading about.

Pregnancy timeline

■ First day of last period   ■ Likely date of conception   WEEKS IN PREGNANCY

1	2	3	4	5	6	7	8	9	10	11	12	13	14	15	16	17	18	19	20	21	22	23	24	25	26	27	28	29	30	31	32	33	34	35	36	37	38	39	40

| FIRST TRIMESTER | SECOND TRIMESTER | THIRD TRIMESTER |

CONCEPTION

Q WHEN DOES CONCEPTION TAKE PLACE?

A You are most likely to conceive if sexual intercourse takes place when you are at your most fertile, that is, just after an egg has been released from a follicle in one of your ovaries; this usually happens around the middle of your menstrual cycle (see p. 12).

Q WHAT HAPPENS TO THE EGG WHEN IT IS RELEASED?

A Once the egg has been released from your ovaries, it is swept into the Fallopian tube and then slowly propelled down the tube by fine hairs (called cilia) that line the inside. These cilia act like a moving carpet, brushing the egg towards the womb.

HOW IS THE BABY'S SEX DETERMINED?

Chromosomes contain all the information needed to determine the genetic structure of the new baby. All human beings normally have two sex chromosomes – a combination of either an X and a Y (male), or an X and an X (female). The woman's egg always has an X chromosome, but sperm can have an X or a Y, so the sex of the baby will depend on whether it is an X or a Y sperm that penetrates the egg.

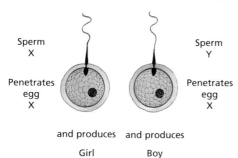

Sperm X · Penetrates egg X · and produces Girl XX

Sperm Y · Penetrates egg X · and produces Boy XY

X AND Y SPERM
The diagram above shows the penetration of the eggs by sperm containing either an X or a Y chromosome. The egg with an X sperm produces a girl, and with a Y sperm produces a boy.

Q HOW DOES FERTILIZATION TAKE PLACE?

A Once sperm are inside the vagina, they use their long tails to swim very rapidly through the cervix, along the inside of the womb, into the Fallopian tube, and then towards the released egg. The sperm are attracted to the egg by chemicals the egg produces. Several sperm may meet the egg at more or less the same time but, although many sperm cling to the egg's surface, only one sperm actually penetrates the egg's membrane; this is the point at which fertilization takes place.

Q WHERE DO THE SPERM AND EGG MEET?

A The sperm and egg normally meet in a Fallopian tube and this is where fertilization takes place. Occasionally, the sperm and egg meet and fertilize in other places, for example, at the ovary where the egg is released; this can cause an ectopic pregnancy (see p. 18), that is, a pregnancy that develops outside the womb. Fertilization usually has to take place within 36 hours of the egg being released from the ovary; after this time the egg is too old, and conception is unlikely to occur. Sperm can survive for up to three days in the womb.

Q WHAT HAPPENS AFTER FERTILIZATION?

A Once the sperm has penetrated the egg, the two cells fuse. The egg's outer membrane prevents any other sperm entering the egg. The fertilized egg then moves down the Fallopian tube into the womb and within a few days becomes a cluster (called a blastocyst) of about 60 cells. At around the time of your missed period, the blastocyst starts to glue itself to the inside wall of your womb; this is called implantation (see opposite). From here the cluster of cells will begin to develop into an embryo.

Q WHAT IF THE FERTILIZED EGG DOES NOT IMPLANT?

A Sometimes, in the complex events of fertilization and cell division, something goes wrong and a "non-viable" embryo (one that is unlikely to survive) is produced. When this occurs, the fertilized egg does not implant properly in the wall of the womb but continues on out of the womb. The only clue that this has happened may be a slightly late and heavy period.

What happens at conception?

Life begins with the miracle of conception, when one sperm penetrates an egg's outer membrane and fuses with the egg. When the sperm and the egg (each of which has 23 chromosomes) fuse, the fertilized egg then has the full 46 chromosomes necessary to form a human being. Twins or multiple births occur when two or more eggs are fertilized at the same time. Identical twins occur when one fertilized egg divides into two and becomes two babies (see p. 70).

The journey of the egg

When the egg is first fertilized, as it journeys down the Fallopian tube to the womb, it is like a self-contained space capsule that survives on its own energy stores. At this stage, the egg is still microscopically small and can only just be seen by the human eye. After six days, just as the egg begins to exhaust its supply of energy, it attaches itself to the wall of the womb.

The beginning of life
The fertilized egg divides rapidly into two cells, then four, then eight, and so on. These early cells, when the fertilized egg (morula) is fewer than than 32 cells, have the ability to form any part of the baby's body and are known as "totipotential" cells.

Two cells

Four cells

Eight cells

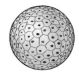
Multi-celled

The moment of conception
Normally, only one sperm can break through the tough outer membrane of the egg; once the sperm enters the egg, the sperm loses its tail.

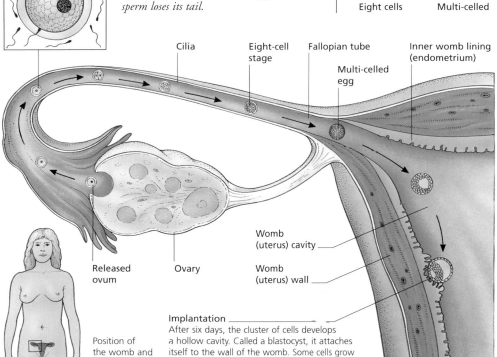

Cilia

Eight-cell stage

Fallopian tube

Multi-celled egg

Inner womb lining (endometrium)

Womb (uterus) cavity

Released ovum

Ovary

Womb (uterus) wall

Position of the womb and area enlarged (right)

Implantation
After six days, the cluster of cells develops a hollow cavity. Called a blastocyst, it attaches itself to the wall of the womb. Some cells grow into the womb's lining, and the baby's life-support system (the placenta) begins to form.

THE FIRST SIX WEEKS

YOUR BABY'S SIZE

Length (crown to rump)
4mm (⅛in)

Weight Less than 1g (⅓₀oz)

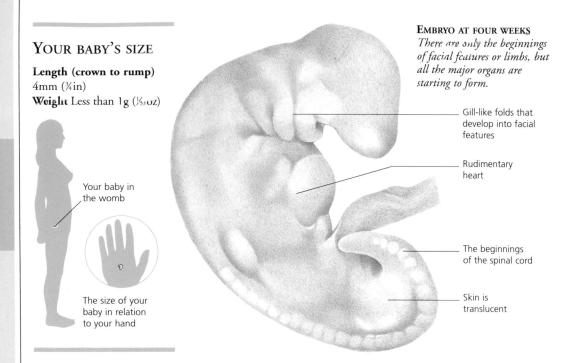

Your baby in the womb

The size of your baby in relation to your hand

EMBRYO AT FOUR WEEKS
There are only the beginnings of facial features or limbs, but all the major organs are starting to form.

Gill-like folds that develop into facial features

Rudimentary heart

The beginnings of the spinal cord

Skin is translucent

HOW IS MY BABY GROWING?

What does my baby look like?

By the time you are six weeks pregnant, the cluster of cells (blastocyst) that will become your baby has developed into what is known as an embryo. Around 4mm (⅛in) in length (crown to rump) and weighing less than 1g (⅓₀oz), the embryo looks like a tadpole.

■ **Head and face** A "blob-like" head curves down towards the tip of a pointed tail. At the head's base there are gill-like folds that develop into facial features.

■ **Limbs** Little buds appear at each side of the embryo; these are the beginnings of arms and legs, and will develop nodules that will become hands and feet.

■ **Skin** The skin, a thin layer of cells, is translucent and permeable to fluids. The follicles that produce hair develop later.

How are my baby's internal organs developing?

At six weeks, although the embryo is only about the size of your fingertip, the beginnings of all the major organs will have formed.

■ **Heart** The embryo has its own tiny heart, which circulates blood through new blood vessels.

■ **Nervous system and brain** A "row" of darker cells runs down the embryo's back – this is the basis of the spinal cord and nervous system. These cells form a lengthwise fold which, when it closes, becomes the neural tube and the brain. At the top of this row of cells are two large lobes for the brain, which is out of proportion to the rest of the body.

■ **Digestive system** The beginnings of a system are in place; there is a tube that runs from the mouth to the tail, from which the stomach and bowels will develop. However, it will be many weeks before it begins to function as a digestive system.

The embryo's life-support system

The cells of the fertilized egg burrow into the womb lining where little "fingers", or villi, form with tiny blood vessels to provide a blood supply for the embryo. The embryo's needs are simple at first, requiring just energy and protein obtained from its yolk sac (see box, opposite) as its cells rapidly divide.

WEEKS IN PREGNANCY

1	2	3	4	5	6	7	8	9	10	11	12	13	14	15	16	17	18	19	20
					FIRST TRIMESTER														SECOND

Q WHAT HAPPENS AFTER THE CELL CLUSTER REACHES THE WOMB?

A Once the blastocyst has implanted itself in the womb wall, it releases chemicals that send signals to stop your menstrual cycle and let your body start to prepare itself for the pregnancy. These chemicals also send messages to your immune system to ensure that the blastocyst is not rejected by your body but is allowed to develop.

Q HOW DOES THE CLUSTER OF CELLS DEVELOP INTO AN EMBRYO?

A The rapidly dividing cells eventually develop different functions, probably around the time of the thirty-second cell division, and just before the cluster of cells (blastocyst) embeds itself in the wall of the womb. The cells can then be divided into three different types: endoderm (forming the lining of the bowel, digestive system, and organs); ectoderm (forming the skin, nervous system, and brain); and mesoderm (forming the bones, muscle, and cartilage). Once a cell has a specific function, it cannot change to become another cell type.

Q WHEN DOES THE EMBYRO START TO TAKE A HUMAN FORM?

A In the fifth to sixth weeks of pregnancy, the embryo grows quickly and can be seen on a scan. After the sixth week, the head, chest, limbs, and spinal cord begin to form, and by week eight, the embryo has a recognizable human form.

Q WHEN DOES THE HEART START TO BEAT?

A The heart starts to form in the fifth week of pregnancy and begins to "flutter" or beat. An early scan, at around six weeks, may show the heart fluttering. Initially, the heart is simply a tube, and throughout the following six weeks this develops into the complicated structure that is the definitive four-chambered human heart.

Q DO EARLY DEVELOPMENTAL STAGES FOLLOW ANY PARTICULAR PATTERN?

A In the first 12 weeks, all embryos develop at the same rate. In fact, their growth rate is so predictable that your pregnancy can be dated precisely by measuring the embryo's exact length from crown to rump. Only in the second trimester do differences in growth appear.

WHAT YOU CAN SEE

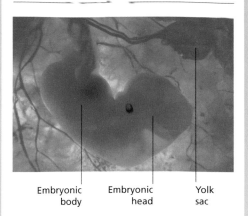

| Embryonic body | Embryonic head | Yolk sac |

AT SIX WEEKS
At this early stage, the embryo floats in a fluid-filled bubble that will develop into the amniotic sac. This sac is covered by a protective layer of cells, called the chorion. The yolk sac, which looks rather like a balloon attached to the embryo, supplies the embryo with all its nutrients until the placenta is fully developed and takes over at around the twelfth week.

Q HOW CAN I AVOID HARMING MY BABY IN THE WOMB?

A During the first 12 weeks the embryo will develop all the features and major organs of a little human being and be particularly susceptible to harmful environmental influences. You can help the embryo to develop healthily in this vital time by, for example, taking supplements of folic acid, avoiding certain foods (see p. 102), and completely cutting out, or at the very least reducing, alcohol, cigarettes, and any unnecessary drugs or medicines (see p. 106).

Q CAN THE EMBRYO EXPERIENCE PHYSICAL SENSATIONS?

A It is unlikely that the embryo can feel anything until the nervous system is fully developed and the nerves and muscles are connected, which occurs at around the thirteenth week. Even then, physical sensations are unlikely to be experienced until the brain is developed sufficiently to process information from the nerves.

WEEKS IN PREGNANCY

21	22	23	24	25	26	27	28	29	30	31	32	33	34	35	36	37	38	39	40

TRIMESTER | THIRD TRIMESTER

UP TO NINE WEEKS

YOUR BABY'S SIZE

Length (crown to rump)
3cm (1¼in)
Weight 3g (¹⁄₁₀ oz)

Your baby in
the womb

The size of your
baby in relation
to your hand

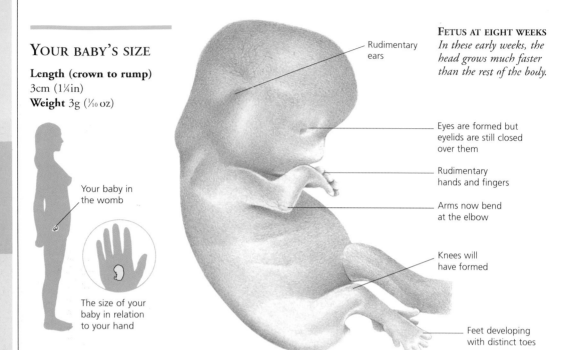

Rudimentary
ears

FETUS AT EIGHT WEEKS
*In these early weeks, the
head grows much faster
than the rest of the body.*

Eyes are formed but
eyelids are still closed
over them

Rudimentary
hands and fingers

Arms now bend
at the elbow

Knees will
have formed

Feet developing
with distinct toes

HOW IS MY BABY GROWING?

What does my baby look like?

By nine weeks your baby is about 3cm (1¼in) long
(crown to rump) and weighs about 3g (¹⁄₁₀ oz). The body
has begun to straighten, the head has a more defined
shape, though it is tucked forward over the chest. Limbs
have developed and the little tail has almost completely
disappeared. Your baby is four times the size it was at six
weeks – and is known as a fetus, meaning "young one".

■ **Head and face** There is a high forehead and you can
see ears, nose, and mouth, as primitive bones form the
framework of facial features. Even now, tooth buds for
all the teeth are in place, and tastebuds are developing.

■ **Arms and legs** The arm buds at first sprout wrists
and fingers, and then grow longer to form arms,
complete with a bend for each elbow. Little touchpads
appear at the end of each stubby finger. The same
process takes place with the legs, feet, and toes.

■ **Skin and hair** The skin is still fine and transparent,
but is now in two layers. Sweat glands have started to
develop, and light downy hair has begun to sprout.

What is happening inside my baby's body?

By nine weeks the basic structure of all the major
organs is in place.

■ **Heart** This is now a four-chambered and fully
formed organ; it beats about 180 times per minute –
twice the speed of the average adult heart.

■ **Brain and nervous system** The brain is four times
the size it was at six weeks. Cells, called glial (glue)
cells, are being formed within the neural tube; these are
vital because they allow nerve cells to be joined so that
messages can be transmitted from the brain to the body.

■ **Digestive system** The mouth, intestine, and stomach
are developing very rapidly, but do not function yet.
The middle part of the intestine grows so quickly that
it briefly protrudes from the baby's stomach.

The baby's life-support system

The placental tissue that initially surrounds the baby
and the amniotic sac is becoming concentrated in one
circular area on the wall of the womb to form the
placenta, but does not yet perform all the placental
functions of breathing, digesting, and excreting.

WEEKS IN PREGNANCY

1	2	3	4	5	6	7	8	9	10	11	12	13	14	15	16	17	18	19	20
				FIRST TRIMESTER														SECOND	

Q WHY IS THE HEAD SO LARGE IN RELATION TO THE BODY?

A The developing fetus appears to have a small body dominated by a large head; this is simply because the brain and head grow far more rapidly than the rest of the body in the first few weeks after conception. The back portion of the head grows even faster than the front, and so the head can appear to be nodding forward or curled around over the body.

Q WHEN WILL THE LIMBS DEVELOP?

A These grow more slowly than the brain and other internal organs. At about five weeks the limbs begin as little buds, or folds of skin. These buds begin to condense into cartilage (the origin of bone) until, at about eight to nine weeks, distinct fingers and toes have formed. Gradually (by about 12 weeks) the cartilage develops ossification centres, where calcium is deposited. These eventually become hard bone, a process that continues long after your baby is born. At this stage, the hands and feet look quite similar, it is only after about 12 weeks that they are distinguishable from each other.

Q DO THE ARMS AND LEGS GROW AT THE SAME RATE?

A At first the arms develop more rapidly than the legs; this is a natural progression that carries on into babyhood when a baby can grasp things long before learning to crawl or to walk.

Q WHEN WILL THE BABY BE ABLE TO SEE AND HEAR?

A At six weeks very primitive eyes and ears appear as little swellings on the head. They look more recognizable at about nine weeks when the development of the eyes and inner ears is complete, but the eyes are still hidden behind sealed eyelids and they won't function until the nervous system is fully formed later in the second trimester.

Q IS IT POSSIBLE TO TELL THE SEX AT THIS STAGE?

A No, the vagina and male organs are not yet visible externally, although there is some swelling in the genital area. After 12 weeks, this swelling becomes the penis in a boy or the clitoris in a girl.

WHAT A SCAN SHOWS

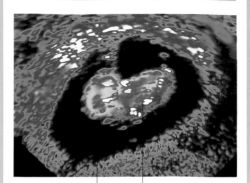

Lining of the womb — Fetus

AT NINE WEEKS
This scan shows that by nine weeks the fetus is beginning to resemble a human being. The facial features are becoming more distinct, and the "tail" has disappeared. The muscles are also developing, so movement is visible on the scan.

Q HOW IS THE BABY'S BLOOD MADE?

A In the first few weeks, the blood is formed from cells in the yolk sac (see p. 52). Towards the end of the first trimester, at around 10 to 12 weeks of pregnancy, the liver is properly formed and takes over the manufacture of blood cells. The liver does this until the bone marrow (the final site of blood production) starts to produce blood cells later in the second trimester.

Q HOW DOES THE HEART DEVELOP?

A At six weeks, the heart is a single tube bent in an S-shape. Over the next few weeks this tube divides into four chambers, two of which are called atria and receive blood; the other two are called ventricles, which pump blood out to the lungs and the rest of the body. At around nine to ten weeks, special valves have developed at the outflow of each atrium and ventricle; these ensure that the blood is only pumped in one direction and does not leak back into the heart. The baby's circulation is quite separate from that of the mother.

WEEKS IN PREGNANCY

21	22	23	24	25	26	27	28	29	30	31	32	33	34	35	36	37	38	39	40

TRIMESTER   THIRD TRIMESTER

UP TO TWELVE WEEKS

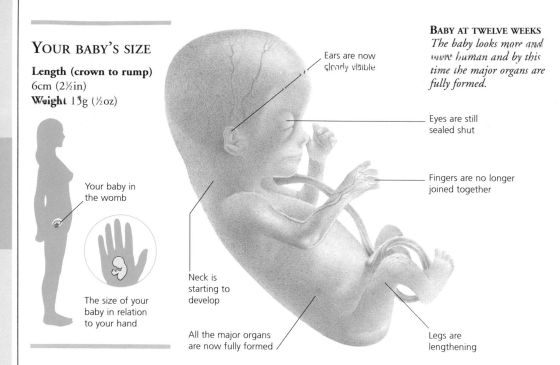

YOUR BABY'S SIZE

Length (crown to rump)
6cm (2½in)
Weight 15g (½oz)

Your baby in the womb

The size of your baby in relation to your hand

Ears are now clearly visible

Neck is starting to develop

All the major organs are now fully formed

BABY AT TWELVE WEEKS
The baby looks more and more human and by this time the major organs are fully formed.

Eyes are still sealed shut

Fingers are no longer joined together

Legs are lengthening

HOW IS MY BABY GROWING?

What does my baby look like?

At twelve weeks the fetus looks like a tiny human being; it is about 6cm (2½in) long (crown to rump) and weighs about 15g (½oz). It has miniature arms and legs, with fingers, toes, and more defined facial features. The body is straighter and the first bone tissue appears. The head is still relatively large (about one third of the entire length of the body) but it is now supported by the suggestion of a neck.
■ **Face** The face is completely formed, with a chin, high forehead, and the small button nose of a young baby. The eyes are further developed and are at the front of the face, rather than the sides, but they are still widely spaced and shut tight by sealed eyelids. The ears are now higher on the side of the head.
■ **Arms and legs** These are now beginning to move.
■ **Skin and hair** The fetus' skin is red, translucent, and permeable to amniotic fluid.
■ **Feet and hands** The fingers and toes are by now more defined, and nails are starting to grow.

What is happening inside my baby's body?

By the end of the eleventh week of pregnancy, the main organs are completely formed but not all are fully functional.
■ **Heart** The heart is now completed and working, pumping blood to all parts of the body.
■ **Digestive system** The stomach has formed and is linked to the mouth and the intestines.
■ **Sexual organs** Ovaries or testes have formed inside the body, but although external sexual organs are developing, the baby's sex cannot yet be established visually on a scan.

The baby's life-support system

At around 12 weeks, the placenta has achieved its final shape and takes over from the yolk sac to become your baby's life-support system (see opposite). Much larger than the baby at this stage, the placenta is a thick disc-shaped organ attached to one area of the womb. After its initial rapid enlargement, the placenta's growth slows; by the time the baby is born, it weighs about one sixth of the baby's weight.

WEEKS IN PREGNANCY

1	2	3	4	5	6	7	8	9	10	11	12	13	14	15	16	17	18	19	20

FIRST TRIMESTER	SECOND

Q WHAT IS THE UMBILICAL CORD?

A The cord, which connects the placenta to the baby's navel, consists of three blood vessels that wind around each other. Two of the vessels are arteries taking blood from the baby to the placenta and one is a vein returning blood from the placenta to the baby. These vessels are surrounded by a thick protective substance called Wharton's jelly and encased in a further covering.

Q CAN KNOTS OCCUR IN MY BABY'S CORD?

A Yes, the cord can occasionally become knotted, but because the cord is very rubbery and slippery, the knot or knots are usually loose and cause no problem. Should the knot become tight during the birth, it can cause the baby distress by cutting off the supply of oxygen and nutrients. This is a rare occurrence but it can be linked to stillbirth before labour has started.

Q WHEN CAN I HEAR A HEARTBEAT?

A Your baby's heart can be heard by ten weeks with a device called a sonicaid. This uses Doppler ultrasound waves (see p. 38), which are high-frequency sound waves and quite harmless to your baby. At this early stage of development, your baby's heart rate is very fast, around 160 beats per minute. This rate slows as the baby grows.

Q WHEN DO THE BONES DEVELOP?

A The cartilage foundations are laid down in the body at about six weeks. Although the joints and bones are all formed in outline by 12 weeks, the process by which cartilage turns into hardened bone (ossification) takes far longer. Centres of hard bone are created while your baby is in the womb but at and after the birth the bones are still forming and will not be fully complete unril adolescence.

WHAT IS THE PLACENTA AND WHAT DOES IT DO?

The placenta is a marvellous piece of biological engineering. Attached to your womb wall and connected to your baby by the umbilical cord, it has several functions: it produces hormones that are vital to maintain the pregnancy; it acts as a filtering membrane, rather like the lungs, to breathe, digest, and excrete for your baby. Without ever mixing the maternal and fetal blood, it takes in oxygen and nutrients from your blood, and expels your baby's carbon dioxide and waste products.

HOW THE PLACENTA WORKS
Where the placenta adheres to the womb wall, it consists of very fine blood vessels containing the baby's blood. These are enveloped by pools of the mother's blood and this is where fluids, nutrients, and gases are exchanged.

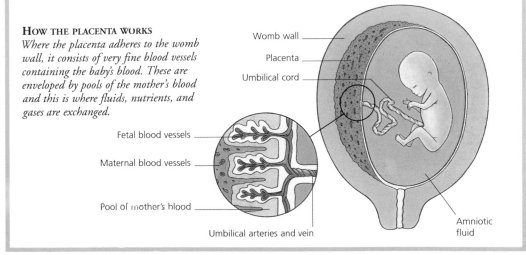

Womb wall
Placenta
Umbilical cord
Fetal blood vessels
Maternal blood vessels
Pool of mother's blood
Umbilical arteries and vein
Amniotic fluid

WEEKS IN PREGNANCY

21	22	23	24	25	26	27	28	29	30	31	32	33	34	35	36	37	38	39	40
TRIMESTER					THIRD TRIMESTER														

Up to Sixteen Weeks

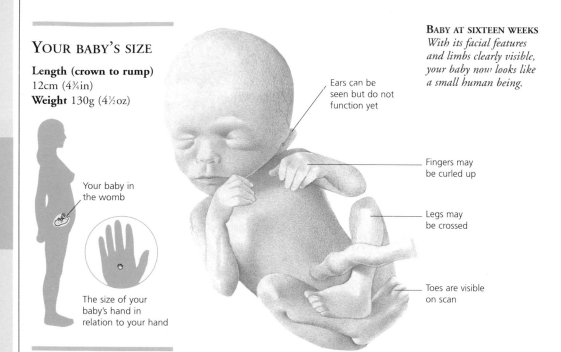

Your baby's size

Length (crown to rump)
12cm (4¾in)
Weight 130g (4½oz)

Your baby in the womb

The size of your baby's hand in relation to your hand

Baby at sixteen weeks
With its facial features and limbs clearly visible, your baby now looks like a small human being.

Ears can be seen but do not function yet

Fingers may be curled up

Legs may be crossed

Toes are visible on scan

How is my baby growing?

What does my baby look like?
By 16 weeks your baby is about 12cm (4¾in) long (crown to rump), and weighs about 130g (4½oz). Although the baby is still very small, all the limbs and features are formed, and are more in proportion. Because there is no layer of fat, the baby will look thin; the skin is so fine and translucent that underlying blood vessels can be clearly seen. The baby is also very active and can make a fist, suck a thumb, swallow fluid, and excrete into the amniotic fluid.
■ **Head** The facial bones have formed, so a scan at this stage may reveal more delicate features, such as the nose or mouth. Because the facial muscles have developed, the baby can make – but not control – expressions. The eyes are becoming sensitive to changes in light, even though they are still shut tight. Very fine eyebrows and eyelashes have started to grow; tastebuds appear on the tongue. By 16 weeks, the small bones in the ear harden and your baby hears some first sounds.

■ **Arms and legs** The legs have now caught up with arm development, and become longer than the arms. Tiny fingernails are appearing at the end of delicate fingers, but the toenails begin to grow later.

What is happening inside my baby's body?
The baby's range of movements greatly increases due to the development of the nervous system.
■ **Nervous system** A layer of fat (myelin) is beginning to coat the nerves that link muscles to the brain. This is important because once the connections are complete, messages can be passed to and from the brain, allowing co-ordinated movement.

The baby's life-support system
Inside the sac of membranes, your baby is surrounded by protective amniotic fluid, which means that he or she can move about freely and develop muscle tone. Your baby may be head down one minute and feet down the next but you are unlikely to feel any of the movements yet because the fluid cushions you from these tiny sensations.

WEEKS IN PREGNANCY

1	2	3	4	5	6	7	8	9	10	11	12	13	14	15	16	17	18	19	20
FIRST TRIMESTER																		SECOND	

Q WHY IS MY BABY SURROUNDED BY FLUID?

A The amniotic fluid protects your baby from knocks, and keeps the temperature in your womb steady. Until 14 weeks the amniotic fluid is absorbed through the baby's delicate skin. After this time, as the kidneys start to work, the baby swallows and excretes the fluid back into the amniotic cavity. Although the amount of fluid around your baby is relatively stable, it is constantly absorbed and replaced and never becomes stale. Until around the thirty-fourth week there is enough to allow your baby to move around and develop the muscles.

Q WHY DOESN'T A BABY DROWN IN THE SURROUNDING FLUID?

A Your baby cannot actually breathe yet and instead obtains all its oxygen from the blood in the placenta. Imagine the baby as a diver immersed in water, and using the placenta as an oxygen tank; the only difference between your baby and a diver is that the baby's oxygen is passed directly into the circulatory system via the placenta, by-passing the lungs.

Q WHAT CAN MY BABY DO AT THIS STAGE?

A All the connections between your baby's brain, nervous system, and muscles are established by now, allowing for a far more intricate range of movements. He or she will be able to flex and extend fingers, arms, and legs. If you have a scan, you may even be able to see your baby sucking his or her thumb, or appearing to grasp the umbilical cord. The baby's bladder is filling and emptying with amniotic fluid as a rehearsal for its eventual role.

Q CAN I FEEL MY BABY'S MOVEMENTS THIS EARLY ON?

A It is rare to feel any movement as early as this because although your baby can move in a reasonably co-ordinated way from about 13 weeks, the surrounding amniotic fluid cushions these small movements. Some women say that they can feel very light sensations like "butterflies" in their lower abdomen at around 16 weeks, but this is unusual. As your baby grows, you will be able to feel the movements become more and more definite.

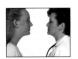

DISCUSSION POINT

WHAT AFFECTS MY BABY'S SIZE?

Family and medical reasons

Your baby's size is dependent on many different factors, although genetics usually determine the size of a baby, which is related to the size of the mother. Therefore, if you are small in stature, your baby is also likely to be small, and if you are tall, you are likely to have a larger baby. You will probably have a small baby if you yourself are small but your partner is very tall. If you have already had a baby, subsequent babies will tend to be heavier than the earlier one and boys tend to weigh more than girls at delivery. However, the birthweight does not necessarily relate to the eventual size of the adult. Medical conditions can also have a major effect on your baby's size; pre-eclampsia, for example (see p. 138), can result in a small baby, and diabetes can cause a baby to be large (see p. 136).

Other factors

Your lifestyle and environment can also affect the size of your baby. What and how you eat is important for your baby's welfare. If you eat a balanced diet, your baby should receive all the necessary nutrients to be able to grow to the optimum size. However, if you are malnourished, you can have a low birthweight baby and there may be problems with the baby's health. Regular heavy smoking can cause small babies because smoking reduces the amount of oxygen and nutrients reaching the baby. For each cigarette smoked per day, the baby's weight will be reduced on average by 13g (½oz). Your ethnic origin can also influence the size of your baby; for example, for genetic and dietary reasons, women from Asia tend to have smaller babies than those of Scandinavian and American origin.

WEEKS IN PREGNANCY

21	22	23	24	25	26	27	28	29	30	31	32	33	34	35	36	37	38	39	40

TRIMESTER · THIRD TRIMESTER

UP TO TWENTY WEEKS

YOUR BABY'S SIZE

Length (crown to rump)
16cm (6⅓in)
Weight 340g (12 oz)

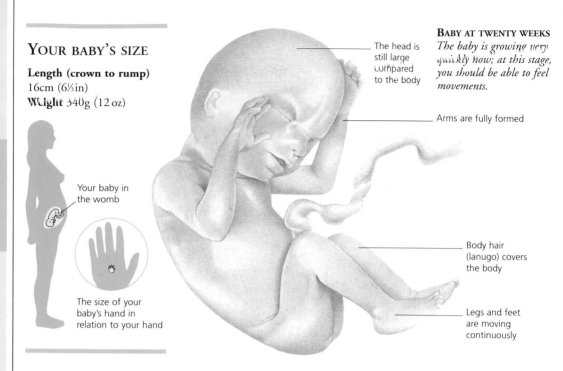

Your baby in the womb

The size of your baby's hand in relation to your hand

The head is still large compared to the body

BABY AT TWENTY WEEKS
The baby is growing very quickly now; at this stage, you should be able to feel movements.

Arms are fully formed

Body hair (lanugo) covers the body

Legs and feet are moving continuously

HOW IS MY BABY GROWING?

What does my baby look like?

By 20 weeks your baby will be about 16cm (6⅓in) long (crown to rump), and weigh approximately 340g (12oz). The growth rate, which has so far been very fast, now slows down to allow the lungs, digestive system, and immune system more time to mature. Your baby can now hear acutely and loud bangs will make him or her jump. You should feel these movements very clearly.

■ **Head and face** The eyes are still shut but eye movements have developed enabling your baby's eyes to move slowly from side to side. The taste buds are very well developed and the first teeth have now formed within the gums.

■ **Body** Your baby is not quite as thin as last month because it has developed a layer of fat. Some of this is brownish-coloured (brown fat) and appears around the nape of the neck, the kidneys, and behind the breastbone. Layers of ordinary (white) fat are also building up on the rest of the body.

■ **Skin and hair** The skin is covered by fine downy hair known as lanugo, and a protective waxy coating of thick white cream known as the vernix (see p. 67).

What is happening inside my baby's body?
Movements are far more co-ordinated and the baby's own reproductive organs are developing rapidly.

■ **Movements** Your baby will be much more active and have far greater control because the muscles and nervous system are more developed. Most of the major organs are now functioning.

■ **Sexual organs** These are now well developed and are usually visible on a scan. In a girl, the ovaries will now hold all her eggs (about seven million at this stage) and the nipples and mammary glands appear.

Your baby's life-support system
From now on, the fully developed placenta will provide all your baby's needs until birth; in addition to providing oxygen, nutrients, and protective antibodies, it disposes of waste products. Although the placenta continues to grow, it is now smaller than the baby.

WEEKS IN PREGNANCY

1	2	3	4	5	6	7	8	9	10	11	12	13	14	15	16	17	18	19	20
				FIRST TRIMESTER														SECOND	

Q WHEN WILL I BE ABLE TO FEEL MY BABY MOVING?

A You may not be able to feel your baby moving properly before 22 weeks, although you may sometimes detect occasional "flutterings" from about 16 weeks onwards. If you have had a baby before, you may be more aware of these light movements. However, you will not notice any regular movements until about 24 weeks, so you should try not to worry about how much your baby is moving at this stage.

Q WHEN DOES MY BABY START TO GROW ANY HAIR?

A The first hairs appear around the baby's eyebrows and upper lip from about 14 weeks onwards. By around 20 weeks, the baby is covered all over by fine hair. This hair, called lanugo, is shed at birth. Both lanugo and the baby's head hair (which may be scarce or plentiful at birth) are entirely replaced by new, coarser hair growing out of new hair follicles within the first three months.

Q WHEN WILL I KNOW WHETHER MY BABY IS NORMAL OR NOT?

A Most babies are born perfectly normal and healthy. An ultrasound scan at 18 to 20 weeks, is usually detailed enough to allow many major abnormalities to be detected; this scan will also allow your doctor to check the major organs such as the brain and heart. If there is any question of a chromosomal or genetic problem (see p. 39), further tests are usually done during this trimester. If all these tests are clear, it is very likely that your baby is normal. However, it is important to understand that no test can guarantee a problem-free baby, as some minor defects cannot be detected before birth (see p. 144).

QUESTIONS TO ASK

Is my baby the right size for my dates?

Is my baby moving enough?

Where is the placenta situated?

Are my baby's major organs developing well?

Is there enough amniotic fluid around my baby?

WHAT YOU CAN SEE

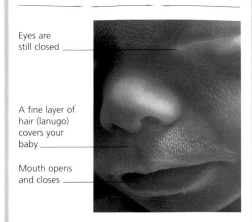

Eyes are still closed

A fine layer of hair (lanugo) covers your baby

Mouth opens and closes

AT TWENTY WEEKS

If you were to see a photograph or have a scan of your baby at around 18 to 20 weeks, you would see that the facial features are very clear. It may even be possible to see the baby's tongue poking out through parted lips.

Q CAN MY BABY FEEL COLD IN THE WOMB?

A This is unlikely because your baby is protected by your body, and also bathed in warm amniotic fluid so that there is a consistent, temperature-controlled environment.

Q IS MY BABY AWARE OF ANYTHING OUTSIDE THE WOMB?

A Babies can hear, and do respond, to acoustic (sound) stimulation from the end of the first trimester; they respond by moving, or their heartbeats can change. Some mothers report that their babies change the pattern of their movements in response to different kinds of music.

Q CAN MY BABY SEE ANYTHING?

A Until about 22 weeks, your baby's eyelids are shut. After this time your baby can't see much, partly because it is very dark, and also because babies have a limited visual range until a few weeks after birth. However, it is thought that babies are aware of sunlight and darkness in the womb.

WEEKS IN PREGNANCY

21	22	23	24	25	26	27	28	29	30	31	32	33	34	35	36	37	38	39	40

TRIMESTER | THIRD TRIMESTER

UP TO TWENTY-FOUR WEEKS

YOUR BABY'S SIZE

Length (crown to rump)
21cm (8in)
Weight 630g (1lb 6 oz)

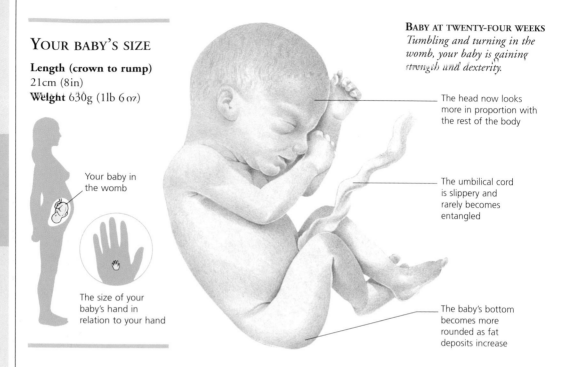

Your baby in the womb

The size of your baby's hand in relation to your hand

BABY AT TWENTY-FOUR WEEKS
Tumbling and turning in the womb, your baby is gaining strength and dexterity.

The head now looks more in proportion with the rest of the body

The umbilical cord is slippery and rarely becomes entangled

The baby's bottom becomes more rounded as fat deposits increase

HOW IS MY BABY GROWING?

What does my baby look like?
By 24 weeks, your baby has become less delicate and has probably gained about 500g (1lb) in weight in the last month; it is now about 21cm (8in) long (crown to rump) and weighs about 630g (1lb 6oz).
■ **Skin** Still fine, but no longer translucent, the baby's skin is now reddish in colour and, because layers of fat have yet to form, rather wrinkly.
■ **Eyes** At 22 to 24 weeks, your baby's eyes open.

What is happening inside my baby's body?
Surrounded by about 500ml (18fl oz) of amniotic fluid your baby can move around inside your womb with great mobility. He or she can kick, suck a thumb, open and close the mouth, and will respond to movement or loud noises. The heart rate has dropped to about 140–150 beats per minute, and it is now possible to get a print-out of your baby's heart rate on a CTG (cardiotocograph) machine. All the major organs (except the lungs) are now functioning.

■ **Brain and nervous system** If the brain waves of your 24 week-old baby are viewed on a special monitoring machine called an EEG (electro-encephalogram), they would resemble those of a newborn infant. The cells that control conscious thought are developing, and your baby becomes much more sensitive to sound and movement and, by this stage, is also thought to have developed a cycle of sleeping and waking.
■ **Lungs** The lungs, which are still full of amniotic fluid, are the least mature organs and still have several weeks before all the small air exchange sacs (alveoli) are completely formed.
■ **Digestive system** Your baby is constantly swallowing and excreting amniotic fluid.

The baby's life-support system
The walls of the tiny blood vessels (villi) of the placental tissue become thinner and more permeable as the pregnancy progresses, so that the amount of nutrients passed to the baby increases and greater quantities of waste are eliminated.

WEEKS IN PREGNANCY

1	2	3	4	5	6	7	8	9	10	11	12	13	14	15	16	17	18	19	20
					FIRST TRIMESTER													SECON	

Q WHAT IS THE EARLIEST AGE AT WHICH BABIES CAN SURVIVE IF BORN EARLY?

A The legal definition of viability (the age at which a baby can survive outside the womb) is 24 weeks and after. A baby born before this time is unlikely to survive and the mother will be considered to have had a miscarriage. At 24 weeks, there is a possibility of damage to the baby's internal organs during labour and the baby may be physically or mentally disabled. If you give birth after 24 weeks, you are considered to have had a premature labour and your baby may be put in a special care unit, possibly in an incubator (see p. 228). After 28 weeks, the risks decrease and the prospects for the baby's survival are very good (over 90 per cent).

Q CAN MY BABY DEVELOP IMMUNITY TO INFECTIONS WHILE IN THE WOMB?

A Your body provides certain antibodies that cross the placenta and provide your baby with immunity during the pregnancy and for several months after delivery (breastfeeding augments this protection). Your baby can produce antibodies while in the womb, but this usually only happens if you contract an infection to which you and your baby have no immunity.

Q IS IT QUIET IN THE WOMB?

A On the contrary, evidence suggests that the womb is very noisy. With the sound of your blood whooshing through your arteries and through the placenta, the continuous humming of blood along major veins, as well as the gurgling of your bowels, it is probably comparable to being underwater in a swimming pool. Your baby can also hear voices, and learns to identify your voice and that of your partner.

Q WHY IS MY BUMP BIGGER/SMALLER THAN THOSE OF OTHER WOMEN?

A Some women have a large bulge at 24 weeks, others seem to hide the pregnancy completely until 30 weeks or later! It all depends on your body shape and how thin or overweight you are, the strength of your abdominal wall muscles, and the size of your baby or babies. If your doctor or midwife confirms that your baby is growing normally, don't worry about comparisons with other bumps – it really does not matter.

WHAT YOU CAN SEE

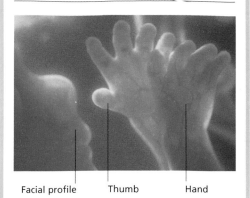

Facial profile   Thumb   Hand

AT TWENTY-ONE WEEKS
A photograph taken of your baby in the womb at this time (like the one above) would show that your baby's fingers are now fully formed and can grasp. This baby seems to be holding on to the umbilical cord.

Q WILL MY BABY GROW BIGGER AND HEALTHIER IF I EAT MORE?

A Unless you have been severely malnourished, and you suddenly start eating a tremendous amount of food, the answer is no. As long as your diet is providing the basic nutrients, your baby will continue to grow at a steady rate regardless of what you actually eat (see p. 103). However, it is important not to eat too much during your pregnancy; if you become seriously overweight, you increase the risk of developing a condition called gestational diabetes (see p. 136). Also, if your baby has to be delivered by a Caesarean section, being very overweight can make the operation more complicated.

Q WHY ARE SOME BABIES MORE ACTIVE IN THE WOMB THAN OTHERS?

A This is a difficult question to answer. Some babies do seem to move more than others, but the reason for this is not clear. However, it is also true that some women simply feel their babies moving more, whereas other women do not feel their babies moving even when they have done a complete somersault in the womb.

WEEKS IN PREGNANCY

21	22	23	24	25	26	27	28	29	30	31	32	33	34	35	36	37	38	39	40

TRIMESTER   THIRD TRIMESTER

UP TO TWENTY-NINE WEEKS

YOUR BABY'S SIZE

Length (crown to rump)
26 cm (10in)
Weight 1.1kg (2lb 7oz)

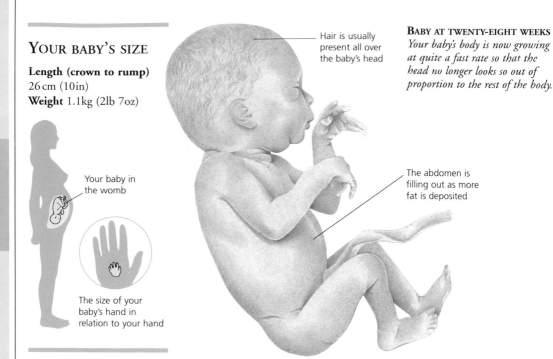

Your baby in
the womb

The size of your
baby's hand in
relation to your hand

Hair is usually
present all over
the baby's head

The abdomen is
filling out as more
fat is deposited

BABY AT TWENTY-EIGHT WEEKS
*Your baby's body is now growing
at quite a fast rate so that the
head no longer looks so out of
proportion to the rest of the body.*

HOW IS MY BABY GROWING?

What does my baby look like?
By 29 weeks your baby is about 26cm (10in) long
(crown to rump) and weighs about 1.1kg (2lb 7oz);
a greasy substance called vernix covers and
insulates the baby's skin (see p. 67). If born now,
your baby should be physically developed enough
to survive, but would require special care.

What is happening inside my baby's body?
Your baby moves around regularly in the womb.
■ **Brain** This grows much larger, and a fatty
protective sheath covers the nerve fibres; this
important development allows brain impulses
to travel faster, enhancing the ability to learn.
■ **Movements** Your baby is now more cramped in
the womb due to the increase in length and weight.
However, your baby can still change position; less
cushioning fluid means that you will begin to feel
these movements more and they may even be
visible from the outside.

■ **Lungs** At 29 weeks, the lungs have developed most
of their smaller airways and tiny air sacs (alveoli).
Equally important is the development of a substance
called surfactant, which is produced by cells in the
lungs. Surfactant assists with breathing by reducing
the surface tension of the lining of the lungs; this
prevents the airways in the lungs from collapsing
when breath is exhaled. A premature baby may have
problems with breathing because this substance has
not been produced. In a premature birth, either a
steroid injection is given to the mother to stimulate
the baby's lungs to produce surfactant, or the baby
is given artificial surfactant at birth.

The baby's life-support system
At this stage the placenta grows at a slower rate than
your baby. It receives about 400ml (14fl oz) of blood
from your circulation every minute and exchanges
nutrients, gases, and waste products. The placenta
is quite selective in what it allows to pass from the
mother to the baby's blood, stopping some harmful
substances, such as certain drugs, from crossing over.

WEEKS IN PREGNANCY

1	2	3	4	5	6	7	8	9	10	11	12	13	14	15	16	17	18	19	20
				FIRST TRIMESTER														SECOND

Q SHOULD MY BABY STILL BE MOVING?

A Yes, at 29 weeks your baby should feel very active. It is only after 36 weeks that your baby will quieten down because, by this stage, there will be less space and therefore less amniotic fluid to move around in. You may see your baby move if your bump heaves and bulges, and you can often feel him or her moving under your hand.

Q CAN MY BABY DAMAGE ME BY KICKING AND MOVING?

A Although vigorous movement is common after about 28 weeks, your baby will not injure you because the amniotic fluid will absorb any kicks, and the thick muscular wall of the womb will protect your stomach, liver, and bowels.

Q I SOMETIMES FEEL A SHARP PAIN UNDER MY RIBS. SHOULD I BE CONCERNED?

A If your baby is head down (cephalic) and he or she kicks, it can sometimes hurt you just below the ribs. Occasionally, pain beneath your ribs can be caused by your baby's head bobbing around in the breech position (see p. 67). This isn't dangerous but it can be uncomfortable. Sometimes a sharp pain under the ribs is the only sign that your baby is breech.

Q IF MY BABY IS HEAD DOWN AT THIS STAGE, IS IT GOING TO STAY THAT WAY?

A No, not necessarily. At this stage, the baby is still able to move around and will continue to move until about 35 to 36 weeks; after this time, your baby is too big to move easily and usually settles into one position ready for labour.

Q WHY DO BABIES GET HICCUPS?

A Babies do have occasional short, jerky "hiccups" which you can sometimes feel. They are probably caused by the baby moving the chest in an attempt to practise breathing. These movements can be seen on an ultrasound scan, and are thought to allow the baby's lungs to expand and develop properly. However, the baby doesn't need to breathe in the proper sense until born because oxygen is carried through the placenta straight into the baby's blood system via the umbilical cord.

WHAT A SCAN SHOWS

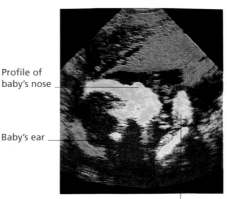

Profile of baby's nose

Baby's ear

Arm

AT TWENTY-FOUR WEEKS
This ultrasound scan shows the profile of a baby around six months. By this stage, all facial features are formed, so that he or she will look much the same now as at birth, only smaller. The eyes are still shut, but will open in the next few weeks.

Q DO BOYS AND GIRLS WEIGH THE SAME?

A Boy babies during the third trimester of pregnancy usually weigh slightly more than girls at the same number of weeks.

Q WHAT DOES IT MEAN IF MY BABY IS SAID TO BE SMALL FOR ITS DATES?

A This means that your baby is smaller than is typical for its number of weeks. The most common reason for this is genetic: your baby was never meant to be big in the first place. This is especially true if you and/or your partner are short or underweight. Another possible cause is that the placenta isn't functioning properly, therefore the baby is not getting enough nutrients and oxygen. This is called "placental insufficiency" and is sometimes, but not always, linked to the development of pre-eclampsia (see p. 138). A possible but less likely reason is that your dates are wrong and you are, in fact, less far advanced in pregnancy than everyone thinks. Rarely, an infection, chromosomal, or genetic problem can hinder a baby's growth (see p. 59).

YOUR DEVELOPING BABY

WEEKS IN PREGNANCY

21	22	23	24	25	26	27	28	29	30	31	32	33	34	35	36	37	38	39	40
TRIMESTER									THIRD TRIMESTER										

UP TO THIRTY-FIVE WEEKS

YOUR BABY'S SIZE

Length (crown to rump)
32cm (13in)
Weight 2.5kg (5lb 8oz)

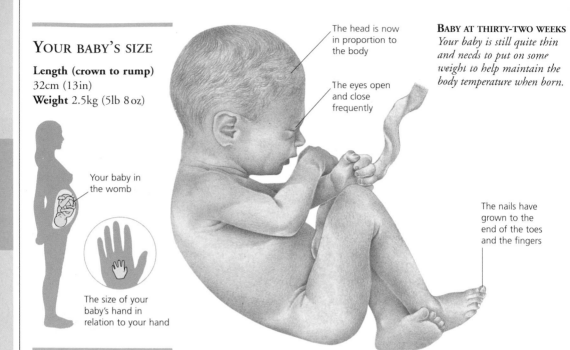

Your baby in the womb

The size of your baby's hand in relation to your hand

The head is now in proportion to the body

The eyes open and close frequently

BABY AT THIRTY-TWO WEEKS
Your baby is still quite thin and needs to put on some weight to help maintain the body temperature when born.

The nails have grown to the end of the toes and the fingers

HOW IS MY BABY GROWING?

What does my baby look like?
At this stage of the pregnancy your baby is 32cm (13in) long (crown to rump), weighs 2.5kg (5lb 8oz), and is fully formed, with the head more in proportion with the body. More fat has accumulated under the skin, which will help to regulate body temperature after the birth, although the skin is still quite thin on top of it.
■ **Face** The skin on your baby's face is much smoother, having lost many of its wrinkles. If you have an ultrasound scan around this time, the structure of the baby's face should have formed sufficiently for you to see its profile quite clearly. The baby's eyes now open and close a lot, and can sense changes in light through the wall of the abdomen; if you were to have a premature delivery at this stage, your baby's eyes would open and close automatically.
■ **Arms and legs** These are developed and the muscles and nerves are linked, allowing relatively co-ordinated movements. The baby tends to lie with the arms and legs drawn up and can now grip with the fingers.

■ **Skin and hair** The skin loses its transparent quality as fat is deposited, becoming pinker as the blood vessels become harder to see. The vernix increases and there may be some hair on the baby's head.

What is happening inside my baby's body?
Most of the major organs have developed and your baby starts gaining weight in preparation for the birth.
■ **Lungs** These are still developing. However, if your baby was born now, there would be a very good chance of survival with assisted breathing.
■ **Brain and nervous system** These are now fully developed although, if born now, the reflexes, such as the sucking reflex, and co-ordination would be poor.
■ **Digestive system** Meconium, a dark green, thick, substance made up of dead cells and secretions from the bowel and liver, fills the intestine. Your baby may pass meconium (the first faeces) if distressed during labour.

The baby's life-support system
The placental supply of nutrients to the baby is at its most efficient as the placenta reaches maturity.

WEEKS IN PREGNANCY

1	2	3	4	5	6	7	8	9	10	11	12	13	14	15	16	17	18	19	20
			FIRST TRIMESTER															SECON	

Q IS MY BABY'S SKIN NOT WATERLOGGED BY THE AMNIOTIC FLUID?

A During the third trimester your baby's skin is impermeable to the amniotic fluid that surrounds it, unlike the first and early second trimesters (see p. 59). This is because, at around 28 weeks, a thick, white, waxy covering called the vernix develops, which is protective and stops the skin becoming thick and soggy – as your skin would if you spent several hours in water. Also, the level of some salts and minerals in the amniotic fluid, which are not easily absorbed through a baby's skin, increases at this time.

Q HOW MUCH DOES A BABY SLEEP?

A As you have probably noticed, whenever you lie down, your baby often wakes up and starts to kick and move around. Babies may lie quietly in the womb or sleep for several hours and then be awake and move for several hours. Studies on babies' movements and heart rate changes reveal that they appear to have alternating sleep/waking cycles. This pattern of sleep can also persist in newborn babies until a more regular sleep pattern has been established.

Q CAN I INFLUENCE WHETHER MY BABY IS AWAKE OR ASLEEP?

A Your baby's sleep pattern is quite separate to your own. Often it is possible to wake a baby up by pressing gently on your abdomen, getting up and moving around, or even eating a high carbohydrate meal. Loud noises can often provoke some activity, and some mothers say that their babies wake up and/or react to certain types of music. Obstetric researchers use vibro-accoustic stimulation applied directly to the abdomen; this wakes a baby up so that changes in the heart rate when asleep and awake can be investigated.

Q MY BABY IS SITTING HEAD UP IN MY WOMB, IS THIS COMMON?

A Babies often lie head up (breech) until the last weeks of pregnancy and this is why premature babies are often born in this position. About 30 per cent of premature babies are breech but only 3–4 per cent of babies born at 37 weeks are in this position. The breech position is more common with very large or small babies or, if you are expecting twins, one baby is often breech. It is possible for your baby to be in the breech position up to 36 weeks, but to turn before the birth.

YOUR DEVELOPING BABY

HOW IS MY BABY POSITIONED IN THE WOMB?

The way your baby's body is positioned within your womb is called the "lie" of your baby. The presentation of your baby is described in terms of the part of your baby – head or bottom – that lies closest to the pelvis.

How the position can affect the birth
The normal way for a baby to lie in the womb is "up and down" (longitudinally). However, very rarely, the lie may be across the womb (transverse), or between transverse and longitudinal (oblique). If your baby is in one of these positions or is breech (see right) when you start labour, you are more likely to need a Caesarean delivery (see p. 196).

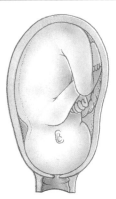

Head down

CEPHALIC PRESENTATION
This is the most common position for a baby at birth, with the head on the cervix.

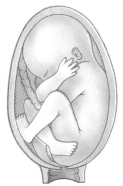

Bottom down

BREECH PRESENTATION
This is much less common; only about 3–4 per cent of babies are breech at term.

WEEKS IN PREGNANCY

21	22	23	24	25	26	27	28	29	30	31	32	33	34	35	36	37	38	39	40
TRIMESTER											THIRD TRIMESTER								

BY FORTY WEEKS

YOUR BABY'S SIZE

Length (crown to rump)
36cm (14in)
Weight 3.5kg (7lb 11oz)

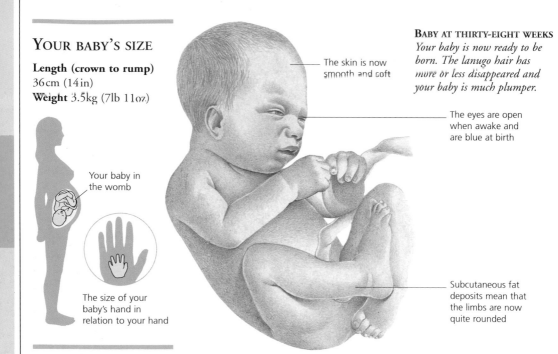

Your baby in
the womb

The size of your
baby's hand in
relation to your hand

The skin is now
smooth and soft

BABY AT THIRTY-EIGHT WEEKS
*Your baby is now ready to be
born. The lanugo hair has
more or less disappeared and
your baby is much plumper.*

The eyes are open
when awake and
are blue at birth

Subcutaneous fat
deposits mean that
the limbs are now
quite rounded

HOW IS MY BABY GROWING?

What does my baby look like?
The average baby is about 36cm (14in) in length
(crown to rump) and weighs about 3.5kg (7lb 11oz).
At 36 weeks, your baby is almost fully mature and
would survive if born, without needing to spend time
in a special care baby unit. In the last four weeks of
pregnancy your baby puts on a lot of weight and in
particular, develops a thick layer of subcutaneous fat,
so is relatively plump at birth.
■ **Face** At birth, the face is quite rounded and the
eyes always blue, although the colour may change
up to six months after the birth.
■ **Arms and legs** These are fully grown and, by week
36, your baby's fingernails and toenails should also
be fully grown.
■ **Skin and hair** The lanugo hair (see p. 61) has
almost completely disappeared by this stage, although
a few patches may remain at birth. The skin may be
pale, peeling, and cracked, and have deeply indented
creases, especially over the palm of the hand.

■ **Sexual organs** In girls, breast tissue is present and
the nipples are raised. In boys, the testicles have
usually descended into the scrotum.

What is happening inside my baby's body?
Your baby is plump and ready to be born; his or her
consciousness and co-ordination are well established.
■ **Lungs** These should be fully formed by now,
although they still need to mature; your baby is now
producing the hormone, cortisol, which helps the
lungs to develop in preparation for the birth.
■ **Heart** The heart is beating at a rate of 110–150
beats per minute. Once your baby is born, major
changes will occur in his or her circulation as the lungs
expand, allowing blood to flow into the lung tissue.

The baby's life-support system
The placenta, which has been providing your baby
with nourishment and oxygen during the pregnancy,
reaches maturity at around 34 weeks. It then stops
growing and starts to age. At birth, it weighs about
one sixth of your baby's weight.

WEEKS IN PREGNANCY

1	2	3	4	5	6	7	8	9	10	11	12	13	14	15	16	17	18	19	20
				FIRST TRIMESTER														SECON	

YOUR DEVELOPING BABY

Q WHEN ARE MY BABY'S LUNGS FULLY MATURE?

A By 37 weeks the cells lining the airways of the lungs have developed, and the many dividing branches of the lungs are present, ensuring adequate gas exchange at birth. Crucially, at this stage, the lungs have produced enough surfactant to allow the lungs to function normally.

Q IS MY BABY'S SKULL FULLY FORMED AT 40 WEEKS?

A A baby's brain is surrounded by a series of "flat" bones, but unlike an adult's skull, they are not yet fused. The bones of a baby's skull are quite soft and can slide over each other and overlap, allowing the head to pass through the birth canal and vagina without damage. There are spaces called fontanelles at the top of the head where bones meet. Fontanelles remain soft until several months after the birth.

Q WHY DOES MY BABY MOVE LESS NOW THAT I AM 38 WEEKS PREGNANT?

A It is normal to feel less activity from your baby after 36 weeks. Now that your baby is mature enough to be born, there is less amniotic fluid and less room for big turns or kicks inside your womb, and you will be less aware of its smaller gestures.

Q SHOULD I BE CONCERNED IF MY BABY DOESN'T MOVE AT ALL?

A Although it is common for babies to move less vigorously around the time they are due (see above), if there are no movements at all, or suddenly much less than you are used to, then you should contact your doctor or midwife. If you can't contact either of them, go to your labour ward where the baby's heart rate can be checked using a monitoring system called a CTG (cardiotocograph).

Q HOW DO I KNOW IF THE BABY HAS ENGAGED?

A Some women experience a definite decrease in pressure around their diaphragm and stomach, which makes it is easier to breathe deeply and eat a large meal. There is also an increase in discomfort in the bladder and perineal area, so you may urinate more frequently. Your doctor or midwife will confirm engagement by an external examination of your abdomen.

WHAT IS ENGAGEMENT, AND WHEN WILL IT TAKE PLACE?

When the head moves down from high in your abdomen and settles deeper into your pelvis in preparation for the birth, it is said to have engaged. Engagement is also referred to as the head "dropping".

When will my baby engage?
This can happen any time between 36 weeks and labour. It is more likely to engage early if this is a first baby. If the baby does engage, this doesn't mean that labour is about to begin; you may have several weeks to go. Also, if the baby does not engage, do not worry that you won't be able to have a normal delivery because it can occur any time up to your labour. Indeed, with second or subsequent babies, the baby often doesn't engage until labour has started.

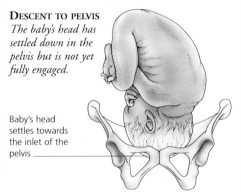

DESCENT TO PELVIS
The baby's head has settled down in the pelvis but is not yet fully engaged.

Baby's head settles towards the inlet of the pelvis

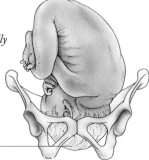

ENGAGEMENT POSITION
When engaged, the head is usually down, fitting in the hollow of the pelvis.

Soft skull bones compress to fit through the birth canal

YOUR DEVELOPING BABY

WEEKS IN PREGNANCY

21	22	23	24	25	26	27	28	29	30	31	32	33	34	35	36	37	38	39	40
TRIMESTER											THIRD TRIMESTER								

TWINS AND MULTIPLE BIRTHS

Q AM I MORE LIKELY TO HAVE TWINS IF THERE ARE TWINS IN MY FAMILY?

A Yes, you are. Non-identical twins are more likely if a close relative has had twins or triplets, or if you are a non-identical twin. However, the incidence of identical twins is more random and not always linked to your family history.

Q HOW COMMON ARE TWINS?

A Twins are more common in women who conceive after the age of 35, or have had fertility treatments, such as IVF and ICSI (see p. 16); over half of triplets result from assisted conception techniques. Although the reason for this is not clear, multiple pregnancies are also more common in certain parts of the world such as Nigeria, where 45 per 1,000 births are twins. In Europe the rate is about 10 per 1,000.

Q WHEN WILL MY DOCTOR CONFIRM THAT I'M EXPECTING TWINS?

A It is possible to see twins on an ultrasound scan at about eight weeks. However, because there is a higher risk of miscarriage (of one or both babies), a diagnosis of "viable" twins is rarely made until the beginning of the second trimester, at 12 to 14 weeks.

Q WHAT ARE THE RISKS INVOLVED IN HAVING TWINS?

A If you are expecting twins, you are considered to be a high-risk pregnancy. Extra demands are placed on the mother and the placental system on which the babies rely. In turn this can slow the growth of one or both the babies, and cause high blood pressure in the mother. There is also a strong chance of premature birth. These risks are further compounded with triplets or even higher multiple pregnancies (see p. 142).

HOW DO TWINS DEVELOP?

Twins develop at an early stage when, or just after, the egg and sperm meet. Twins are either non-identical (more common, accounting for about 80 per cent of twins) or identical (less frequent, about 20 per cent). The twins below are in a vertex (head down) position, but they can also occupy other positions in the womb (see p. 185).

IDENTICAL TWINS

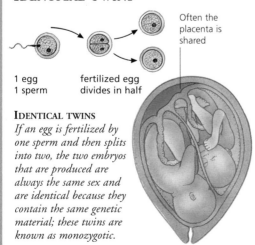

Often the placenta is shared

1 egg
1 sperm

fertilized egg divides in half

IDENTICAL TWINS
If an egg is fertilized by one sperm and then splits into two, the two embryos that are produced are always the same sex and are identical because they contain the same genetic material; these twins are known as monozygotic.

NON-IDENTICAL TWINS

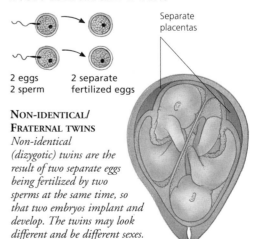

Separate placentas

2 eggs
2 sperm

2 separate fertilized eggs

NON-IDENTICAL/ FRATERNAL TWINS
Non-identical (dizygotic) twins are the result of two separate eggs being fertilized by two sperms at the same time, so that two embryos implant and develop. The twins may look different and be different sexes.

Q IS A MULTIPLE PREGNANCY ALWAYS HIGH-RISK?

A Yes, you will be under the very close eye of an obstetrician, and have regular scans and clinic visits. A home birth will not be recommended.

Q WILL TWO BABIES BE ABLE TO DEVELOP PROPERLY IN MY WOMB?

A Your womb is amazingly stretchy and it is quite possible for two, and sometimes three (or more) babies to grow and develop quite normally; there is usually no problem in their development as long as each is surrounded by a separate protective sac of amniotic fluid. It is, however, much more likely that you will go into labour before 40 weeks because the amount of space in your womb is limited.

Q CAN THE TWINS KNOCK INTO OR HURT EACH OTHER IN THE WOMB?

A Your twins can bump into each other in your womb, because they will be quite active and even playful. However, they cannot hurt each other because they each have their own sac and fluid.

Q HOW DO I KNOW IF MY TWINS ARE IDENTICAL, AND WHY DOES IT MATTER?

A The only way to know for sure is to have an ultrasound scan at 10 to 14 weeks. The thickness and degree of folding of the separating membranes allows a diagnosis. If they are identical and share the same placenta, they may have more problems with their development and delivery than non-identical twins. If you are pregnant with identical twins, you will be closely monitored and you can expect frequent scans.

Q WHY DID MY EARLY SCAN SHOW TWINS, AND NOW ONLY ONE BABY SHOWS?

A Twin pregnancies may develop more often than we think, but at an early stage one twin dies or doesn't develop. As the surviving twin grows, the non-viable twin is "reabsorbed" and disappears with almost no trace. In the first trimester this shouldn't cause problems, but if a twin dies later in pregnancy, difficulties may occur (see p. 142).

Q DO TWINS AND TRIPLETS DEVELOP AT THE SAME RATE AS SINGLE BABIES?

A Yes, they develop in exactly the same way, at the same rate except that they may not grow quite as large as single babies, even taking into account the fact that they are usually born earlier.

Q DO TWINS SHARE THE SAME SAC OF AMNIOTIC FLUID?

A Non-identical twins, being the result of two eggs fertilized by two separate sperm that develop independently of each other, have separate umbilical cords, placentas, and amniotic sacs. Identical twins, which are the result of one egg fertilized by a single sperm that has divided to form two or more embryos, share a placenta, but always have their own cord and usually their own amniotic sac.

Q I'M TOLD THAT MY TWINS ARE GROWING AT DIFFERENT RATES, WHY IS THIS?

A Twins may be different sizes to start off with, and can also grow at different rates. This is why if you have twins, you are offered frequent scans. It isn't usually a problem if both babies start off at different sizes but grow at normal rates; however, it may become a problem if they were both the same size initially, and one suddenly starts to grow much slower than the other (see below).

Q WHAT HAPPENS IF ONE TWIN IS GROWING MORE SLOWLY?

A If there is "discrepant growth", you will be scanned frequently and, depending on the well-being of the smaller, less healthy twin, the twins may be delivered early. In identical twins, a big difference in size may suggest a rare condition called "twin-to-twin transfusion syndrome", caused by an abnormal blood vessel connection (see p. 143).

Q IS IT TRUE THAT I WILL BE ABLE TO FEEL MY TWINS MOVING SEPARATELY?

A Because of each baby's own specific patterns of movement and relative position in the womb, many mothers can identify which baby is moving at a particular time. Twins do move separately; often one can be fast asleep or not moving much while the other is bouncing around.

QUESTIONS TO ASK

Are my babies growing at the same rate?

Are my twins identical or non-identical?

Is there a normal amount of amniotic fluid around each twin?

Are they the same sex or different sexes?

Have I got one or two placentas?

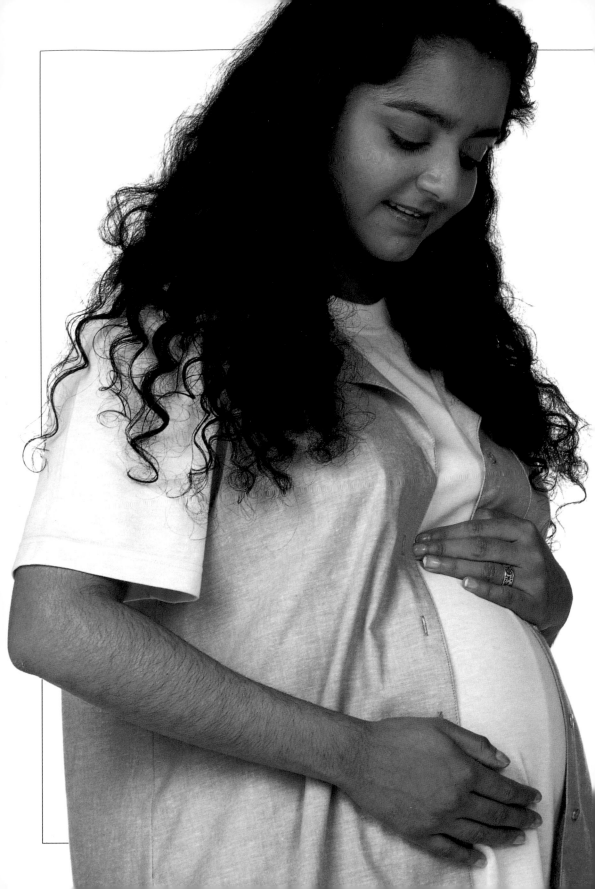

YOUR CHANGING BODY

In pregnancy, powerful forces are at work changing your body to allow your baby to grow and develop. You will experience new symptoms and feelings that may give you some discomfort even as you revel in the positive signs of your advancing pregnancy; or you may feel better than ever before – and look a picture of health. To reassure you that all is progressing normally, this chapter discusses and explains the physical and emotional upheavals that you are undergoing, sometimes offering possible solutions and remedies; it also reminds you that these changes serve one purpose only – to benefit the new life inside you.

HOW YOUR BODY CHANGES

As soon as you become pregnant, your body begins to change so that it can support your growing baby over the coming weeks. Because your body will eventually be supporting two systems, all of your body functions start to work much harder. Your heart has to cope with pumping more blood around your body, in particular to and from your womb, placenta, and baby, so your pulse rate increases by about ten beats per minute; your breathing rate speeds up to take in more oxygen for your baby and to exhale more carbon dioxide; and your metabolic rate accelerates to deal with the increased workload. As well as these physical demands, pregnancy also causes a range of emotional reactions that varies from woman to woman. Below, you can see how much your body is likely to change, the details of which are charted in the following pages.

STAGES OF DEVELOPMENT

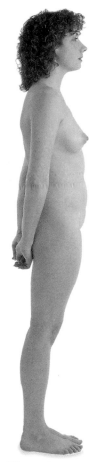 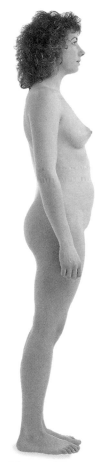 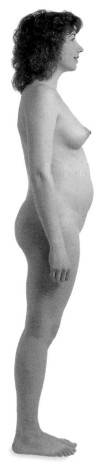 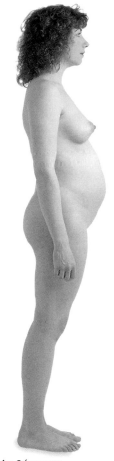

AT 12 WEEKS
Although your baby is growing rapidly, you will not see a bump yet.

AT 16 WEEKS
Your nipples start to darken as your skin becomes more pigmented.

AT 20 WEEKS
Your bump is expanding quickly but you may have lots of energy.

AT 24 WEEKS
Your face, hands, and upper body may swell because of fluid retention.

The Stages of Pregnancy

The 40 weeks, or approximately nine months, of pregnancy are discussed by trimester because each three-month period has distinct characteristics. In the first trimester, the first 12 weeks, little is visible but a great deal is happening; your baby's major organs are fully formed. The second trimester, weeks 13 to 25, is when your bump becomes obvious and you begin to feel your baby move. In the third trimester, from 26 weeks until delivery, as your baby grows and matures, your bump expands enormously so that at term you find even simple tasks tiring and sleeping comfortably at night hard.

Pregnancy timeline   WEEKS IN PREGNANCY

1	2	3	4	5	6	7	8	9	10	11	12	13	14	15	16	17	18	19	20	21	22	23	24	25	26	27	28	29	30	31	32	33	34	35	36	37	38	39	40

FIRST TRIMESTER	SECOND TRIMESTER	THIRD TRIMESTER

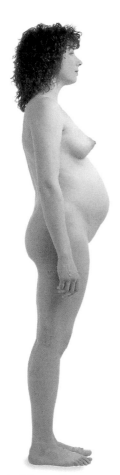 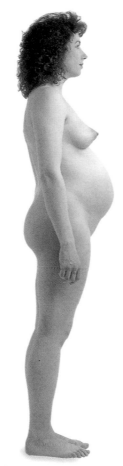 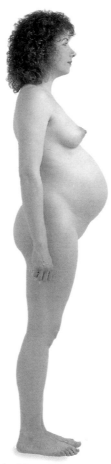 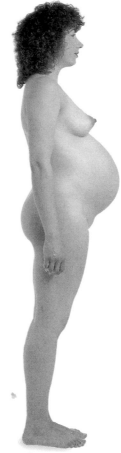

At 28 weeks
Your baby is now very active with much kicking and turning.

At 32 weeks
Your growing womb presses on internal organs and may cause discomfort.

At 36 weeks
By this stage, your baby's head may have dropped down into your pelvis.

At 40 weeks
Your bump is now so large that it is difficult to get comfortable at night.

THE FIRST TRIMESTER

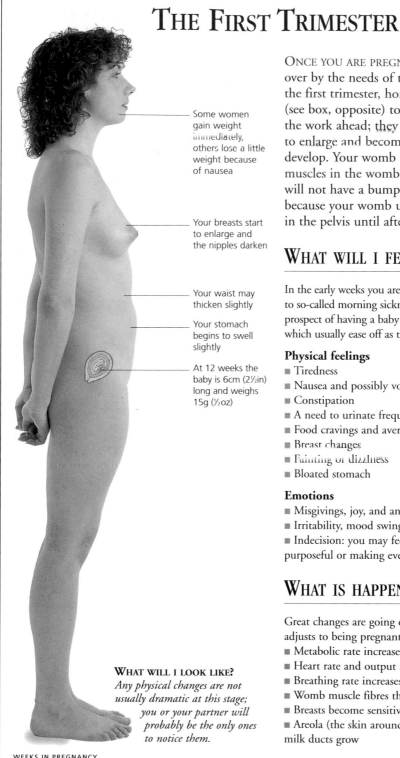

Some women gain weight immediately, others lose a little weight because of nausea

Your breasts start to enlarge and the nipples darken

Your waist may thicken slightly

Your stomach begins to swell slightly

At 12 weeks the baby is 6cm (2½in) long and weighs 15g (½oz)

WHAT WILL I LOOK LIKE?
Any physical changes are not usually dramatic at this stage; you or your partner will probably be the only ones to notice them.

ONCE YOU ARE PREGNANT your body is taken over by the needs of the developing baby. In the first trimester, hormones are produced (see box, opposite) to prepare your body for the work ahead; they also cause your breasts to enlarge and become tender as milk ducts develop. Your womb begins to grow and the muscles in the womb wall thicken, but you will not have a bump in the first weeks because your womb usually remains tucked in the pelvis until after the third month.

WHAT WILL I FEEL?

In the early weeks you are likely to be tired and prone to so-called morning sickness. Excitement at the prospect of having a baby often offsets these symptoms, which usually ease off as the pregnancy progresses.

Physical feelings
- Tiredness
- Nausea and possibly vomiting
- Constipation
- A need to urinate frequently
- Food cravings and aversions
- Breast changes
- Fainting or dizziness
- Bloated stomach

Emotions
- Misgivings, joy, and anxiety (or a mixture)
- Irritability, mood swings, weepiness
- Indecision: you may feel incapable of being purposeful or making even simple decisions

WHAT IS HAPPENING TO MY BODY?

Great changes are going on inside you as your body adjusts to being pregnant.
- Metabolic rate increases by 10–25 per cent
- Heart rate and output rise by up to 40 per cent
- Breathing rate increases
- Womb muscle fibres thicken and lengthen
- Breasts become sensitive and increase in size
- Areola (the skin around your nipples) darkens and milk ducts grow

WEEKS IN PREGNANCY

1	2	3	4	5	6	7	8	9	10	11	12	13	14	15	16	17	18	19	20

FIRST TRIMESTER | SECOND

HOW WILL THE CHANGES AFFECT ME?

Q I DON'T FEEL OR LOOK AT ALL PREGNANT YET. IS THIS NORMAL?

A This is perfectly normal. Some women breeze through the early weeks of their pregnancy without experiencing any nausea, tiredness or other problems. If you are one of these lucky ones, just try to relax and enjoy it. After about 12 weeks, at the start of the second trimester, when your womb has expanded into your abdomen, you will start to see and feel that your bump is growing.

Q WHY DO MY CLOTHES ALREADY FEEL TIGHT AROUND MY WAIST?

A This can happen early on, but your baby is probably not the cause. Unless you are expecting twins or triplets, your bowels rather than your baby are the reason. The increase in progesterone in pregnancy affects the bowels and causes wind and constipation, which can make you feel bloated. This condition should improve during pregnancy but eating high-fibre foods and drinking plenty of fluids will help (see p. 104). However, do not overeat in the early weeks – the baby does not need it and you may put on unwanted weight.

WHAT PART DO HORMONES PLAY?

The production of some hormones greatly increases in pregnancy, and new hormones are produced. The pituitary gland (at the base of the brain) controls some of these, while others are produced by the ovaries, thyroid gland, and later the placenta; their purpose is to prepare your body for pregnancy. Hormonal changes can cause side-effects, but they show that the pregnancy is progressing normally.

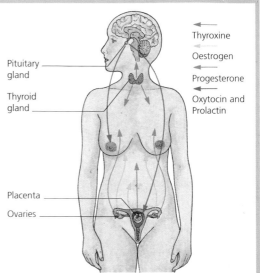

Progesterone
This hormone is important for the maintenance of your pregnancy and eventually for the onset of labour. Its most significant action is to relax certain muscles in your body, which has several effects: it prevents preterm labour; blood vessels dilate, which lowers blood pressure and can cause you to feel faint; the digestive system slows down causing indigestion and constipation. Progesterone affects moods, raises body temperature, increases breathing rate, and can cause nausea. It also contributes to the preparation of the breasts for breastfeeding.

Oestrogen
This hormone causes your nipples to enlarge and stimulates the development of milk glands. It strengthens the womb wall to cope with the powerful contractions of labour and softens body tissues, which allows the ligaments and joints to stretch. This can lead to varicose veins and backache.

HORMONAL INCREASES
The arrows show the origin of the major pregnancy hormones. Progesterone and oestrogen are produced by the ovaries and later by the placenta. Oxytocin and prolactin are produced by the pituitary gland, and thyroxine is controlled by the thyroid gland.

Other hormonal changes
Human chorionic gonadotrophin (hCG) and human placental lactogen (hPL) are produced by the placenta and are unique to pregnancy. HPL is associated with breast enlargement while hCG stimulates your thyroid gland to produce extra thyroxine, which can affect your metabolism. Prolactin and oxytocin help produce breast milk. Oxytocin also stimulates contractions in labour.

WEEKS IN PREGNANCY

1	22	23	24	25	26	27	28	29	30	31	32	33	34	35	36	37	38	39	40

RIMESTER | THIRD TRIMESTER

COMMON COMPLAINTS

Q WHY I AM HAVING HOT FLUSHES?

A As your metabolism speeds up extra heat is generated, and your blood vessels, especially those in the skin, dilate with extra blood. You may feel flushed and warm, particularly during the summer. You may not be able to prevent hot flushes but it helps to wear loose, layered clothing that you can take off when you need to cool down.

Q WHY DO I GET NOSEBLEEDS?

A An increased volume of blood and changes in blood's ability to clot, can cause nosebleeds. When your nose bleeds, sit down and pinch the soft part of your nose below the bridge until it stops.

Q WHY DO I NEED TO PASS URINE SO OFTEN BUT PASS ONLY A TINY AMOUNT?

A This happens because your womb expands and presses on your bladder. You should get some relief in the middle trimester, as the womb expands higher into the abdomen and eases the pressure on the bladder. However, in late pregnancy, the growing baby presses on the bladder from above (see p. 128) and the need to urinate frequently returns.

Q I HAVE A STINGING FEELING WHEN I URINATE, WHY?

A A stinging feeling as you pass urine, low abdominal pain, or blood in your urine could mean that you have a urinary tract infection (UTI) (see p. 127). Such infections are common in pregnancy and you should see your doctor, midwife, or antenatal clinic as soon as you can. You may be given antibiotics to clear the infection.

Q I SEEM TO BE BREATHING VERY QUICKLY THESE DAYS, IS THIS NORMAL?

A Your lungs are adapting to your body's extra energy needs. As your metabolism speeds up, more carbon dioxide is produced, which has to be cleared by your lungs. At the same time, your body takes in more oxygen increasing your lung capacity by about 40 per cent. Therefore, as well as a larger volume of gas inhaled and exhaled per breath, your breathing rate speeds up.

HOW DO I COPE WITH TIREDNESS?

Why am I so tired?
Even though you may not be aware of it, your body is now working harder than it ever has before. To make this possible, your metabolic rate has increased by one fifth to support it. Your heart is pumping more blood more quickly around your body and your breathing rate has also increased. With this major increase in your body's workload, it is not surprising that you are feeling tired.

How tired should I feel?
Anything from feeling mildly tired to absolutely drained is normal. As well as all the changes mentioned above, you may also be feeling sick and find it difficult to eat anything or to keep food down.

What can I do to reduce general fatigue?
Don't fight it, give in to it. As your pregnancy progresses, you should gradually feel more energetic; in the meantime, just take it easy and, if possible, try to get more rest during the day or early evening.

How can I get a good night's sleep?
Try to rest during the day so that you are not totally exhausted by bedtime or, if this is not possible, go to bed much earlier than usual. Get yourself into a pleasantly relaxed state by the end of the day, perhaps by having a warm bath and a warm milky drink (unless you are feeling nauseous) (see p. 116). Getting a full night's undisturbed sleep is unusual during the first and last trimesters as you may need to urinate in the night. You should therefore avoid drinking tea, coffee, or avoid alcohol; also avoid taking sleeping pills, which may leave you feeling groggy.

Should I see a doctor about feeling tired?
If after several weeks you feel increasingly exhausted, see your doctor who may check your blood to make sure that you are not anaemic. Anaemia is a blood condition that can usually be treated by taking iron supplements (see p. 128).

WEEKS IN PREGNANCY

1	2	3	4	5	6	7	8	9	10	11	12	13	14	15	16	17	18	19	2
				FIRST TRIMESTER														SECON	

Q WHAT ARE THE SPIDERY RED LINES ON MY LEGS, AND WILL THEY GO AWAY?

A These are called spider naevi and are small blood vessels in the skin that have expanded. Caused by the oestrogen surge of pregnancy, they should (but don't always) fade after the pregnancy, and are not a sign that anything is wrong.

Q WHY CAN'T I BEAR THE TASTE OF COFFEE WHEN I USED TO LOVE IT?

A The change in hormones and blood chemicals that your body undergoes during pregnancy affects your saliva; this in turn can cause certain foods and drinks to taste odd, sometimes to the point where you can no longer enjoy them. It has been suggested that this may be nature's way of steering you away from harmful substances, such as alcohol, during your pregnancy. Some women report that they suddenly want to drink tea or coffee when they never liked it before, which illustrates the contrary nature of cravings.

Q I FEEL CONSTANTLY SICK, IS SOMETHING WRONG WITH ME OR MY BABY?

A No, unpleasant though it is, morning sickness or nausea is one of the most common symptoms of early pregnancy. Despite its name, morning sickness can occur at any time of the day and can last all day. It usually occurs in the first trimester (before 14 weeks) and is thought to be due to the presence of human chorionic gonadotrophin (hCG), a hormone that is only produced during pregnancy (see p. 77).

Q I AM VOMITING EVERY DAY AND CANNOT KEEP FOOD DOWN, WHAT CAN I DO?

A If you are almost constantly sick and this stops you from keeping fluids as well as solids down, you should see your doctor; you may be given anti-nausea tablets or injections. If, after a course of these, you are no better, you may be advised to spend one or two days in hospital where you will be given re-hydration treatment and vitamin supplements.

WHAT CAN I DO TO STOP NAUSEA OR MORNING SICKNESS?

If you feel most ill in the morning, try to eat something plain, such as a biscuit or dry toast, before you get out of bed. If your nausea persists throughout the the day, try to eat and drink little and often, and avoid fatty foods and milky drinks. Some women report that glucose drinks or sweets reduce their nausea, others are soothed by herbal remedies such as ginger, peppermint, or camomile teas (see p. 109).

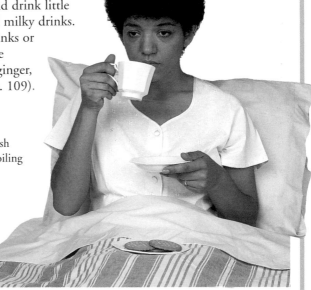

Recipe for ginger tea
Place one teaspoon of ground or grated fresh ginger into a teapot or small bowl. Pour boiling water over it, allow it to steep for a few minutes, then strain into a cup or a glass. Add brown sugar or honey to taste.

BEFORE YOU GET UP
Eating dry biscuits or toast before you get up in the morning may help prevent or reduce morning sickness.

WEEKS IN PREGNANCY

1	22	23	24	25	26	27	28	29	30	31	32	33	34	35	36	37	38	39	40
RIMESTER											THIRD TRIMESTER								

THE SECOND TRIMESTER

THIS MAY BE THE most enjoyable part of your pregnancy. You will become more energetic and will feel your baby move for the first time. The nausea and tiredness of the early weeks usually eases by this stage and, as your thickening waistline rapidly grows into a noticeable bump, you start to look pregnant.

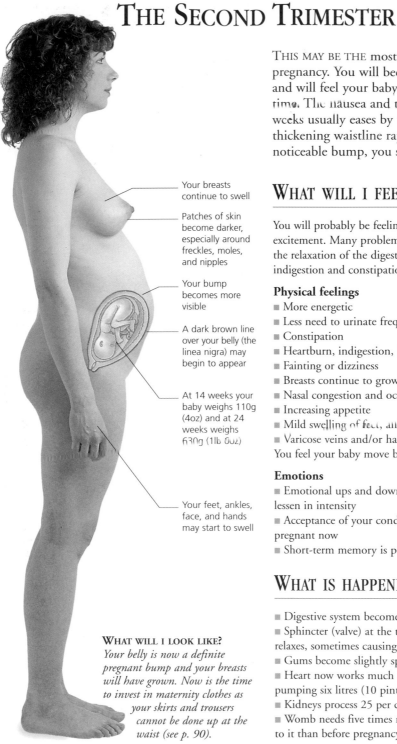

Your breasts continue to swell

Patches of skin become darker, especially around freckles, moles, and nipples

Your bump becomes more visible

A dark brown line over your belly (the linea nigra) may begin to appear

At 14 weeks your baby weighs 110g (4oz) and at 24 weeks weighs 630g (1lb 6oz)

Your feet, ankles, face, and hands may start to swell

WHAT WILL I LOOK LIKE?
Your belly is now a definite pregnant bump and your breasts will have grown. Now is the time to invest in maternity clothes as your skirts and trousers cannot be done up at the waist (see p. 90).

WHAT WILL I FEEL?

You will probably be feeling full of vitality and excitement. Many problems at this stage are due to the relaxation of the digestive system, which causes indigestion and constipation.

Physical feelings
- More energetic
- Less need to urinate frequently
- Constipation
- Heartburn, indigestion, flatulence
- Fainting or dizziness
- Breasts continue to grow
- Nasal congestion and occasional nosebleeds
- Increasing appetite
- Mild swelling of feet, ankles, face, and hands
- Varicose veins and/or haemorrhoids may develop
You feel your baby move by 22–24 weeks

Emotions
- Emotional ups and downs may be the same or may lessen in intensity
- Acceptance of your condition – you really feel pregnant now
- Short-term memory is poor

WHAT IS HAPPENING TO MY BODY?

- Digestive system becomes sluggish
- Sphincter (valve) at the top of your stomach relaxes, sometimes causing heartburn
- Gums become slightly spongy and may bleed
- Heart now works much harder than normal, pumping six litres (10 pints) of blood a minute
- Kidneys process 25 per cent more blood
- Womb needs five times more blood supplied to it than before pregnancy

WEEKS IN PREGNANCY																			
1	2	3	4	5	6	7	8	9	10	11	12	13	14	15	16	17	18	19	2
FIRST TRIMESTER												SECON							

YOUR CHANGING BODY

HOW WILL THE CHANGES AFFECT ME?

Q MY SKIN HAS CHANGED COLOUR AND LOOKS PATCHY, IS THIS NORMAL?

A Extra amounts of oestrogen in pregnancy affect the melanin-producing cells of the skin: the cells that produce the pigment that darkens the skin. This can result in a colour change where your skin is already darker, for example where you have freckles or birthmarks. You may also develop a darker area around your forehead, nose, mouth, and chin; this is known as chloasma or "the mask of pregnancy". Some women also find that they tan more readily and unevenly in the sun. These colour changes are normal and will usually fade once the baby is born.

Q WHY AM I NOT FEELING THE NEED TO URINATE AS URGENTLY AS BEFORE?

A By the time you have reached the second trimester, your womb has expanded upwards into your abdomen, which means that the pressure on your bladder is reduced.

Q I FAINTED THIS MORNING, DOES THIS MEAN THERE'S SOMETHING WRONG?

A Fainting is quite common in the second trimester. Although disconcerting, it seldom means that there is anything wrong with you or your baby. It usually happens when you stand for a long time: blood vessels, especially in your legs, dilate, causing blood to pool in the lower parts of the body; as a result your heart works harder to pump blood around your body. You are more likely to faint when you are tired and have not eaten enough. Mention it to your doctor or midwife who may give you a test to exclude anaemia (see p. 128).

Q IS THERE ANYTHING I CAN DO TO STOP MYSELF FAINTING?

A Yes, you could try to avoid standing for long periods of time. Remember not to get up too quickly from your bed, from a chair, or from the floor. Make sure you eat regularly or carry a supply of food such as plain biscuits, nuts or fruit with you. If you feel light-headed, sit or lie down until you feel better. Take several deep breaths.

WHY ARE MY BREASTS SO BIG AND SORE?

The hormones oestrogen, progesterone, human placental lactogen, oxytocin, and prolactin prepare your body for feeding your baby and cause your breasts to enlarge, become tender, or painful. However, this tenderness may not continue for the entire pregnancy. It is important to wear a good bra to support your breasts.

What is happening
Visible dark blue veins appear as a result of the increased blood flow to the breast tissue, and new milk ducts grow. The dark skin around the nipple (areola) usually becomes larger and darker; the bumps around the nipple (called Montgomery's tubercles) also enlarge and secrete a fluid to lubricate the nipples. Your breasts may sometimes leak a clear fluid called colostrum, which is an early form of milk (see p. 207); this is nothing to worry about.

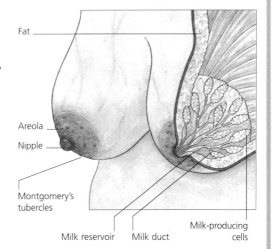

Fat

Areola

Nipple

Montgomery's tubercles

Milk reservoir   Milk duct   Milk-producing cells

BREAST CHANGES
Progesterone causes the main changes in your breasts in pregnancy, while oestrogen is primarily responsible for the growth of milk ducts. Some women find that their breasts become very sensitive.

WEEKS IN PREGNANCY

1	22	23	24	25	26	27	28	29	30	31	32	33	34	35	36	37	38	39	40

RIMESTER   THIRD TRIMESTER

COMMON COMPLAINTS

Q I OFTEN HAVE A BURNING PAIN IN MY STOMACH, IS THIS HEARTBURN?

A Very probably. Heartburn occurs in pregnancy when high levels of the hormone progesterone relax the valve that normally stops the contents of your stomach moving back into your oesophagus (food pipe). The stomach contents irritate your oesophagus, causing heartburn. Later in pregnancy, heartburn can occur because your enlarged womb squashes your stomach and gastric acids seep out.

Q IS THERE ANYTHING I CAN DO TO PREVENT HEARTBURN?

A Try to eat little and often and preferably long before you go to bed. Some women find that a glass of milk eases acute heartburn (although it can cause nausea, see p. 79); there are also various herbal remedies (see p. 109). Sit up straight when you eat to prevent your stomach being squashed. Also, avoid eating highly spiced food unless you are used to it. If you suffer from heartburn at night, do not lie completely flat in bed but use pillows to prop up your upper body. If these solutions don't work, your doctor may prescribe an antacid to neutralize the acidity of your stomach.

Q WHY DO I HAVE INDIGESTION ALL THE TIME?

A Indigestion is common in pregnancy because high levels of the hormone progesterone slow the rate of digestion; food therefore remains in the stomach for longer. Try eating little and often; large heavy meals may cause an uncomfortable, heavy feeling in your stomach, and occasionally burning pain like heartburn.

Q HOW CAN I CURE MY CONSTIPATION?

A The hormones that slow down your digestive system also make your bowel action sluggish. Eat plenty of fruit, vegetables, and other high-fibre foods (see p. 104), and drink plenty of water (about 2 litres/4 pints a day). Some iron supplements cause constipation; if taken for a prolonged period they may cause piles (see haemorrhoids, p. 86); if this is a problem, and you are anaemic, ask your doctor about changing your iron tablets.

Q DO ALL PREGNANT WOMEN GET VARICOSE VEINS?

A Women are more likely to get varicose veins if they run in the family. Varicose veins are caused by the weight of the womb pressing on the veins in the pelvis; this increases the pressure in the veins in your lower body. Progesterone also makes the veins dilate (open up) so that blood pools in your legs, vulva, and anus. You may notice that your veins bulge or your legs ache when you stand for a long time. Very rarely, redness, swelling, or pain in your calves may be a serious condition called venous thrombosis (see p. 141); if you have these symptoms you should seek prompt medical advice.

Q MY LEGS HAVE BECOME SWOLLEN AND UNCOMFORTABLE, IS THIS NORMAL?

A The same pressure that causes varicose veins can also cause your legs to swell with fluid, especially if you are carrying more than one baby. This is usually noticeable around 24 weeks and can be very uncomfortable near the end of pregnancy. Rarely, leg swelling is a sign of pre-eclampsia (see p. 138), particularly if it develops rapidly; talk to your midwife or doctor if you notice this.

Q WHAT CAN I DO TO HELP PREVENT VARICOSE VEINS AND SWOLLEN LEGS?

A Wear support tights or stockings and rest with your legs raised whenever possible. Try to avoid excessive salt intake, weight gain, and standing still for long periods. Gentle daily exercise (see p. 110) also improves the circulation.

Q MY VAGINAL DISCHARGE HAS BECOME HEAVY, HAVE I GOT AN INFECTION?

A Vaginal discharge does increase in the second trimester but it should be clear and mucus-like. If there are other symptoms, such as itching, soreness, or an unusually strong smell, you may have an infection that needs treatment (see p. 127).

Q MY GUMS BLEED AFTER I BRUSH MY TEETH, WHAT DOES THIS MEAN?

A Hormonal changes cause gums to thicken and soften; this makes you prone to gum injury from hard toothbrushes or sharp foods, which can cause bleeding and infection (gingivitis). Make sure you brush gently, and regularly use dental floss. In the UK, NHS dental care in pregnancy is free.

WEEKS IN PREGNANCY

1	2	3	4	5	6	7	8	9	10	11	12	13	14	15	16	17	18	19	2
					FIRST TRIMESTER													SECON	

WEIGHT GAIN

YOUR CHANGING BODY

Q HOW MUCH WEIGHT GAIN IS NORMAL?

A This depends on your body type. A weight gain of between 11kg and 16kg (24lb and 35lb) by the end of pregnancy is normal. However, there are major variations and some women may gain very little weight in a normal pregnancy. With a multiple pregnancy your weight gain does not double and the average weight gain is 18kg (40lb).

Q IF I GAIN A LOT OF WEIGHT WILL MY BABY BE LARGE AND HARDER TO DELIVER?

A Probably not, because it is you, not the baby who gains the excess weight. Whether you have a large or a small baby is usually determined by factors other than how much you eat (see p. 59).

Q IS IT EASY TO LOSE THE WEIGHT AFTER THE BIRTH?

A The time it takes to regain your figure varies. Some women are slim again within weeks of delivering, others find that it takes much longer (see p. 240). Following a healthy, balanced diet before, during, and after the birth, and doing post-natal exercises, should all help. You may also lose weight faster and more easily if you breastfeed.

Q HOW CAN I KEEP MY WEIGHT UNDER CONTROL DURING PREGNANCY?

A There is no magic formula, apart from eating a balanced, nutritious diet and taking regular exercise. This can be especially hard during pregnancy, when food cravings and a faster metabolic rate make you hungrier. If you gain weight gradually, you should find it easier to keep it to a minimum (see p. 104).

CAN MY WEIGHT GAIN CAUSE CONCERN?

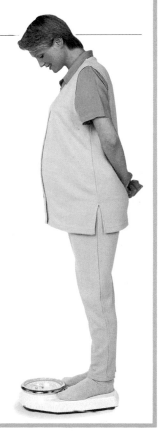

Professional opinion is that an average weight gain of 11.5 kg (26–28lb) by the time of the birth is ideal – but you may gain more or less than this. In fact, your doctor or midwife will probably show little concern about your weight unless you gain too little weight or far too much. A poor diet (resulting in low weight gain) can cause your baby to have a low birth weight; excessive weight gain can cause you back problems, varicose veins, or indicate pre-eclampsia. Ideally, your weight gain should be gradual until the third trimester, but there are no hard and fast rules to go by.

Average weight distribution
The fetus, placenta, and amniotic fluid account for just over a third of your weight gain. The remaining weight comes from your enlarged breasts and womb, extra body fat, increased blood volume, and fluid retention. You should experience your most dramatic weight gain in the third trimester (see p. 84).

AVERAGE WEIGHT GAIN

Blood volume	1.3kg	(2lb 15oz)
Breasts	0.4kg	(14oz)
Womb	1kg	(2lb 3oz)
Fetus	3.4kg	(7lb 8oz)
Placenta	0.7kg	(1lb 8oz)
Amniotic fluid	0.8kg	(1lb 13oz)
Fat	3.5kg	(7lb 11oz)
Retained water (This can be as much as 4.5kg (10lb))	1.5kg	(3lb 5oz)
TOTAL	**12.6kg**	**(27lb 13oz)**

WEEKS IN PREGNANCY

1	22	23	24	25	26	27	28	29	30	31	32	33	34	35	36	37	38	39	40

RIMESTER | THIRD TRIMESTER

THE THIRD TRIMESTER

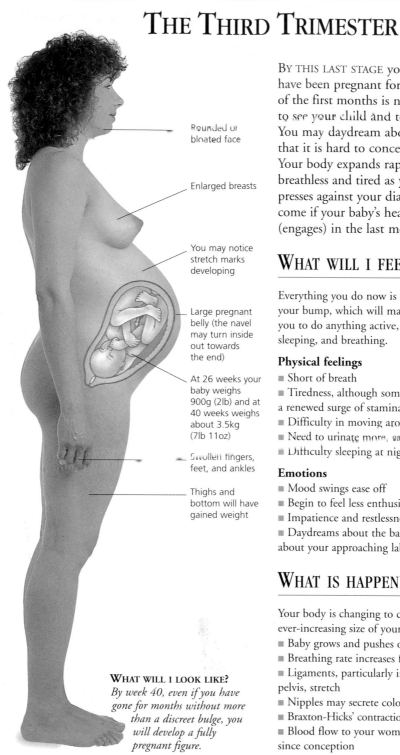

Rounded or bloated face

Enlarged breasts

You may notice stretch marks developing

Large pregnant belly (the navel may turn inside out towards the end)

At 26 weeks your baby weighs 900g (2lb) and at 40 weeks weighs about 3.5kg (7lb 11oz)

Swollen fingers, feet, and ankles

Thighs and bottom will have gained weight

WHAT WILL I LOOK LIKE?
By week 40, even if you have gone for months without more than a discreet bulge, you will develop a fully pregnant figure.

BY THIS LAST STAGE you probably feel as if you have been pregnant forever and the excitement of the first months is now an impatient desire to see your child and to get rid of your bump. You may daydream about your baby so much that it is hard to concentrate on other things. Your body expands rapidly and you feel breathless and tired as your womb enlarges and presses against your diaphragm. Relief may come if your baby's head drops into the pelvis (engages) in the last month (see p. 69).

WHAT WILL I FEEL?

Everything you do now is affected by the sheer size of your bump, which will make it increasingly hard for you to do anything active, even bending over, sleeping, and breathing.

Physical feelings
- Short of breath
- Tiredness, although some women experience a renewed surge of stamina just towards the end
- Difficulty in moving around
- Need to urinate more, especially if the head engages
- Difficulty sleeping at night

Emotions
- Mood swings ease off
- Begin to feel less enthusiastic about being pregnant
- Impatience and restlessness for the birth to be over
- Daydreams about the baby and possible anxiety about your approaching labour

WHAT IS HAPPENING TO MY BODY?

Your body is changing to cope with the ever-increasing size of your womb and the baby in it.
- Baby grows and pushes out your lower ribs
- Breathing rate increases further
- Ligaments, particularly in the hips and pelvis, stretch
- Nipples may secrete colostrum
- Braxton-Hicks' contractions (see opposite) may begin
- Blood flow to your womb has increased tenfold since conception

WEEKS IN PREGNANCY

1	2	3	4	5	6	7	8	9	10	11	12	13	14	15	16	17	18	19	20
				FIRST TRIMESTER														SECON

HOW WILL THE CHANGES AFFECT ME?

Q CAN I DO ANYTHING TO PREVENT STRETCH MARKS?

A Unfortunately, there are no pills or creams that make any difference to whether or not – and how badly – you get stretch marks. Stretch marks are not directly related to how much your stomach has had to expand; they are probably connected with the collagen and elastin content of your skin. The marks can be red and livid in pregnancy, but in the weeks and months after the delivery, they lose their colour, usually become silvery-white and less obvious.

Q MY BUMP TIGHTENS SEVERAL TIMES A DAY, WHAT DOES IT MEAN?

A You may feel your abdomen tightening for about 30 seconds, several times a day during the last trimester. This tightening, called Braxton-Hicks' contractions, means that your womb is "practising" for labour: the contractions don't mean that you are in – or about to go into – labour. Real labour contractions are very different; they are regular, usually more powerful and painful, and do not go away (see p. 166). As your due date approaches, you may experience Braxton-Hicks' contractions often; if so, try to relax and use the contractions to practise your breathing (see p. 161).

Q MY FINGERS HAVE BECOME SWOLLEN, WILL THEY STAY LIKE THIS?

A Many women suffer from mild swelling of the fingers, hands, and ankles towards the end of their pregnancy. It's a good idea to remove your rings until after your baby is born, when the swelling will go down.

Q WHY HAS MY FACE BECOME SWOLLEN AND ROUND?

A This is caused by the effect of the hormone oestrogen and a steroid hormone, cortisol, which change the distribution of fat in your body. Extra fluid also collects under the skin in a normal pregnancy. Occasionally, general but marked swelling of the legs, arms, and face are symptoms of pre-eclampsia (see p. 138), which is a serious condition that needs medical attention. Mention signs of swelling to your doctor or midwife.

Q WHAT IS THE FLUID LEAKING FROM MY BREASTS?

A This watery discharge is called colostrum and it is the first milk you produce, usually just after giving birth. Sometimes, in second and subsequent pregnancies, colostrum is produced well before you go into labour.

Q I LEAK URINE WHEN I LAUGH, SNEEZE, OR COUGH, HOW CAN I STOP THIS?

A The weight of the womb pressing on your bladder and pelvic floor means that a little urine may escape because of the extra pressure: this is called stress incontinence (see p. 126). Doing exercises to strengthen the muscles of the pelvic floor is important and will be of great benefit both during and after pregnancy (see p. 111). While this problem persists, you may feel more comfortable if you wear a sanitary pad or liner.

IS IT SAFE TO BE ACTIVE?

If you are enjoying a healthy pregnancy and have the energy, motivation, and will-power, it is certainly safe for you to be active, but you will find it harder to move fast. Gentle exercise, such as walking or swimming, is beneficial and there is no reason why you shouldn't do house-hold chores or go to work. However, do not overdo it or tackle difficult jobs such as climbing ladders or lifting heavy boxes on your own.

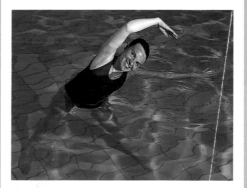

STAYING FIT AND ENJOYING LIFE
You can enjoy being physically active if you feel energetic – just rest whenever you feel the need.

	WEEKS IN PREGNANCY																		
21	22	23	24	25	26	27	28	29	30	31	32	33	34	35	36	37	38	39	40

TRIMESTER | THIRD TRIMESTER

COMMON COMPLAINTS

Q MY BUMP IS NOW HUGE AND I AM VERY UNCOMFORTABLE – WHAT CAN I DO?

A There is little you can do about the discomfort in the final phase of your pregnancy because your baby is now very large and takes up a lot of space in your abdomen. Lying on your back may no longer be possible or advisable because the weight of your womb presses on the main blood vessel. This causes your blood pressure to drop, which in turn can make you feel faint. By this stage of pregnancy, your baby is probably also pushing out your ribs, causing them to ache. There are positions you can adopt to ease some of the pressure (see p. 117). It may also help to know that if your baby engages, a few of these discomforts should ease.

HOW CAN I RELIEVE CRAMP?

Cramp is the excruciating pain of muscles in spasm. The causes of cramp are uncertain but may be linked to low calcium levels. Cramp often occurs in bed at night, and particularly if you point your toes.

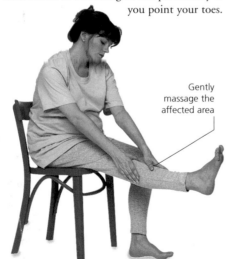

Gently massage the affected area

WHAT TO DO
To help relax the muscle that is in spasm, try extending the leg and then bringing the toes towards your body. Having a glass of milk (which contains calcium) can ease leg cramps.

Q IS IT NORMAL TO BE SHORT OF BREATH ALL THE TIME?

A It is normal to feel that you are not breathing deeply enough. Also, as your womb continues to expand into your abdomen, it presses against your diaphragm and your lungs, and this also makes it more difficult for you to take deep breaths. The increase in the hormone progesterone may also speed up your breathing (see p. 77).

Q WHY ARE THE PALMS OF MY HANDS RED AND BURNING?

A You have what is called palmar erythema; this occurs because of the increased blood flow through the skin tissues. It is not serious, but is just a result of the changes in your blood vessels.

Q I SEEM TO BE CONSTANTLY ITCHING ALL OVER – IS THERE SOMETHING WRONG?

A As your belly expands, your skin stretches to accommodate the growing baby; this stretching can make the skin itchy. Creams, calamine lotion, and bath oils can moisturize the skin, helping to reduce this itching. Rarely, severe generalized itching, especially late in pregnancy, needs to be seen by your doctor because it could indicate a liver disease (see p. 133).

Q I'VE DEVELOPED PILES, CAN I DO ANYTHING TO RELIEVE THEM?

A Piles (haemorrhoids) are varicose veins in the back passage that swell when the weight of the baby puts pressure on the main veins in the pelvis; this pressure in turn reduces the return of blood from the pelvic organs to the heart. Piles can be painful and delivery of your baby is really the only cure. Avoid constipation as this will add to your discomfort. Your doctor can prescribe soothing ointments for piles; if they ache, sit for ten minutes on an ice pack or bag of frozen peas wrapped in a towel. Pelvic floor exercises may help to reduce piles (see p. 111).

Q MY HEARTBEAT FEELS UNEVEN SOMETIMES – IS THIS UNUSUAL?

A "Missed" beats are also called palpitations, and normally they are nothing to worry about. However, if your heart starts missing beats very frequently, or you feel breathless or have chest pain with these palpitations, you should see your doctor.

1	2	3	4	5	6	7	8	9	10	11	12	13	14	15	16	17	18	19	20
					FIRST TRIMESTER													SECON	

WHY DO MY BACK AND HIPS ACHE?

Throughout your pregnancy, hormones relax the ligaments and joints, particularly those in the pelvis, causing the ligaments to soften and stretch to allow the baby an easier passage in labour. Added to which, the weight of your growing baby can weaken your stomach muscles and put pressure on your lower back. As your centre of gravity changes, you may also tend to lean backwards, which can result in further strain. If your back pain is constant or severe, consult your doctor: it may be necessary to see a physiotherapist or an osteopath for help with pain relief.

TYPES OF BACK AND JOINT ACHE

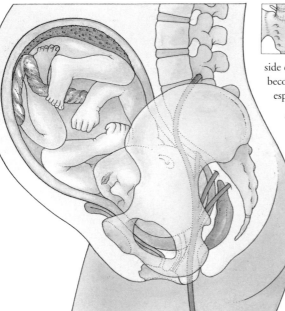

Sacroiliac joint
Steady pain in middle/low back
Where your pelvis meets the lower spine (the sacrum), there are joints on either side called sacroiliac joints. In pregnancy, these can become unstable, which can be very painful, especially when walking, standing or bending.

Treatment Wear low-heeled shoes and ensure correct posture (see p. 114). If in severe pain, see your doctor, a physiotherapist or an osteopath.

Coccyx
Pain in the lower spine
The coccyx can become slightly displaced from the sacrum, causing excruciating pain especially when sitting. This type of pain usually results from previous injury.

Treatment You can take a pain-relieving drug, such as paracetamol. After pregnancy, an osteopath may be able to help.

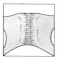
Pubic joint
Pain in the front of the pelvis
The pelvis is made up of fused bones which form a ring-like structure; at the front, where the bones meet, is the symphysis pubis. If the ligaments around this joint loosen in late pregnancy, the pubic bones rub against each other, causing severe pain when you walk. Rarely, these bones separate: this is called diastasis of the symphysis pubis.

Treatment This usually requires consultation with a doctor or physiotherapist. You may have to wear a special support belt to relieve the pressure, or you may need further treatment.

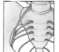
Sciatic nerves
Sharp/constant/intermittent pain in the back, buttocks, and legs
As your baby's head moves down into your pelvis, it often presses directly on the pelvic bones, which may affect the sciatic nerves in your lower back and legs. This can cause severe back and leg pain, or your legs may feel numb. This is called sciatic nerve pain (see p. 126).

Treatment The best way of dealing with this is to spend some time lying down on a firm mattress. Your baby's head may move and relieve the pressure on the nerves; the pelvic tilt exercise may also help (see p. 112).

YOUR CHANGING BODY

WEEKS IN PREGNANCY

21	22	23	24	25	26	27	28	29	30	31	32	33	34	35	36	37	38	39	40

| TRIMESTER | | | | | THIRD TRIMESTER | | | | | | | | | | | | | | |

FAMILY CHANGES

Q HOW SHOULD I PREPARE MY CHILD FOR THE NEW BABY'S ARRIVAL?

A First, tell your child that a new baby is on the way and explain what this will mean; then prepare for changes in your child's routine. You need to handle these issues positively but with great care and sensitivity. What you say and how you say it will obviously depend on the age of your child (see opposite).

Q WHY IS IT IMPORTANT TO PREPARE MY CHILD FOR THE NEW BABY'S ARRIVAL?

A After the birth of your baby, your child will undergo a major change in his or her life. After all, your first child has been an only child for all of his life and has enjoyed not only all your attention but also that of close family and friends. Whatever the age of your child, he or she has been your "baby" for some time and is now expected to relinquish that role to become a big brother or sister. This can seem a very poor deal.

Q HOW IS MY CHILD LIKELY TO REACT?

A The chances are that you will be faced with mixed emotions, ranging from excitement at having a new playmate, to worry that the new baby will be your favourite child. Your child may appear to be unaffected by the news but then go through a bout of naughtiness, or be unable to comprehend that a new baby is on its way and not react until after the birth. Or you may hear your child proudly tell friends that he or she is going to have a sister or brother. Whatever the reaction, your child will need reassurance and understanding from you.

Q HOW DO I CHANGE MY CHILD'S ROUTINE TO MANAGE THE NEW BABY?

A If you are planning any major changes in your child's routine, try to do this months before your baby is born. For instance, if you want your child to move from a cot to a bed, to start at nursery, or to go to bed earlier every night, try to establish these new routines months ahead of the birth or these upsets will become inextricably linked with the baby's arrival. Alternatively, you could leave any changes in your child's routine until a few months after the birth.

Q I HAVE A TEENAGE CHILD – WILL A NEW BABY CAUSE PROBLEMS?

A Some teenagers will have no trouble coping with the fact that you are pregnant; others may feel deep embarrassment at seeing the proof that their mother or parents still have an intimate sexual relationship. There may be some resentment towards the baby because they see the newcomer as a definite rival for your time and attention. These reactions are very common and you could try to discuss the situation with them as adults; perhaps by reassuring him or her that you have no intention of remaining heavily pregnant for longer than is necessary and by reminding them of the special place they occupy in the family.

Q CAN MY OTHER CHILD/CHILDREN BE PRESENT AT THE BIRTH?

A This depends on many factors. The first and most important consideration is whether you feel confident that your child could cope with seeing you in pain. Many children find this very upsetting and it may therefore be better not to put them through the experience. If you are having a hospital birth it would also be difficult to have your child waiting around for many hours. Furthermore, should any complications develop, your partner would have to take the child outside when you may prefer that your partner stay with you. With a home birth, things are easier because you can call the child in at the appropriate moment to witness the actual birth (see p. 154).

Q HOW CAN I GET TIME ALONE WITH MY BABY WITHOUT UPSETTING MY CHILD?

A You could try to encourage a strong, loving attachment between your child and another adult who can occasionally stand in for you. This will not only give you more time for the baby but also enrich the emotional life of your child. You can do this by making sure your partner, a grandparent or a friend is part of your everyday routine. However, you must also make time to give your older child some special attention without a demanding baby around. For instance, you could try asking your partner or another adult to take the baby out for walks so that you can establish a regular time alone with your child.

PREPARING YOUR CHILD

The arrival of a new baby can be a difficult time for your existing child, who may feel left out and so demand more attention. Making plans and preparing your child for the new arrival could spare you the trauma of an unhappy older child. How you tell your child about the new baby can make a difference to how they view the event.

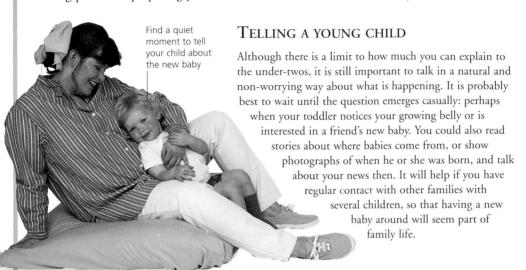

Find a quiet moment to tell your child about the new baby

TELLING A YOUNG CHILD

Although there is a limit to how much you can explain to the under-twos, it is still important to talk in a natural and non-worrying way about what is happening. It is probably best to wait until the question emerges casually: perhaps when your toddler notices your growing belly or is interested in a friend's new baby. You could also read stories about where babies come from, or show photographs of when he or she was born, and talk about your news then. It will help if you have regular contact with other families with several children, so that having a new baby around will seem part of family life.

TELLING AN OLDER CHILD

The older the child, the more you can explain and the earlier you can break the news. An older child may be interested in what is happening to you and how the baby grows; encourage him or her to feel the baby move inside you. You could involve your child in choosing a name for the new baby. All this will help to make the coming birth a family event.

Family and friends can help

Encourage family and friends to make a fuss of the older child. Discuss your concern that your child should not feel that all the attention is focused on the new baby.

Presents

Your new baby will receive plenty of presents, which may make your other child feel left out. When you pack for the hospital, wrap up a gift for your child from the new baby. Ask grandparents and close family to bring something for the older child when they come to see the new baby.

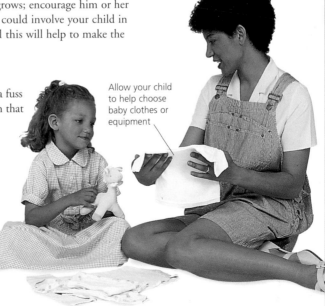

Allow your child to help choose baby clothes or equipment

DRESSING FOR THE OCCASION

How you dress during your pregnancy obviously depends on your own personal taste and your lifestyle. When it comes to buying maternity clothes, you will find that there is a large choice available: department stores, specialist shops, mail order catalogues, and even some fashion chain stores now offer up-to-date and fashionable maternity wear. You may not wish or need to buy many special maternity outfits; a selection of large shirts or jumpers, a few loose-fitting dresses, and some maternity leggings could easily carry you through most of your pregnancy.

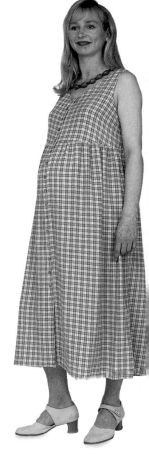

WHAT TO BUY

You don't need to spend a fortune on expensive maternity clothes. Instead, you can buy just a few basic items, such as those listed below, and then treat yourself to a few special garments.

- Maternity trousers or leggings
- Maternity dresses
- Loose-fitting shirts
- Large sweaters or cardigans
- Support bras
- Maternity support tights or stockings
- Cotton socks
- Comfortable low-heeled shoes
- Nightdresses (preferably with a front opening so that you can wear them for breastfeeding afterwards)

Optional extras
- Smart jacket
- A dressy outfit for evenings out
- Maternity swimsuit
- Maternity exercise leotard
- Trainers

WHEN TO BUY

Most women start looking at looser clothing in the third or fourth month when their waistbands can no longer be fastened. However, don't buy everything at once: you'll need to buy clothes in stages to cope with your changing size and shape, and with different seasons.

SEASONAL CLOTHES
Bear in mind the changing seasons: you become pregnant in one season, but by the time you need big dresses, the weather will have changed.

WHY COMFORT COMES FIRST

Whatever style you prefer, make sure your clothes feel comfortable as well as look good. There is nothing worse than squeezing into a dress that cuts under the arms and is tight across your breasts or bump. During pregnancy you are likely to feel much warmer and perspire more, so it is best to wear natural fibres, such as cotton, wool, or linen, that allow heat and moisture to escape.

BIG IS BEST
Large sweaters or shirts and layers of clothing work well in pregnancy, because they allow plenty of air to circulate and you can peel off a layer when you get too warm.

YOUR CHANGING BODY

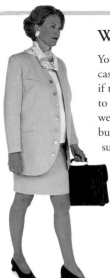

WHAT TO WEAR AT WORK

Your job may require a smarter wardrobe than the casual clothes you can wear at home, particularly if there is a strict dress code, so that you may have to invest some money in more formal maternity wear. You will get the most value out of separates: build different outfits around a smart jacket or suit, a skirt and/or trousers with elasticated waists, loose-fitting shirts, and a few dresses that can be mixed and matched.

FITTED ELEGANCE
You do not have to wear loose clothes. Fitted and tailored suits are fine, as long as you are comfortable.

SHOES

Low-heeled, comfortable shoes are best in pregnancy. The feet, ankles, and calves need good support because the ligaments (like those in the pelvis) can easily become stretched. As you get bigger, your balance is altered; high heels can make you feel unsteady on your feet. Also, high heels encourage bad posture, which could cause back problems. In late pregnancy, feet and ankles can swell and you may need a larger shoe size temporarily. Choose shoes with a non-slip sole.

UNDERWEAR

The most important items in your maternity wardrobe should be new bras; be sure to invest in ones that are well-fitting and supporting.

Support Bras
Your breasts enlarge almost at once and can become very swollen and heavy; they will sag without support, especially after the baby is born or is weaned. A good support bra is essential but do not guess your size; measure yourself or have a proper fitting done at a lingerie shop or department store each time you buy. For comfort, choose cotton-rich maternity bras with wide shoulder straps and a deep band under the cups. Buy only two at first, then more as your breasts grow. When you have had your baby, buy two or three nursing bras for breastfeeding. Some women like to wear a sleep bra for night-time support.

Briefs
It is best to avoid briefs with a tight waistband and leg elastic that may feel constricting. Choose small mini-briefs that fit under the bump, or maternity briefs that cover your bump; these have an expanding front panel in stretch fabric (see right).

Support tights and stockings
Support hosiery can help prevent or reduce tired, aching legs, swollen ankles, and varicose veins, particularly if you are working through your pregnancy.

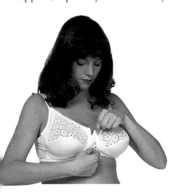

NURSING BRAS
An ordinary bra is awkward to undo at the back when breastfeeding, so a nursing bra with cups that can be opened individually at the front is essential. Some have cups that unzip, others unhook from the strap.

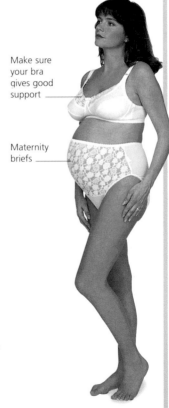

Make sure your bra gives good support

Maternity briefs

BASIC NEEDS
Well-fitting maternity underwear should support you and increase your comfort.

TWINS AND MULTIPLE BIRTHS

Q WILL I NEED TO TAKE EXTRA CARE OF MYSELF?

A Being told you are expecting twins or more can be a shock, particularly if you have no family history of twins. You will get more antenatal care (see p. 26), and you will also need to take more care of yourself than if you were having one baby, but there is no reason to consider yourself an invalid. Making sure that you have enough rest and eat a healthy diet are important because your body has to work even harder. You probably won't go to full term, so if you have a job, you might leave work earlier than planned; if you have other children, try to arrange for help so that you don't feel overtired.

WHEN WILL I FIND OUT?

Your doctor or midwife may suggest an early scan if you look large for your due date or have a history of twins in your family. However, you are most likely to be told that you are having twins at your first routine scan, at 12 to 14 or 18 to 22 weeks, depending on the hospital. On rare occasions, the second baby is missed in an earlier scan as it is hidden behind the first; in the past, some mothers have been told they were expecting two babies as late as 24 weeks.

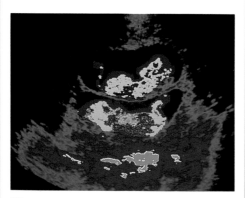

ULTRASOUND SCAN OF TWINS IN THE WOMB
Taken after the first trimester, this scan shows each twin (red and yellow) enclosed in its own amniotic sac; they are non-identical.

Q HOW MUCH LARGER WILL I BECOME WITH A MULTIPLE BIRTH?

A It is not just the weight of the babies that makes you bigger, but also the fact that you are carrying an extra or larger placenta, twice the normal amount of amniotic fluid, as well as extra body fluids. Your bump will show earlier if you are carrying more than one baby, becoming visible at 11 weeks, a week or two earlier than if you were expecting one baby. At 20 weeks, your bump may start to enlarge quite rapidly, and as early as 32 weeks, your womb will start to press against your ribcage. However, it is unlikely that you will reach the full 40 weeks of pregnancy; most twins or triplets are born at 36 to 37 weeks, because of the womb's capacity. They are also usually smaller than single babies.

Q WILL I HAVE TO EAT MORE IF I AM EXPECTING MORE THAN ONE BABY?

A If you are expecting twins or more, you may not necessarily have to eat more, but you will have to pay special attention to what you do eat. You are providing nutrients for two or more growing babies, maintaining your own energy levels, and also coping with the extra physical demands that are being made on your body, so it is very important that you obtain the essential nutrients from your diet (see p. 104). You may also feel extremely tired, sometimes perhaps too tired to cook. Enlist your partner's help with the shopping and cooking so that you are able to get enough rest during the day and do not miss meals.

Q CAN HAVING TWINS HARM MY BODY?

A The idea of carrying and giving birth to more than one baby can seem a daunting one and you may be concerned about the effect of this on your body. Some women worry that their womb, or even their abdomen, may be damaged by carrying more than one baby. This is unlikely; as your womb becomes stretched in the final part of your pregnancy, you are more likely to go into early labour. Another worry is that having more than one baby means worse stretch marks. Stretch marks are probably linked more with the collagen and elastin content of your skin than the size of your bump.

Q DOES HAVING TWINS MEAN I SHOULD EXPECT TWICE THE DISCOMFORT?

A With twins, you experience all the "normal" pregnancy problems, but the symptoms may be exaggerated and occur earlier in pregnancy.

■ **Morning sickness** This may be more severe with a multiple pregnancy and last beyond the first trimester.

■ **Anaemia** You will be more prone to this blood condition, which is caused by a deficiency of iron, because of the extra demands on your iron supplies. Your doctor will test your blood for anaemia, and usually prescribe extra iron and folic acid supplements.

■ **Breathlessness and abdominal pain** As your womb presses against your diaphragm, and your heart works harder pumping more blood around your body, you may find that you are short of breath and experience abdominal pains. This will be more pronounced if you are expecting twins, so you should avoid over-exerting yourself. Sitting in one position for too long is inadvisable because it can further aggravate abdominal pain. Try to eat little and often rather than eat big meals that will bloat your abdomen or give you indigestion.

■ **Backache** This may be worse with twins, because of the extra weight you are carrying.

■ **Varicose veins and piles** These are more likely with twins, because of the extra pressure on your veins. Avoid standing for too long, get regular, gentle exercise, and wear pregnancy support tights.

Q AM I MORE LIKELY TO SUFFER FROM SERIOUS CONDITIONS?

A Yes, in a multiple pregnancy, you are more likely to suffer from complications such as pre-eclampsia and oedema (see p. 138), and these may occur at an earlier stage of the pregnancy than is usual. The chances of premature labour are increased if you are expecting more than one baby; if your babies are premature, they will probably be placed in special care or in an incubator after the birth (see p. 228). However, because you and your babies are at a higher risk with a multiple pregnancy, you will receive extra attention from your doctor and midwife, and will have more check-ups than you would if you were expecting only one baby. Any potential problems should, be picked up at an early stage and the relevant action taken. Your doctor will probably suggest extra rest.

Q WHERE CAN I GET HELP AND ADVICE?

A There may be an organization in your area that offers support, and that can put you in touch with mothers of twins or triplets or provide useful brochures. Talk to other parents who will understand your feelings and offer practical help; they may also be able to offer advice on how to cope with the financial burden of having more than one child. You will also be able to see and hear how they managed with two or more babies after the birth and manage their children now (see p. 256).

DISCUSSION POINT

DO I NEED TO REST MORE?

Resting in hospital
Women expecting twins used to be routinely admitted to hospital several weeks before the birth because it was thought that this reduced the incidence of premature labour and meant that the babies were able to grow more. However, studies have shown that enforced bed rest does not necessarily prevent premature labour or increase the chances of the babies' survival. In some special cases, if you are expecting triplets or quadruplets, admission to hospital for rest and observation is still advised, especially if you have had complications during your pregnancy, but it is no longer routine medical advice.

Making sure you take it easy
Getting enough rest and relaxation is especially important with a multiple pregnancy because you will be much more tired. If you get plenty of rest you will feel better; this may also keep problems, such as varicose veins and backache, at bay. Rest and relaxation are also important because you are more likely to suffer from high blood pressure if you are having more than one child, which can lead to pre-eclampsia (see p. 138). Gentle exercise, such as swimming and walking, is an ideal way to relax. Swimming can also be very effective in relieving backache and any general aches and pains that you experience.

SEX DURING PREGNANCY

Q WE ENJOY OUR SEX LIFE – BUT IS IT SAFE TO MAKE LOVE WHILE I'M PREGNANT?

A It is usually perfectly safe for couples to enjoy a sexual relationship throughout pregnancy. In fact, a healthy sex life is positively beneficial, because as well as maintaining your relationship with your partner, it helps you to unwind, reminds you that you are a sensual woman as well as a mother-to-be, and it can also be a good form of exercise. Sexual intercourse cannot hurt your baby, who is safely cushioned in a bag of fluid within your womb; even deep penetration is not harmful, except in certain rare situations.

Q WHEN IS SEX NOT A GOOD IDEA DURING PREGNANCY?

A You may be advised not to have sex if you have a history of miscarriage or premature labours. It may also be sensible to avoid intercourse if there is unexplained bleeding, and after your waters have broken. Sex is also not advised in cases of placenta praevia, or where the placenta has partially dislodged itself from the womb wall (see p. 140) – penetration could increase the risk of bleeding. If you have an infection, such as thrush, this is not a reason to stop having sex as your baby is protected by the membranes and a mucous plug that seals the cervix.

WHICH SEXUAL POSITIONS ARE COMFORTABLE?

If you needed an incentive to be more adventurous in lovemaking, pregnancy will provide it. Most positions are feasible in the first months, but once your bump grows, you will not want your partner to rest on it.

Later on in pregnancy you may find moving difficult, so try more comfortable positions that take your bump and tender breasts into account. Not all the positions below will suit you, but it could be fun finding those that do.

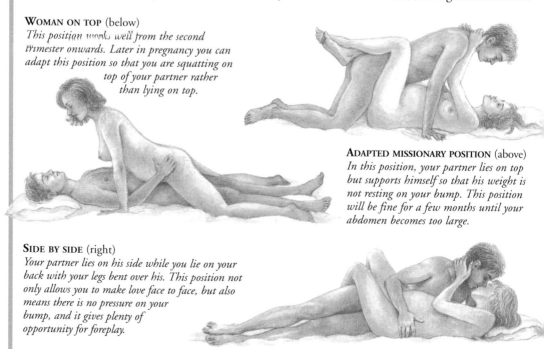

WOMAN ON TOP (below)
This position works well from the second trimester onwards. Later in pregnancy you can adapt this position so that you are squatting on top of your partner rather than lying on top.

ADAPTED MISSIONARY POSITION (above)
In this position, your partner lies on top but supports himself so that his weight is not resting on your bump. This position will be fine for a few months until your abdomen becomes too large.

SIDE BY SIDE (right)
Your partner lies on his side while you lie on your back with your legs bent over his. This position not only allows you to make love face to face, but also means there is no pressure on your bump, and it gives plenty of opportunity for foreplay.

Q WHY HAS MY PARTNER LOST INTEREST IN SEX NOW THAT I'M PREGNANT?

A To some men there is nothing sexier than a woman bearing his child, to others it can all seem rather worrying and brings out a strong protective instinct. Some men fear that sex will hurt you or harm the baby, or bring on premature labour. Try talking to your partner about his fears and anxieties, and reassure him about how safe and natural sex is during pregnancy.

Q WHY AM I SUDDENLY MORE KEEN ON SEX THAN BEFORE?

A This is a perfectly normal way to feel during pregnancy. Some women feel at their most sensual when they are pregnant and their sex life can become more enjoyable than ever. This may be because hormonal changes have created a great sense of well-being and contentment, and your body has become more sensitive to touch. An increased blood flow to the genital area can also enhance your sensitivity and sexual response.

Q I HAVE GONE OFF SEX COMPLETELY, IS THIS NORMAL?

A The changes that make one woman feel more sensual can make another want to avoid sex altogether. Some women feel too sick or tired even to think of sex in the first months. Later on, the bump gets in the way and you may find the whole business too awkward. All of this is normal and reasonable. It is only a problem if your partner is not sympathetic to the physical and psychological changes you are undergoing.

Q I'VE GONE OFF SEX – HOW CAN I STOP THIS DAMAGING OUR RELATIONSHIP?

A You must be honest with your partner about these feelings, because he may interpret your lack of interest in sex as a lack of interest in him. Also, dutiful or resentful sex is worse for your relationship than no sex at all. You could try being adventurous in your love-making by experimenting with different, more comfortable positions (see left). Remember too that there are other ways to express your love apart from sex; a cuddle or a massage can also provide an intimate way of communicating with your partner (see p. 118).

Q CAN SEX TRIGGER OFF THE START OF LABOUR?

A If sperm comes in contact with the neck of your womb (cervix) when you are near or past your due date, it can help to trigger labour by ripening the cervix and causing it to open up. This is because sperm contains a substance called prostaglandin, and artificial prostaglandins are used to ripen the cervix if labour has to be artificially started off (induced). However, don't worry that having sex during pregnancy will cause you to go into premature labour; the cervix will ripen only when it is ready, at term.

Q CAN AN ORGASM CAUSE A MISCARRIAGE?

A No, there is nothing to link orgasm and miscarriage. However, in late pregnancy, orgasm can set off Braxton-Hicks' contractions (see p. 85), which can last for half an hour. These can seem like labour, but are tightenings of your womb rather than real labour contractions.

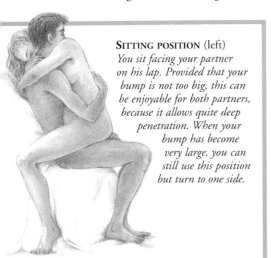

SITTING POSITION (left)
You sit facing your partner on his lap. Provided that your bump is not too big, this can be enjoyable for both partners, because it allows quite deep penetration. When your bump has become very large, you can still use this position but turn to one side.

REAR ENTRY (below)
You kneel on all fours with your partner kneeling and entering from behind. In this position there is no pressure on your bump and your partner is also able to stroke your breasts, clitoris, and abdomen.

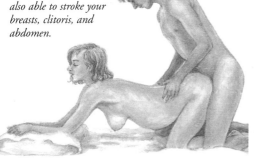

YOUR CHANGING EMOTIONS

Q HOW AM I SUPPOSED TO FEEL NOW THAT I AM PREGNANT?

A Just as no two women are the same, there is no set emotional response to pregnancy. Pregnancy heightens the emotions – you have probably never felt so elated and yet so fearful. You may now find yourself moved at the sight of babies, even if you had little interest in them before, or weeping over bad news on the television. You may daydream about your baby or feel anxious about the future. It can feel like being on an emotional seesaw.

Q WE PLANNED THIS BABY, YET MY FIRST REACTION WAS TO CRY. WHY?

A Mixed emotions are normal, so don't feel that something is wrong if you are not happy all through pregnancy. There is a big difference between wanting a baby and finding out that you are pregnant. A baby changes your lifestyle, and even women who have longed for a child will feel some pangs over the potential loss of freedom.

Q ALL I EVER THINK ABOUT NOW IS MY PREGNANCY – AM I BEING OBSESSIVE?

A As your pregnancy progresses, your thoughts may turn inwards, especially if this is your first baby. It is a natural reaction to be filled with wonder at your growing body. Don't worry about being a "baby bore" – if you enjoy your pregnancy, then revel in it. Share your thoughts with your partner so that he is involved in what is happening.

Q I KEEP FORGETTING THINGS. IS THIS BECAUSE I'M PREGNANT?

A Opinions differ on this. Some health professionals declare that absent-mindedness during pregnancy is largely exaggerated, as many women are able to hold down jobs throughout their pregnancy. Some women report that this mental vagueness is one of their most obvious symptoms. Whether or not you feel this way, there is no need to feel anxious about it. Writing lists and notes to yourself may help.

DISCUSSION POINT

WHY AM I EXPERIENCING SUCH HIGHS AND LOWS?

Huge mood swings are common in pregnancy. If you feel at the mercy of your emotions, it helps to understand why this is happening to you.

Hormonal developments
Your body is being flooded with hormones (see p. 77). These hormonal changes can affect your emotional as well as your physical self. The effects vary with each stage of your pregnancy and differ from woman to woman. You will probably feel at your most erratic in the first months of your pregnancy, settle into a serene mid-pregnancy, then experience more ups and downs in your final weeks.

Facing up to change
Although your hormones may be affecting your moods, it is perhaps unfair to blame your changing emotions entirely on your hormones.

You are also having to come to terms with a momentous life change. Most women with children agree that having their first baby had a far greater impact on their lives than any other event, including marriage. You can't foresee the effect that the experience of looking after and caring for a new baby will have on you and your partner. So together with pleasant daydreams and eager anticipation, you may also experience darker emotions of fear and anxiety. If you feel very depressed, however, talk to your doctor or midwife (see p. 132).

Talking to others
It will seem much worse if you keep your thoughts and emotions to yourself. Talk over with your partner any concerns you may have or discuss your fears at antenatal classes. You may find that other pregnant women, who seem blissfully happy on the outside, are experiencing the same anxieties and mixed emotions.

Q I HAVE VIVID DREAMS, ESPECIALLY OF LOSING MY BABY. IS THIS AN OMEN?

A No, many mothers-to-be report having colourful dreams – some of these are happy, others are more like nightmares. These dreams probably reflect your heightened emotions and uncertainty about the future, but you should not worry about them. It is also probable that your sleep pattern is fairly disturbed, so you are more likely to remember any dreams you have.

Q I'M SURE SOMETHING IS WRONG WITH MY BABY. IS THIS A NORMAL FEELING?

A Anxieties about the future often translate into fears for the health of your unborn child. Most pregnant women worry at some stage that their baby will be born with something wrong, despite having had tests that indicate there are no problems. This may be because they have had a previous miscarriage, or because there is a family history of abnormalities. Some mothers who have already had one normal baby fear they will not be so lucky the next time, others just cannot believe that they will produce a perfect child. If routine tests are all clear, it is unlikely that there is anything wrong. However, you should remember that no matter how many tests you have, there is no absolute guarantee that there will be no problems. If you are particularly worried or concerned, talk to your doctor or midwife about it.

Q I CAN'T WAIT TO HAVE MY BABY. WHY DO I FEEL SO IMPATIENT?

A By the time you have reached the last few weeks, you will probably feel as if you've been pregnant forever. It has been a long nine months' wait and the closer you get to your due date, the more impatient you are likely to be for labour to start and the baby to be born. Try to relax and to wait calmly (see p. 116).

Q WHY DO I WANT TO REDECORATE THE BABY'S ROOM IN MY CONDITION?

A Towards the end of their pregnancy, many women feel an intense urge to redecorate the baby's room, go shopping for baby clothes, or clean the kitchen cupboards. This is known as "nesting" and may be a sign that your baby is due soon. If you have recently stopped working, it may be that you simply feel the need to be active, but you should try to resist tackling any very ambitious projects because you will need to gather your energy for giving birth.

MAINTAINING A POSITIVE RELATIONSHIP

Pregnancy brings changes which can place a strain on emotional and physical relationships. Mutual understanding and a positive attitude can, however, help to enrich your life together.

Offering support

It is important that you both feel you are going through your pregnancy together. Talking about what is happening can help you to understand each other's changing needs and anxieties. Sharing the stresses as well as the joys of pregnancy can create a powerful bond between you.

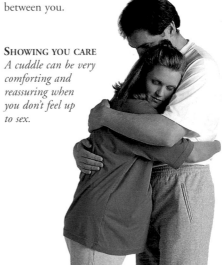

SHOWING YOU CARE
A cuddle can be very comforting and reassuring when you don't feel up to sex.

Making time for each other

Changes in your body and emotions mean that sex is not always top of your agenda in pregnancy; this can sometimes lead to tension. Try not to dwell on how often you have sex, and instead make those times you do make love very special. If you find making love uncomfortable, try new positions (see p. 94) or non-penetrative sex, such as masturbation, oral sex, or massage. Make time to do other things you enjoy together. This can be a special time for you both as you make the transition from life as a couple to life as a family.

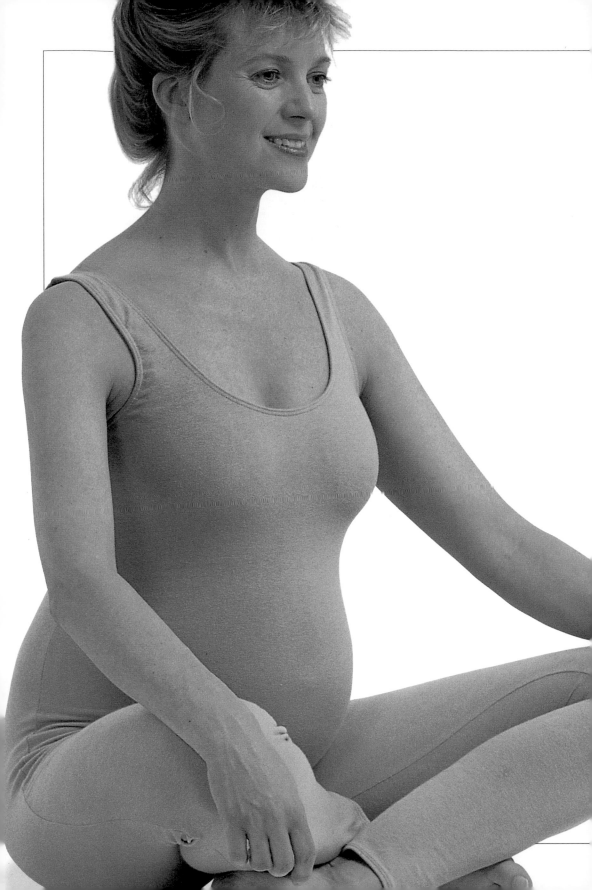

Keeping Fit
and
Healthy

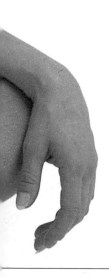

Pregnancy and childbirth place great demands on your stamina and health, so it is important to keep yourself fit and healthy right up to and after the birth of your baby. The focus here is on giving you the knowledge, motivation, and confidence to maintain a healthy pregnancy. To prepare yourself fully for the delivery you need to eat wisely and well, keep supple, and learn how to relax to reduce tension and stress. This chapter discusses ideal pregnancy diets, exercise routines, and healthy lifestyles, which foodstuffs and drugs to avoid, and those complementary medicines and techniques that can benefit you and your baby.

LOOKING AFTER YOURSELF

Q SHOULD I TAKE EXTRA CARE OF MYSELF NOW THAT I'M PREGNANT?

A The more healthy and relaxed you are, the more easily you will be able to cope with the demands of pregnancy. A healthy lifestyle combines many factors: a balanced diet, regular exercise, and plenty of rest. All of these will give you more energy and could mean that you will avoid some of the discomforts associated with pregnancy. For instance, if you eat a balanced diet with plenty of fibre, you will be less likely to suffer from constipation, a common complaint during pregnancy.

Q WHAT CAN I DO TO KEEP HEALTHY?

A Being healthy means eating the right foods (see p. 104) and taking regular exercise. This involves not only antenatal exercises (see p. 110), but also aerobic activities, such as swimming, and going for brisk walks. Remember, however, that this is not the time to embark on a strenuous training programme.

Q WILL MY BABY BENEFIT IF I LEAD A HEALTHY LIFESTYLE?

A Yes, in general, the healthier and happier you are, the better it is for your baby's development. Many things that you eat or drink during your pregnancy can affect your baby, so it is sensible to eat healthily and avoid anything that may be harmful to you or your baby (see p. 102). It is therefore true to say that if you make the effort to have a healthier lifestyle, your baby will ultimately benefit.

Q WHERE SHOULD I BEGIN?

A Take a long, hard look at how you treat your body and then think of ways in which you could be kinder to yourself. If you are a smoker or a heavy drinker, you will need to cut these out or at the very least down (see p. 106). You may have to make a few adjustments to your diet (see p. 104) or plan an exercise routine. Be positive about your new lifestyle – you are not only helping yourself and your baby, but you may also find that you actually enjoy being healthier.

Q WILL MY PREGNANCY AND DELIVERY BE EASIER IF I'M FIT?

A The fitter you are now, the more stamina you will have during labour and the more likely you will be to bounce back after the birth. If you have exercised regularly and eaten well, you will feel more energetic and be better able to look after a new baby. You are also more likely to regain your figure faster. Exercise is also a great reliever of stress; if you feel physically fit and well, you will enjoy your pregnancy more and be less prone to feelings of anxiety.

Q I HAVE PROBLEMS RELAXING AND TAKING IT EASY – WHAT CAN I DO?

A Learning relaxation techniques can help you to unwind throughout pregnancy (see p. 116). Looking after yourself also means ensuring that you do not over-exert yourself, which can lead to exhaustion. This is easier to say than do if you have a demanding job and/or other children, but it is important to make time to relax so that stress does not build up. Taking time out for a massage is another great way to relax (see p. 118).

Q HOW CAN I LOOK MY BEST?

A Pregnancy changes your body in ways you may not expect: as well as your growing bump, it also affects your skin, your hair, your teeth, and even your nails. You need, therefore, to take extra care of yourself during pregnancy (see opposite). Pampering yourself can give you a boost if you are feeling huge and ungainly during late pregnancy. Aromatherapy, massage, and other beauty treatments are just some of the beneficial ways in which you can do this.

Q I FEEL SO HOT AND BOTHERED ALL THE TIME – WHY IS THIS?

A As more blood circulates around your body, you may feel warmer and find that you perspire more. This can make you prone to rashes where the skin creases – in the groin and under the breasts – so keep fresh by washing more frequently. Also try not to put on too much weight (see p. 83), because this will increase your discomfort and make you feel even hotter.

LOOKING GOOD, FEELING GREAT

Hormonal changes in pregnancy can make you look healthy and glowing, or they can have quite the opposite effect.

YOUR COMPLEXION

The extra blood circulating in your body can mean that your skin retains more moisture, is more supple, and less spotty. However, pregnancy hormones can cause problems for certain skins; oestrogen slows oil production, dries skin, and can darken freckles. Because skin texture can change, you may need a different moisturizer. Your doctor will tell you to stop taking any anti-acne drugs during pregnancy. This is important, as these can be harmful.

Greasy skin
If your skin is not usually greasy, don't be too concerned, as this will probably be a temporary condition for the duration of your pregnancy. Use an astringent lotion as part of your daily make-up routine and a special moisturizer for oily skin. If you wear a make-up foundation base, make sure that you use one with an oil-free base.

Dry skin
Avoid using soap, which can dry out your skin by removing its natural moisturizing oils; use a baby lotion, or gentle facial or body wash instead. Using bath oil can help to moisturize your skin, but you should not soak for too long in the bath as this can dry your skin even further.

Gum infection is more likely in pregnancy, so get your teeth checked regularly

Your hair may be thicker and healthier during your pregnancy

Your nails may grow faster and split more easily than usual

Your skin will be affected by increased level of hormones and blood supply

YOUR HAIR

Hair grows in a cycle of loss and regrowth. When you are pregnant, your hair remains in the growth phase, which means it may be thicker and possibly shinier. For some women this is good, as their hair looks better than ever. For others, however, it means more unmanageable hair. If you are among the latter, you may find a shorter haircut easier to look after; changing your shampoo to a gentler variety may also help. For several months after the baby's birth, you may shed a dramatic amount of hair as the growth phase of pregnancy comes to an end. Don't worry, you will not go bald; your hair should re-establish its normal growth-and-loss pattern quite soon.

YOUR TEETH AND GUMS

As soon as you are pregnant, make an appointment to see your dentist. Pregnancy affects your gums, making them spongy and prone to infection, so it is important to have your teeth checked and cleaned regularly. You must tell the dentist you are pregnant, because you should avoid X-rays unless necessary.

YOUR NAILS

These may grow faster during pregnancy, or become brittle and split or break more easily than usual. If this is the case, keep them short and wear gloves when gardening or doing the housework.

EATING FOR HEALTH

Q WHAT SHOULD I BE EATING?

A You do not need a special diet just because you are pregnant but you should eat healthily as your body has to work especially hard during pregnancy. It is now known that what you eat can have a far-reaching effect on your baby's health. You should therefore make sure that you have a well-balanced, varied diet and that you eat regularly and often. In the last three months of your pregnancy, aim to increase your daily calorie intake by about 200 calories – the equivalent of a banana and a glass of milk.

Q WHICH FOODS ARE BEST?

A Often you will find that advice on diet includes foods, such as dried fruits, bran, wheatgerm, and avocado, that are high in nutritional content, but are not the foods you would normally eat – or even like particularly. It is far better to be realistic in your dietary aims and eat what you actually enjoy, because it is likely that if you restrict yourself to an artificial (and possibly unappealing) diet, you will be more tempted to go on an eating binge and put on unwanted pounds. Just make sure that you are getting the basic nutrients in your core diet (see opposite and p. 104)

Q WHAT FOODS SHOULD I CUT OUT?

A Try to cut out very fatty foods such as the fat and crackling on pork, fried bacon, and cream sauces. These are likely to make you feel nauseous in the first three months as well as contribute to weight gain. Look out for the fat in convenience foods such as biscuits, pastries, and cakes. Avoid certain foods that carry the risk of infection and damage to your baby (see chart p. 106).

Q DO I NEED TO TAKE EXTRA VITAMINS?

A If your diet is varied and adequate, you should not need to supplement it with vitamins, unless you are a vegetarian (see below). The exception is folic acid, which is necessary before conception and in the first trimester (see p. 12).

Q SHOULD I DRINK MORE FLUIDS?

A As your blood volume increases, you need to increase your fluid intake. Drink water rather than high-calorie fizzy drinks, which are full of sugar and can make nausea and heartburn worse. Even if you have fluid retention, do not cut your fluid intake; try to drink up to six glasses of water each day. Drinking fluid can also prevent constipation, a common problem in pregnancy.

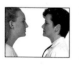

DISCUSSION POINT

HOW HEALTHY IS A VEGETARIAN DIET?

A healthy alternative
Being vegetarian does not necessarily mean that your diet is less healthy. You will, however, need to make up for the lack of meat-derived amino acids by eating a combination of incomplete vegetable proteins that are available in pulses, nuts, tofu, and whole grains such as rice and wholemeal bread. If you do this, your vegetarian diet can be healthy and should not affect your pregnancy. Indeed, you may have lower cholesterol levels than a meat eater and get more fibre from extra vegetables and fruit.

Getting the right nutrients
Your baby takes all the nutrients it needs from you and if you are not getting enough iron, this stresses your body and causes anaemia (see p. 128); therefore, if you do not eat fish, eggs, nuts, and beans, you will almost certainly need iron, and calcium supplements and probably vitamin B12. As well as making you feel very tired, anaemia can affect the baby's growth and your general health. Your body will also be less able to deal with bleeding during the birth.

Q ARE SNACKS AND JUNK FOOD BAD IN PREGNANCY?

A Snacking in itself is not a bad thing (it is much better than feeling faint from going without food for hours) but if you can, you should try to snack on healthy foods. Fresh fruit, nuts, raisins, and raw vegetables are all much better for you than junk foods such as crisps, chocolate, chips, and doughnuts; these are high in calories, fats, sugars, and salt, and although they may produce a fast energy high, they do not contain many nutrients that will help your baby to grow and develop. They may also contain artificial colouring and additives. Of course, the occasional snack now and then will not do you any harm, but snacks shouldn't play a large part in your diet.

Q CAN I STILL EAT FAST FOODS AND GO OUT TO RESTAURANTS?

A Although not as bad for you as junk foods, fast foods can still be high in fat and carbohydrates and, if they are kept heated for long periods of time, many of the vitamins and minerals in the food are destroyed. However, restaurant meals such as freshly made pizza can be nutritious for you, as long as you make sure that you maintain your basic core diet (see p. 104).

Q HOW MUCH WEIGHT SHOULD I GAIN?

A Your weight is not important during pregnancy unless you are very underweight or seriously overweight (see p. 83). What is more important is the growth-rate of the baby; this does not depend on your weight or how much you eat but rather on the efficiency of the placenta and the quality of your food, which supplies the appropriate nutrients. However, you will feel happier if you gain the weight steadily and don't put on large amounts.

Q I HAVE BEEN TRYING TO LOSE WEIGHT – CAN I STAY ON A DIET?

A It is not a good idea to try to slim while you are pregnant, because this is a time when you should be eating a balanced and nutritious diet so that your baby can get all the nutrients he or she needs for healthy development. You will also need plenty of energy to cope with the extra physical demands of pregnancy and labour. Even though you might not want to put on any weight, you will and should if your pregnancy is going well, and this is quite natural and essential.

WHAT BASIC NUTRIENTS DO I NEED?

Protein
This is an essential nutrient which, after being broken down by the liver into amino acids, builds new tissue and is vital for the healthy growth and development of your baby. On top of the normal daily requirement of 45g (1½oz), you need an extra 6g (⅕oz) of protein a day during pregnancy. Protein is found in eggs, fish, meat, cheese, and dairy products.

Carbohydrates
An important food group that gives you most of your fuel or energy, carbohydrates are either sugar or starches. Eat starch-based ones, such as pasta and potatoes, rather than sugar-based ones (see p. 104), because these provide a slower release of energy over a longer period and have fewer calories.

Fats
These build cell walls and are essential for the development of the baby's nervous system, so although you should not eat too much, do not completely cut out fats. The reason why fats are such a dietary taboo is because they contain twice the calories per gram as either proteins or carbohydrates and it is therefore easy to consume large amounts of calories.

Vitamins
Necessary to maintain overall good health, some vitamins such as the B and C vitamins, are not stored by the body, so you need to ensure a daily intake of these. All vitamins are essential, not only for the developing baby but for your immune system, blood production, and nervous system. Folic acid is important in the prevention of spina bifida (see p. 12) in the baby. Avoid eating liver, which is high in vitamin A and can cause problems (see p. 107).

Minerals
Iron is necessary to enable many chemical processes in your body to work and it is essential for the production of haemoglobin in red blood cells. Without iron, your body cannot produce haemoglobin and you will become anaemic (see p. 128). Calcium is needed for healthy bones and teeth and is also important during pregnancy. Zinc is important for healing wounds and for many digestive processes.

WHAT IS A BALANCED DIET?

When pregnant, you should eat sufficient protein, vitamins, carbohydrates, fats, and minerals, as well as fibre every day to ensure a balanced diet. The food pyramid (right), shows the food groups and how much of them you should eat. You will be healthier if you limit your intake of saturated fats and sugars (top), and salt (sodium), but eat more protein for growth, and carbohydrates for energy (bottom). The menu (opposite) shows a nutritious daily diet.

Fats and sugars
Eat these in moderation

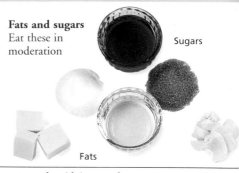

Sugars

Fats

Eggs, meat, fish, nuts, pulses/dairy products
2 servings of protein; 2–4 servings of dairy products a day

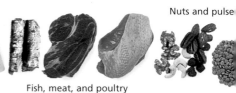

Nuts and pulse

Eggs and dairy products   Fish, meat, and poultry

Fruit and vegetables
4–5 servings a day

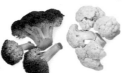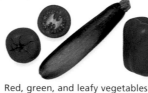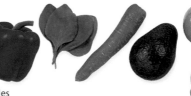

Red, green, and leafy vegetables

Carbohydrates
4–6 servings a day

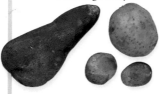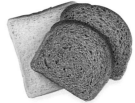

Potatoes   Grains   Rice

YOUR CORE DIET

These are the basic food groups and the quantities that you need for good health during pregnancy. The foods shown above and listed right contain important vitamins and minerals. If you often eat in restaurants or have take-away meals, as long as you make sure that your nutritional needs are met, your diet will be adequate.

Fats and sugars
Eat these in moderation. You must eat fats for your health, but they are high in calories. Of the two types of fat: saturated and unsaturated, eat less saturated fats (animal fat, cheese, cream, and butter) because they are high in cholesterol. Unsaturated fats (poly and mono) such as sunflower, olive, and safflower oils are better for your heart. Avoid sweet snacks: these are high in empty calories.

Eggs, meat, fish, nuts/pulses
2 servings a day of any of the following:
- 85g/3oz red meat or poultry
- 113–170g/4–6oz fish
- 28–57g/1–2oz cheese or 1 egg
- 113g/4oz pulses, grains or cereal
Eggs, meat, fish, and dairy foods are good sources of protein – an essential nutrient when pregnant or breastfeeding. If you are vegetarian, eat tofu, nuts, grains, and pulses.

THE FOOD PYRAMID

Eating sensibly during your pregnancy and afterwards means choosing foods from all the groups shown here. Make sure that you reduce your intake of fats (top) and eat more protein and carbohydrates (bottom).

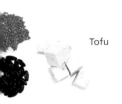
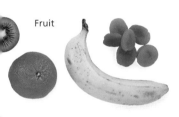

Tofu

Fruit

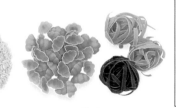

Pasta

A SUGGESTED MENU FOR PREGNANCY

This menu gives you an idea of just how much food your daily diet should contain so that you get enough of the basic nutrients for you and your developing baby.

Breakfast

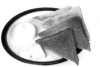

Cereal with semi-skimmed milk

Poached egg and toast

Fruit juice

Morning snack

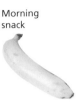

A piece of fruit

Lunch

Pasta with a tomato and tuna sauce

Green salad

Glass of water

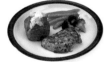

Fruit salad and yogurt

Afternoon snack

Milkshake and cookies

Evening meal

Chicken, jacket potato, and fresh vegetables

Roll and butter

Fruit juice

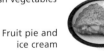

Fruit pie and ice cream

Evening drink

Herbal tea or hot milky drink

Dairy products

2–4 servings a day of any of the following:

- 200ml/⅓pt semi-skimmed milk
- 28–57g/1–2oz cheese
- 1 carton of yogurt

Dairy products provide protein, fat, calcium (for healthy teeth and bones), and vitamins A, B, and D. Semi-skimmed milk contains the same calcium and vitamin content but much less fat than full-fat milk.

Fruit and vegetables

4–5 servings a day of any of the following:

- 85g/3oz vegetables (at least one dark green, leafy vegetable)
- 1 mixed salad
- 1 piece of fruit/dried fruit

These are good sources of fibre and vitamins B, C, and K; some provide potassium and zinc. Dark green vegetables provide iron, magnesium, and folic acid.

Carbohydrates

4–6 servings a day of any of the following:

- 1 slice bread
- 57–113g/2–4oz pasta, rice, or potatoes
- 1 57g/2oz portion of cereal

Starch-based carbohydrates are a source of slow-release energy, fibre, protein, and B vitamins. You need more of these when pregnant or breastfeeding.

HEALTHY YOU, HEALTHY BABY

Q HOW CAN I MAKE SURE I DO NOTHING TO DAMAGE MY BABY'S HEALTH?

A A lot of what you eat, drink, or inhale passes through your body to your baby. It is therefore best to cut out, or down on, things known to be harmful, such as alcohol, smoking, and drugs, and avoid potentially harmful foods (see panel, below).

Q SHOULD I QUIT SMOKING?

A Yes, because smoking and even passive smoking reduces the oxygen and nutrients passing via the placenta to your baby. If you (or your partner) smoke, your baby is more likely to have a low birthweight, and be vulnerable to problems in the first months of life. The risk of bleeding, placental abruption, miscarriage, or premature birth also increases.

Q I WANT TO BUT HOW CAN I GIVE UP SMOKING?

A You may find the decision to stop smoking easy if the queasiness of early pregnancy makes the thought of smoking sickening. If not, then giving up or cutting down can be hard. It will help if you have support from your partner or another smoker who also wants to give up, or you could join a "give-up smoking" group, which will offer you support and advice. Start by gradually cutting down; if you find it impossible to stop smoking altogether, then a maximum of five cigarettes a day is less harmful for you and your baby than smoking ten or more. Other techniques to help you stop smoking include aversion therapy, hypnosis, and acupuncture. Do not use nicotine patches during pregnancy to help you stop smoking.

FOODS THAT MAY CAUSE INFECTIONS

Although the chance of contracting one of these rare infections is limited, you will reduce this likelihood even further if you follow the basic guidelines given here.

Listeriosis
Caused by the bacterium *Listeria monocytogenes*, this is a very rare infection. Its symptoms are similar to flu and gastroenteritis (see p. 128) and it can cause miscarriage or stillbirth.

Toxoplasmosis
Usually symptomless, this can cause serious problems for the baby. Caused by direct contact with the organism *Toxoplasma gondii*, it is found in cat faeces, raw meat (especially undercooked pork), and unpasteurized goats' milk. Soil on fruit and vegetables may be contaminated.

Salmonella
Contamination with Salmonella bacterium can cause bacterial food poisoning. This doesn't usually harm the baby directly, but any illness involving a high temperature, vomiting, diarrhoea, and dehydration could cause a miscarriage or preterm labour.

WHICH FOOD	RISK
Liver and liver pâtés	Listeriosis
Unpasteurized dairy produce, especially soft cheeses such as camembert, brie, and blue-veined cheeses	Listeriosis
Cook-chill pre-prepared meals, especially chicken and seafood	Listeriosis
Undercooked meat, especially pork	Toxoplasmosis
Undercooked eggs and poultry	Salmonella
Offal and offal-based products such as haggis and black pudding. Economy beefburgers and sausages made with dairy beef*	*See below

*Although to date there is no clear evidence that there is an association between BSE (bovine spongiform encephalopathy) and human brain diseases such as CJD (Creutzfeld-Jacob disease), it is probably best to avoid these products.

Q SHOULD I DRINK ALCOHOL AT ALL?

A It is impossible to say if there is a safe limit for alcohol, because its effects vary from woman to woman. What is certain, however, is that regular heavy drinking (more than 14 units of alcohol a week) can lead to mental and physical problems in your baby. To be safe, avoid alcohol in the first three months when the baby's major organs are developing. After this, it is quite safe to have an occasional glass of wine or beer with food.

Q HOW DOES EXCESSIVE ALCOHOL AFFECT THE BABY?

A Regular heavy drinking in pregnancy can cause "fetal alcohol syndrome". This may result in a small baby, and often causes defects. The baby's eyes are often widely spaced, with a flat nose and possibly cleft lip/palate; in addition there may be a degree of learning difficulty.

Q IS IT SAFE TO TAKE ANY DRUGS OR MEDICINES?

A The message is simple: avoid all drugs, particularly in early pregnancy, unless your doctor prescribes them (see panel right). If you buy any medicines over the counter, you must tell the pharmacist that you are pregnant.

Q WHAT IF I HAVE TO TAKE DRUGS THAT ARE POSSIBLY HARMFUL?

A In special situations, your doctor may have to prescribe a drug that could be harmful to your baby. This will occur only if the disease for which the drug is given poses a greater risk to you or your baby's health than the drug. For example, quinine, used to treat malaria, can cause miscarriage or premature labour, but the risks from the actual disease are far greater. If you suffer with epilepsy or a thyroid condition, this will also need thorough treatment, or the consequences for you and your baby can be severe (see p. 130).

Q WHY IS EATING LIVER NOT RECOMMENDED IN PREGNANCY?

A Until recently, pregnant women were advised to eat liver as a source of iron. However, we now know that, in addition to iron, liver contains high levels of vitamin A, which in large doses can cause birth defects. The current advice is to avoid all liver and liver products, such as pâté, especially in the first trimester when the baby's major organs are developing.

ILLICIT DRUGS AND YOUR BABY

Taking illicit drugs is inadvisable when pregnant because it exposes you and your baby to a range of hazards. Even the relatively harmless-seeming cannabis can cause problems to your baby. Apart from the direct risks listed below, you also risk contracting the HIV virus if you inject drugs with shared needles.

Ask for advice

Consult your doctor or a help group about the potential problems of using drugs during pregnancy. If you do regularly use street drugs, you must tell your midwife or the obstetrician about this preferably before labour, because your baby may need special care after the birth.

DRUG	EFFECT
Amphetamines	Causes low birth weight
Cannabis	Causes premature labour. Possible risk of chromosomal abnormality
Cocaine	Causes premature labour, serious placental bleeding, and low birth weight
Ecstasy	Apart from the possible effects on you, such as dehydration and personality changes, taking ecstasy may increase the risk of serious bleeding from the placenta
Heroin and methadone	Causes low birth weight, premature labour, higher rate of twins. After delivery: baby suffers withdrawal symptoms, higher risk of fits, increased risk of cot death (sudden infant death syndrome: SIDS)
LSD	Causes birth defects

NATURALLY HEALTHY

Q WHAT IS NATURAL OR COMPLEMENTARY MEDICINE?

A Any treatment that is not classed as orthodox modern medicine comes under this umbrella (for example, reflexology, homeopathy, acupuncture, aromatherapy, and Chinese medicine, as well as osteopathy, and chiropractic). Complementary therapy can, however, also work alongside orthodox medicine. A complementary therapist aims to treat you as a whole person and, as well as looking at specific symptoms, will consider your lifestyle, diet, and emotional well-being before giving you any treatment.

Q CAN COMPLEMENTARY MEDICINES HELP ME DURING MY PREGNANCY?

A Complementary medicines were developed after centuries of use and observation, and although it can be hard to say exactly how effective these remedies are, they do appear to be successful for many people. You can experience many extra discomforts such as backache, nausea, and constipation, when pregnant; you could find that natural remedies offer you gentle relief and are the ideal alternative to orthodox drugs, which you should avoid at this time.

Q WHERE CAN I GET COMPLEMENTARY MEDICINES?

A You can buy homeopathic and herbal remedies from registered practitioners; some chemists with trained staff also sell homeopathic remedies. You can also prepare your own herbal remedies, but if you do this make sure you follow the recipes carefully and use the correct quantities. If you are considering other therapies, such as reflexology, acupuncture or aromatherapy, see a qualified practitioner for advice and treatment.

Q ARE COMPLEMENTARY MEDICINES SAFE TO USE WHEN I'M PREGNANT?

A Most are safe; however, some herbal remedies and aromatherapy oils are not recommended in pregnancy. If you are in any doubt about what you can or cannot use, always ask a registered practitioner for advice. Also discuss any doubts or worries with your own doctor before starting any complementary treatments.

WHICH THERAPIES CAN BE USED?

Reflexology
To relieve disorders in other parts of the body, reflexologists apply pressure to specific points on the foot to stimulate nerve endings. In pregnancy it can help to ease circulatory problems, backache, and general pains and is used with orthodox medicine for more serious problems such as high blood pressure or pregnancy-induced diabetes. Some women use reflexology in labour as a form of pain relief.

Homeopathy
Homeopathic medicines stimulate your body's own healing mechanisms. Miniscule amounts of plant, animal, and mineral extracts are used: the smaller the dose, the more potent the treatment. Minor pregnancy-related ailments, including nausea, vomiting, heartburn, and indigestion, are amenable to homeopathic treatment, but really potent doses should not be taken during pregnancy.

Acupuncture
This is a branch of Chinese medicine based on the idea that a life-force called "chi" flows through the body, and that disorders are a result of imbalances in this flow. Balance is restored by the insertion of fine needles into specific points on the body to unblock the "chi". Many women find acupuncture helpful in pregnancy to treat complaints such as morning sickness, headaches, allergies, indigestion, and emotional problems such as depression, as well as more serious problems such as high blood pressure. Some women also use acupuncture during labour for pain relief.

Other remedies
Aromatherapy, which involves using essential oils taken from plants and applied with massage, can help you to relax in pregnancy (see p. 118). It is impossible to mention every therapy here, but there are organizations you can contact for more information (see p. 256).

WHICH HERBAL REMEDIES CAN I TAKE IN PREGNANCY?

Medicinal herbs have been part of the healing traditions of certain cultures for thousands of years. Several herbal systems, including the complex Chinese system, have developed around the world. The more familiar Western herbalism, shown in the chart below, provides remedies for pregnancy problems.

How herbal medicine helps

Herbal medicines can help to restore energy, to calm or strengthen the spirit, and to enhance the performance of body organs. In particular, herbal remedies can relieve many pregnancy ailments, including morning sickness, constipation, anaemia, and heartburn. Tonic herbs can help in the preparation of the womb for childbirth: raspberry leaf tea helps to relax the muscles of the womb in preparation for labour.

Using herbal remedies

Herbal remedies come in several forms. Infusions are made by soaking approximately 30g (1oz) dried or 75g (2½oz) fresh herbs in 500ml (1pt) boiling water for ten minutes. The mixture is strained and drunk hot or cold. A tincture, where herbs are preserved in alcohol and drops placed on the tongue, can be bought from a specialist herbalist. Always check with your herbalist whether the herbs you are buying are safe for use in pregnancy.

AILMENT	HERBAL REMEDY	WHAT TO DO	EFFECT
Nausea	Ginger	Drink as an infusion or take 2–5 drops of tincture with water when needed	Has a soothing effect on the digestive system and helps to prevent vomiting
	Peppermint	Drink as an infusion after meals or take in a tincture	Aids digestion, increasing the flow of digestive juices, and reduces nausea
Tension	Skullcap	Drink as an infusion or take in a tincture with water. Can also be taken as a powder in a capsule	Acts as a relaxant and has a calming effect, relieving tension, anxiety, and stress
Depression	St. John's Wort	Drink as an infusion or take in a tincture with water three times a day	Traditionally used to treat nervous complaints, this helps to ease depression
Constipation	Dandelion	Take as an infusion; dandelion leaves can also be eaten in a salad	This is a detoxifying herb that helps to stimulate the liver and the kidneys
Heartburn	Slippery elm	Take as a powder in a capsule or dilute in water. Do not use more than 5g (0.2oz)	Has a soothing effect on the digestive process
Fluid retention	Cornsilk	Drink as an infusion. Can also be taken as a powder in a capsule	Traditionally used as a diuretic, this relaxes the bladder and helps urine flow

KEEPING FIT AND HEALTHY

EXERCISE IN PREGNANCY

Q HOW ACTIVE SHOULD I BE DURING MY PREGNANCY?

A Unless your lifestyle already keeps you very active with normal occupations such as housework, walking, or gardening, you will probably feel better if you take up some form of regular, gentle exercise during your pregnancy. With a fairly inactive daily routine, exercise such as swimming will help to increase your fitness and stamina and will help you to cope with the workload of pregnancy and the demands of labour. Listen to your body and stop exercising when it tells you to. It will probably not be until the final stages of your pregnancy that you feel too uncomfortable to exercise.

Q ARE THERE ANY SPECIAL EXERCISES FOR PREGNANCY?

A Yes, the pelvic floor exercises (see panel, opposite). The weight of your baby places a great strain on the muscles of your pelvic floor. It is important to strengthen these muscles during your pregnancy to prevent tearing in labour, and also after the birth to aid recovery of the pelvic floor area. Exercising your pelvic floor muscles will help to support the weight of the baby and the womb and help control the need to urinate. There are also specific exercises that help to tone up your muscles and improve the suppleness of your joints, making your pregnancy more comfortable (see p. 112) and relieving problems such as backache (see p. 114).

WHICH KIND OF EXERCISE IS BEST?

Swimming is an excellent exercise because the water supports your bodyweight and allows you to tone your muscles without strain. It can also improve your stamina. Some swimming pools or clubs now offer exercise classes particularly aimed at pregnant women. These are ideal for less confident swimmers because they are done while standing in shallow water. Brisk walking, yoga, and dancing are also good ways to keep fit and supple.

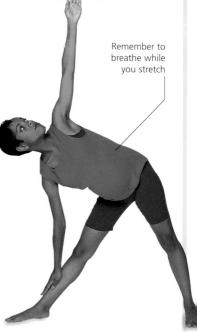

Remember to breathe while you stretch

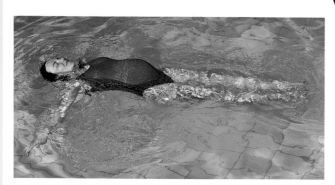

SWIMMING
This can be particularly enjoyable in late pregnancy because you will feel much lighter and the water will keep you cool. Avoid breaststroke if you have pain in the symphysis pubis area or sacroiliac joint problems (see p. 87).

YOGA OR GENTLE STRETCHING
Gentle yoga or stretch exercises are excellent for releasing tension, increasing the mobility of joints, and improving circulation and breathing.

Q HOW OFTEN SHOULD I TAKE EXERCISE?

A Several times a week is ideal but it needn't be the same kind of activity – you could have a varied routine: a swim one day, a walk on another, and perhaps an exercise class or yoga, as you prefer. If you are used to this type of regular exercise, you can continue with it for as long as you feel comfortable, but always listen to your body and slow down if necessary. However, if you are new to exercise, you should start slowly, gradually building up stamina. A little stretching every other day is better than a long hard work-out once a fortnight.

Q ARE THERE SPECIAL EXERCISE CLASSES?

A There are now many classes organized specially for pregnant women. Some offer antenatal exercises, some are for yoga, others are active birth classes. Some pools and clubs also offer exercise classes in water run by qualified professionals.

Q WHAT SHOULD I WEAR?

A Make sure you wear supporting exercise footwear to prevent jarring and damage to the joints. Choose comfortable clothes that won't cause you to overheat. It is a good idea to wear a support bra during any exercise.

Q WHEN SHOULD I AVOID VIGOROUS EXERCISE?

A There are certain times when vigorous exercise is not recommended in pregnancy; these include: if you have previously had problems in pregnancy or your doctor has advised against it; if you have a temperature or feel unwell; in very hot weather. Most importantly, make sure that you do not exhaust or over-exert yourself doing any exercise that you are not used to.

Q ARE THERE ANY PARTICULAR ACTIVITIES THAT I SHOULD AVOID?

A This is not the time to participate in violent or hazardous activities where there is a chance of injury to you or the baby. Activities or sports to avoid include strenuous athletics such as high jumping, or sprinting, and any that require intense training; also, any high-risk activities, such as horse riding and downhill skiing, that could result in physical injury. As always, if you are contemplating doing something you don't normally do, check with a professional first.

THE PELVIC FLOOR

The pelvic floor supports your pelvic organs (the bladder, the womb, and part of the bowels). Pelvic muscles also help to control your bladder and bowels. These muscles can be stretched by the weight of the baby; this causes discomfort and may result in stress incontinence (see p. 126).

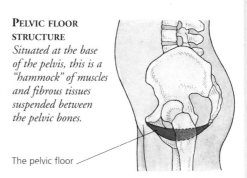

PELVIC FLOOR STRUCTURE
Situated at the base of the pelvis, this is a "hammock" of muscles and fibrous tissues suspended between the pelvic bones.

The pelvic floor

PELVIC FLOOR EXERCISES

Strengthen your pelvic floor muscles by pulling and squeezing in the back passage, vagina, and the urethra as if to stop passing urine. Hold.

Slow pull-ups
Pull up and hold the squeeze as hard as you can and count up to ten. Let go and relax for a few seconds before repeating.

Fast pull-ups
Squeeze tight and let go several times.

How often
Practise several times daily, especially near the end of pregnancy, and as soon as possible after birth. As your muscles strengthen, increase the number of squeezes and length of holding time.

Testing yourself
To check that you are doing the exercise properly, try any of the following tests:
■ When you are urinating, see if you can stop or slow down in mid-flow.
■ Hold a mirror between your legs to see if there is a lift between the vagina and back passage.
■ Put a finger into your vagina and feel it tighten when you practise.

A BASIC STRETCH ROUTINE

Giving birth tests your physical resources to the limit, and looking after a baby can be hard work, so it makes sense to prepare yourself. These non-strenuous stretching and toning exercises can increase your strength and suppleness; they can also help reduce aches and tiredness.

HINTS ON EXERCISING

- Try to exercise as part of your daily routine.
- Exercise with a friend or partner if possible.
- Warm up and cool down when exercising.
- If you are unused to exercise, start gently to build your strength and stamina gradually.
- If you are a beginner in a class, don't try to keep up with more experienced exercisers.
- Make sure that your exercise class teacher knows you are pregnant.
- Exercise should never be painful or make you feel sick, dizzy, or breathless. If any activity causes pain or discomfort, stop immediately.
- Make sure you do not become overheated with vigorous exercise: overheating may be linked with problems in early pregnancy.
- Drink plenty of fluids (preferably water) to avoid becoming dehydrated.

PELVIC TILT

These pelvic tilt exercises help to strengthen your lower back and abdominal muscles, preventing bad posture

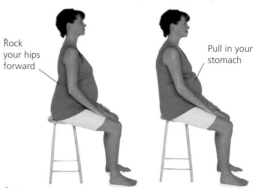

Rock your hips forward

Pull in your stomach

SITTING
Sit on a chair or stool, making sure your feet can rest flat on the floor. Rock your pelvis forward. Then pull in your stomach and rock back on your hips. Repeat.

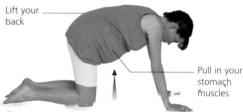

Lift your back

Pull in your stomach muscles

ON HANDS AND KNEES
On all fours, lift your back and pull in your stomach muscles. Imagine your spine is stretching. Return your back to a level position, holding stomach muscles firm.

HIPS AND TRUNK

Mobility can be increased by twisting and circling exercises that loosen the trunk area. You may also find these exercises a comforting movement in the first stage of labour.

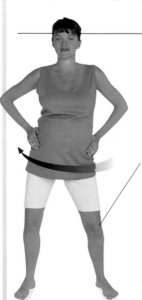

Bend your knees slightly

HIP CIRCLING
With your feet apart and knees slightly bent, place hands on hips. Slowly circle your hips from the waist in one direction five to ten times; then repeat the other way.

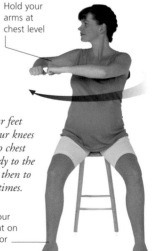

Hold your arms at chest level

TWISTING
Sit on a chair with your feet flat on the floor and your knees apart. Lift your arms to chest level and twist your body to the right as far as you can, then to the left. Repeat several times.

Rest your feet flat on the floor

LEG STRETCHES

The legs carry a lot of extra weight during pregnancy, so stretching and strengthening your leg muscles will be beneficial. The exercises will also improve the circulation in your legs, which could make you more comfortable later in pregnancy.

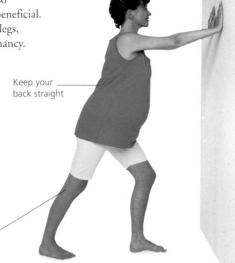

Keep your back straight

LEG STRENGTHENING
Stand with your back to a wall with your feet apart. Slowly bend your legs until you feel some pull on your thigh muscles but before you feel uncomfortable. Hold for a count of 20, then return to standing. Repeat this five times.

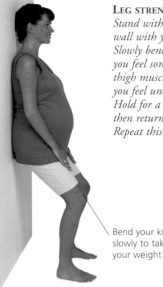

Keep back leg straight and bend front knee

Bend your knees slowly to take your weight

CALF STRETCH
Stand facing the wall, bend your elbows and lean against the wall, resting your weight on your forearms. Now, with both feet facing the wall, place one foot behind the other. Feel the stretch in the calf muscles. Hold the stretch for a few seconds, then repeat with the other leg. Repeat five times.

FEET AND ANKLES

Pregnancy hormones relax the walls of veins; this slows the blood to the heart and can cause varicose veins and swollen ankles and legs. Do these exercises regularly during the day to stimulate the circulation in the legs and help relieve the discomfort of swollen ankles. This is important for women who have to sit at a desk all day or stand for long periods.

You can either sit on the floor or on a chair for this exercise

UP AND DOWN
Move one foot up and down from the ankle, without pointing the toes. Repeat with the other foot. Perform ten to 20 times per foot twice a day.

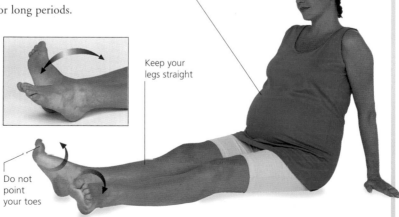

Keep your legs straight

ROTATIONS
Make circling movements with each foot ten times one way and again the other way. Keep the toes relaxed.

Do not point your toes

LOOKING AFTER YOUR BACK

Backache in pregnancy can have several causes. Early in pregnancy, hormones cause the ligaments and joints of the spine to stretch more easily, which makes backache more likely. Added to this, the weight of the baby pulls the spine forward. While prevention is always better than cure with backache, if you are in pain, here are some ways to alleviate the severity (see also panel, below).

YOUR POSTURE

Be conscious of how you sit or stand: your back should always be in a straight line, not arched, and your shoulders should be held back rather than slumped forward.

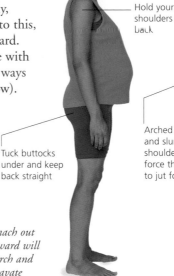
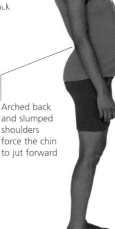

Hold your shoulders back

Arched back and slumped shoulders force the chin to jut forward

Tuck buttocks under and keep back straight

Correct

Incorrect

CORRECT
As your bump grows, it is tempting to lean back and stick your bump out, but this puts pressure on the ligaments and joints of the spine.

INCORRECT
Sticking your stomach out and slumping forward will make your back arch and may cause or aggravate lower backache.

SITTING WELL

It is also important to sit well, especially if you spend a lot of time sitting at a desk or sitting watching television.

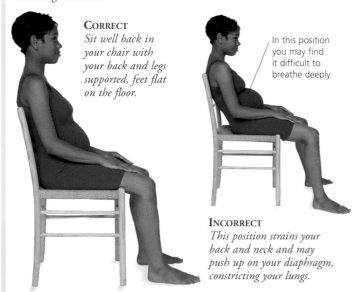

CORRECT
Sit well back in your chair with your back and legs supported, feet flat on the floor.

In this position you may find it difficult to breathe deeply

INCORRECT
This position strains your back and neck and may push up on your diaphragm, constricting your lungs.

ALLEVIATING YOUR BACKACHE

Backache can sometimes be the worst aspect of an otherwise problem-free pregnancy, but there are ways you can help reduce its severity:

■ Improve your posture.
■ A proper back massage can ease some backache (see p. 118).
■ Apply local heat; use a hot water bottle on the aching areas.
■ Gentle stretching exercises (see opposite, above) can keep your muscles and joints supple and may relieve low back pain.
■ Take paracetamol, which is safe to use, for pain relief.
■ Consult your doctor or a physiotherapist or osteopath if symptoms are severe.

STRETCHING YOUR LOWER BACK

You can help reduce low back pain by doing a few simple stretches. The pelvic tilt exercise (see p. 112) also helps strengthen the lower back.

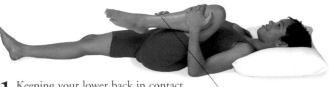

1 Keeping your lower back in contact with the floor, and your other leg straight, bring one knee up to your chest and hug it. Hold for a few moments. Repeat with the other leg.

Clasp your ankle with your other hand for support

2 Bring both knees up to your chest and hug them with both arms. Hold for a few moments. Release slowly. If your bump is too large, bring your legs up either side of it.

Lying in this position is good for the lower back

HOW TO GET UP

It is important to protect your back when you are pregnant. As your stomach muscles are separating to allow your bump to grow, they cannot be used in the same way as before.

Rest one leg over the other

1 First, turn on your side so that you are ready to lever yourself up.

2 Support yourself with your hands, and let your arms take your weight.

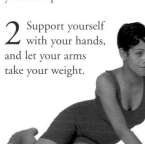

3 Move into a kneeling position. Stand up, one leg at a time, keeping your back straight.

Push up from the floor

LIFTING YOUR CHILD SAFELY

If you lift a small child correctly, it is quite safe. As your lump grows, however, you may find your child difficult to hold. Instead, give your child lots of cuddles while sitting down.

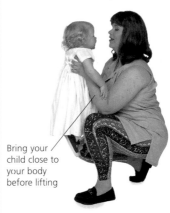

Bring your child close to your body before lifting

1 To lift your child (or a heavy object) bend your knees and lower yourself to his or her level.

Keep your back straight

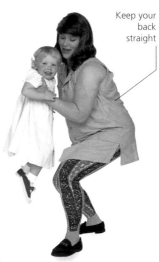

2 When you lift your child, keep your back straight and use your legs, making sure that you hold your child as close to your body as possible.

REST AND RELAXATION

Q WHY IS IT IMPORTANT TO LEARN TO RELAX IN PREGNANCY?

A The more relaxed you are, the more comfortable your pregnancy will be and the more you will enjoy it. Your mind and body will work better, you will feel healthier, and your baby will thrive. You will have more energy without tension and stress, because these are physically draining. You will also sleep better.

Q WHAT IS THE DIFFERENCE BETWEEN RESTING AND RELAXATION?

A During the day when you take a rest, or when you are sitting in a chair watching television, for example, you may be physically resting, but not necessarily relaxed: your mind may be active and your body could feel stiff and tense. Reaching a state of complete relaxation enables you to switch off from worries and achieve a calm, positive frame of mind; this will allow your body and muscles to unwind and any tension to ebb away.

Q WHAT IS THE BEST WAY TO RELAX COMPLETELY?

A You don't have to be sitting still or lying down to relax. Taking regular walks or going for a quiet swim can relieve physical tension and clear your mind. Massage and aromatherapy (see p. 118) are luxurious ways to unwind. However, one of the most effective ways to release stress is by learning relaxation techniques (see opposite).

Q HOW WILL LEARNING RELAXATION TECHNIQUES HELP ME?

A If you practise relaxation techniques regularly, you will find that they provide a short break from physical and mental stress and make it easier to deal with day-to-day pressures. You will be more aware of how your body feels when it is tense, and learn how to relieve the tension. This is particularly useful during pregnancy, when sleep may be difficult; relaxation techniques can also help relieve anxiety and therefore help with pain during labour.

WHAT IS THE BEST POSITION FOR SLEEPING?

A good night's rest can seem an impossible quest, especially in late pregnancy when your baby may kick and turn during the night. Sleeping on your front or your back feels uncomfortable and is inadvisable. Sleeping on your side is best; it takes the weight off your back and thus your circulation, which allows an unrestricted flow of blood to the placenta and baby. This position also allows you to try the relaxation technique opposite.

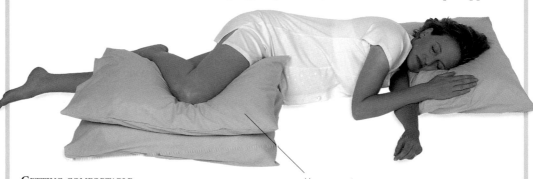

GETTING COMFORTABLE
Lie on your preferred side, put one or two pillows between your legs, and rest your upper leg on the pillows. You may also need a pillow under your bump.

Use one or two pillows to lift your upper leg

TAKING TIME OUT TO RELAX

The only difference in the busy, active life of a pregnant and a non-pregnant woman is that the pregnant woman has the added physical weight and discomfort of a growing baby. As the pregnancy progresses, you may find it is necessary to take time out to relax mentally and physically. This will help relieve tension and tiredness.

GET COMFORTABLE

Make sure you are sitting or lying comfortably. If you prefer to sit in a chair, make sure that your back is supported with a pillow and that your feet are flat on the floor or resting on a cushion or similar support. Alternatively, you could lay your head on your folded arms on top of several pillows placed on a table (see below). You can either close your eyes or leave them open, whichever seems least distracting.

CALM YOUR BREATHING

Begin by slowly blowing out through your mouth to empty your lungs completely. Then close your mouth, and slowly breathe in through your nose. You will find that this makes you take a deeper breath than you might do normally and you should find that this is calming. Breathing in this way will also help to clear stale air from the bottom of your lungs. Repeat this several times. Your body will begin to relax on the out-breath. Continue in this way until you are breathing in a slow, comfortable rhythm.

CALM YOUR MIND

Calming your mind is just as important as relaxing your body, but it does take practice and patience. As far as possible, try to eliminate any distractions from your environment: turn off the TV and any music. Close your eyes and concentrate on steadying your breathing and the way your body feels as you begin to relax. If your mind starts to wander on to familiar nagging worries, gently call it back. Picture a pleasant scene in which you feel happy and relaxed. Explore this scene and conjure up all the details, imagining that you are actually there. Try to do this for at least twenty minutes and then open your eyes and stretch gently to finish the exercise.

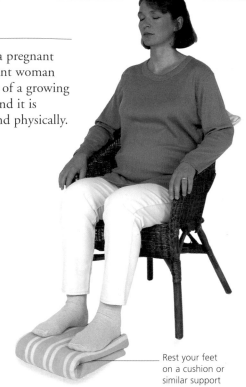

Rest your feet on a cushion or similar support

SITTING IN A CHAIR
If you don't want to lie down, you can practise while sitting in a chair. Support your lower back with a cushion, and rest your feet on a cushion or folded blanket.

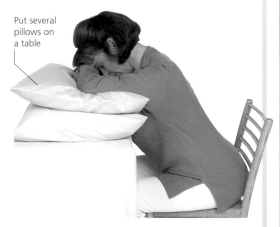

Put several pillows on a table

AT A TABLE
This position, which allows you to stretch out, is particularly comfortable in late pregnancy when your baby is high under your diaphragm and it is difficult to breathe.

KEEPING FIT AND HEALTHY

MASSAGE IN PREGNANCY

Q WHAT BENEFITS WILL I GAIN FROM MASSAGE IN PREGNANCY?

A Recognized for centuries as a method of healing, massage is an aid to relieving pain and stiffness in muscles. Most importantly, it gives you a great feeling of well-being; it releases tension and restores and boosts vitality; your circulation is stimulated by a massage, which can have either a calming or an invigorating effect. Regular massages during pregnancy will help you to relax and will reduce tiredness as well as relieve any aches and pains, particularly backache.

Q HOW IS IT DONE?

A The muscles and soft tissue are stroked, rubbed, and kneaded gently and rhythmically, usually with the hands, sometimes with specialist tools, which is soothing and restorative.

Q IS MASSAGE IN PREGNANCY SAFE?

A It is safe to stroke most of your body but vigorous rubbing or kneading of the abdomen is not advised. You may find that, except in the first trimester, you are not comfortable lying on your front. Certain essential oils should not be used because they are too astringent (see below).

Q WHAT ABOUT BEAUTY PARLOUR MASSAGES?

A These are fine, but tell the masseur or masseuse that you are pregnant, because some restrictions should be observed. However, a physiotherapist, professional masseur, or qualified aromatherapist will probably give you a better massage.

Q WHAT IS AROMATHERAPY?

A Aromatherapy is the treatment of the whole body with essential oils or essences from plants and flowers to regulate the body and relax the mind and spirit. The oils can be absorbed through the skin either in massage, when they are added to creams or oils, or during bathing; they can also be inhaled from vaporizers. Aromatherapists also value herbs and teas as a means of detoxifying the body.

Q WHAT PROBLEMS CAN AROMATHERAPY HELP ALLEVIATE?

A In pregnancy, aromatherapy can be used to help alleviate nausea, painful Braxton-Hicks' contractions, oedema, and heartburn. It can also be of benefit in cases of tiredness, insomnia, depression, and anxiety. When used in conjunction with massage in the first stage of labour, it can be helpful for its relaxing and calming effects, and for pain relief.

WHICH ESSENTIAL OILS CAN I USE?

Oils used in massage are the "essence" of plants or flowers. Each oil has a different action, fragrance, and sometimes colour. Oils can be antiseptic or antibiotic, astringent and stimulating, or calming and aphrodisiac.

The essential oils recommended in pregnancy
Chamomile, citrus (oils), geranium, lavender, neroli, rose, sandalwood.

The essential oils to be avoided in pregnancy
Basil, clary sage, hyssop, juniper berry, marjoram, myrrh, pine, rosemary, sage, thyme, bay.

Recipes for massage treatments
Mix the following oils in a small jar or bottle and apply with warm hands.

For relaxation 50ml grapeseed oil, 5ml wheatgerm oil, 8 drops neroli, 8 drops sandalwood.

To moisturize the skin 25ml avocado, 25ml almond oil, 5ml wheatgerm oil, 10 drops chamomile, 5 drops sandalwood, 5 drops frankincense.

During pregnancy 50ml almond oil, 5 ml wheatgerm oil, 4 drops lavender, 4 drops sandalwood, 2 drops tangerine, 2 drops geranium.

RELAX WITH A MASSAGE

Massage can release tension and restore the body's natural energy levels. During your pregnancy and labour, a comforting massage can help you relax and sleep better. Lie down or sit comfortably in a warm room. It is best, but not essential, to remove your clothes, keeping the areas not being massaged covered with warm towels.

WHERE TO START

Your partner should begin the massage with stroking movements, using the balls of the fingers softly but rhythmically, then using the hands to work more firmly on tense muscles. The palms can be used to apply pressure, or the knuckles for really tense spots.

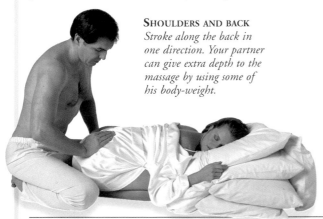

SHOULDERS AND BACK
Stroke along the back in one direction. Your partner can give extra depth to the massage by using some of his body-weight.

EASING TENSION
Rubbing in small, circular movements on the face and around the forehead and temples can relieve tension headaches.

MASSAGE TIPS

- Warm the hands; remove jewellery.
- Scented oils, powder, or creams will allow the hands or massage tool to slide easily over the skin.
- Don't knead the belly or breasts.

KEEPING FIT AND HEALTHY

MASSAGE FOR BACKACHE

The best position for back massage in early pregnancy, when you can lie on your stomach, is face down on a bed or the floor. Later on, sit on the edge of a sofa or chair and support your arms on the back of a chair, or lie on your side on a firm bed or comfortable floor surface.

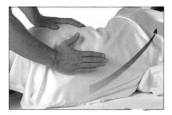

STROKING
Start the back massage with firm, stroking movements from the base of the spine up to the neck, using one or both hands.

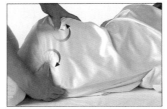

CIRCULAR MOVEMENTS
Gentle pressure applied in circular movements at the base of the spine with the thumbs, relieves muscle tension and relaxes the whole back.

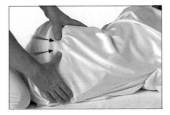

DEEP PRESSURE
Steady, direct pressure applied to either side of the spine is especially good for easing lower back pain in pregnancy and labour.

WORK AND TRAVEL

Q CAN I CONTINUE TO WORK?

A It can be good to work for some, if not most, of your pregnancy. This may be a physical strain, especially in later months, but there are benefits: you will have company during the day; you will be leading a normal life, even if your body is changing. In fact, carrying on with your normal routines will confirm that you are not abnormal or ill because you are pregnant.

Q IS THERE ANY WORK I SHOULD NOT DO IN MY CONDITION?

A The law states that if you are pregnant or are breastfeeding, your employer must ensure that the work you do is not likely to put your or your baby's health at risk. This may mean that your working conditions have to be changed, or that a suitable alternative be found. You can't be sacked just because you are pregnant (see p. 254).

Q WHEN SHOULD I TELL MY EMPLOYER?

A It is a good idea to tell your employer and your colleagues as soon as possible, so that they will be understanding about any late starts if you suffer from morning sickness, for time off to attend antenatal appointments (without any loss of pay), and about rest if you feel tired. Before you stop work, you have a legal obligation to confirm in writing to your employer: your date of departure; when your baby is due; and when you plan to return (see p. 254).

Q WHY DOES MY EMPLOYER NEED TO BE INFORMED IN WRITING?

A This means that you will have it on record that you gave advance notice that you are pregnant and that you wish to return. This is a legal requirement which protects your rights to receive Statutory Maternity Pay (SMP), and return to work.

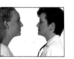

DISCUSSION POINT

MATERNITY LEAVE

When to give up work
This depends on how you feel, how far you have to travel, and how stressful your work is, but you can leave work eleven weeks before the week your baby is due – SMP and Maternity Allowance are paid from this date. You will have to stop earlier if you have a pregnancy-related illness or medical problem; your doctor will give you a medical certificate for this. Otherwise you can continue for as long as you want. Most women stop work at 34 to 36 weeks, but if you are expecting twins, you may wish to stop earlier (see p. 92).

Once you've left work
Your priorities may change as you prepare for your new life. This can be a creative period with lots of time to think, but you may also be at a loss as to how to fill the hours. Try to make the most of this time to yourself. As you get bigger you will probably wish to be less active and take more rest.

Returning to work – it's your decision
Many women enjoy their work and wish to pursue their careers after the baby arrives. You may also have to return to work for financial reasons, or you may return because you feel more fulfilled doing a job and having a family to look after. You must decide what is best for you and try not to let other peoples' opinions influence your decision. Even if you ultimately change your mind after your baby arrives you can still do so, although you should make sure that you know your legal obligations.

Worry about leaving your baby
Before the birth you cannot know how you will feel about leaving your baby. Inevitably, it will be a wrench after being with your baby every day for a few months. Whatever you decide, be prepared to feel guilty from time to time. However, what is good for you is also usually good for your baby.

Q WHAT ARE MY RIGHTS AND BENEFITS IN PREGNANCY?

A It is important to get help and advice as soon as you become pregnant because the rights and benefits situation is constantly changing. Consult your local Department of Social Security to confirm the latest rules and collect any forms you may need (see p. 254).

Q CAN I TAKE TIME OFF FOR MY VISITS TO THE ANTENATAL CLINIC?

A All pregnant women have a right to take paid time off for antenatal visits, including antenatal classes, no matter how long you have worked for your employer, or how short your hours of work.

Q I FEEL SICK AND TIRED – SHOULD I GIVE UP OR TRY TO WORK THROUGH IT?

A The early trimester is usually the hardest to get through, but this phase of nausea and tiredness will pass. Many women find that the middle trimester and later weeks are a good period for work because they do not feel as tired.

Tips for working through pregnancy

■ By law, employers should provide rest facilities for pregnant or nursing mothers. If your company has a rest room, try to take a short rest or nap every day.

■ If possible, avoid standing for too long. Do not work for prolonged periods without breaks, and try to make sure that you eat at lunch-time rather than going shopping.

■ Try to find a few minutes during the day to do some light exercises for your neck, legs, ankles, and shoulders (see p. 108).

■ If your job is particularly stressful or you are having medical problems, it may be a good idea to suggest working shorter hours or even from home.

■ Ease up on your daily workload, perhaps by being less fastidious about the housework or perhaps by asking your partner to help out more around the home.

QUESTIONS TO ASK

If I continue to work, will I find it more difficult to cope with my pregnancy?

What maternity benefits am I entitled to?

Must I return to work in order to get Statutory Maternity Pay (SMP)?

GETTING OUT AND ABOUT

Is it safe for the baby if I continue to drive?
It is as safe for the baby as it is for you. However, after 37 weeks it is advisable, particularly on long journeys, to have someone with you, and preferably to drive you. Being driven will also help to reduce your fatigue level; having someone with you, in the event of you going into labour, is prudent. Also, some women report that getting behind the wheel is difficult in the last few weeks.

Should I wear a seat belt when I'm in a car?
It is now a legal requirement for drivers and passengers to wear seat belts. Being pregnant does not exclude you from this legislation – unless you have obtained a certificate from your doctor. Seat belts may be uncomfortable because of the bump, but wearing a properly fitted belt best protects the mother and baby in the event of an accident. If you are in an accident, even if you do not feel you have been hurt, you must be checked out at your local obstetric unit: in rare cases, the belt can cause injury to the placenta or the womb.

Can I travel by train?
Yes, there is no reason why not. But long trips can be stressful, especially in overcrowded trains. To minimize stress, book your ticket in advance, travel at times that avoid commuter rushes, and making sure that you have someone to meet you at your final destination.

Can I continue to cycle to work?
As long as you are comfortable, there is no problem with this early in pregnancy. But most women find cycling uncomfortable after 16 weeks or so. And bear in mind that although serious cycle accidents are rare, falling off your bike could damage not just you but also your womb, placenta, and baby.

What should I do for long trips?
If you are driving, break your trip every one or two hours, walk around, and exercise your legs. Take a drink with you and make sure that you have some snacks – fruit or cereal bars – in case you get hungry. Remember to take your mobile phone and maternity records with you.

KEEPING FIT AND HEALTHY

TRAVELLING ABROAD

Q CAN I FLY IN PREGNANCY?

A There is normally no reason why you can't fly, unless of course you have developed a medical condition such as pre-eclampsia (see p. 138) Most airlines set a "cut off" time of around 32 weeks (this varies with each airline) after which they will not allow you to travel. This is because of the (albeit remote) risk of you going into labour on board the aeroplane. Also, long haul flights are extremely uncomfortable after about 24 weeks.

Q SHOULD I TAKE ANY PRECAUTIONS WHEN FLYING?

A Ensure that you have plenty of leg-room and easy access to the toilet (an aisle seat is usually best). Carry some bottled water with you in case you feel a little dry, and some easily digestible fibre/carbohydrate such as fruit or cereal bars. Avoid alcohol, as this will make you dehydrated, which coupled with the demands of your pregnancy, and slightly lower oxygen content in the cabin, may make you light-headed.

Q I AM PREGNANT. IS THERE AN INCREASED RISK OF DVT DURING A FLIGHT?

A The link between increased risk of deep vein thrombosis (DVT) and long flights is not proven, but the concern is serious enough for many airlines to provide exercise sheets and advice on how to reduce the risk while on board. Because of changes occurring to your blood composition in pregnancy, you may be more at risk of DVT but you can take steps to reduce this. Wear comfortable, supportive shoes, keep hydrated with water or clear fluids, avoid alcohol, eat snacks, and try to move around every two hours or so. Follow the exercise advice onboard. Flex, extend and rotate each foot ten times and massage the calves of your legs every hour or so.

Q DO I NEED EXTRA TRAVEL INSURANCE WHEN ABROAD?

A Usually not, but you should tell your insurance company that you are pregnant, especially if you have any other condition as well, such as high blood pressure or diabetes.

VACCINATIONS DURING PREGNANCY

If you're likely to be making a big trip abroad, ideally you should make plans for this before you get pregnant. While in a perfect world, pregnant women would avoid taking any drugs, this is not practical in real life. Your own health is of paramount importance so the benefits of vaccinations or prophylactic treatments should be weighed against the small, often hypothetical, risk of possible harm to your baby.

Should I have any vaccinations before travelling to a foreign country?
It depends. In general, vaccines that provide passive immunity (sometimes called immunoglobulins) are safe in pregnancy (including immunoglobulin for hepatitis A). Those vaccinations that stimulate an immune response (active immunity) are also usually considered safe, as long as they do not contain live, inactivated viruses. Vaccines that contain live inactivated viruses (for example, the vaccine for rubella, or German measles) should normally be avoided during pregnancy as there is a risk that these viruses could cross to your baby and affect him or her.

Which vaccines can I have?
Recommendations change on a month by month basis as new information comes to light and new vaccines become available, so it is really important to get the latest advice from medical experts in foreign travel. Tetanus, diptheria, and polio vaccines may be given safely during pregnancy. Rabies vaccination should be considered if you intend travelling to a high-risk area. Cholera vaccine is not regarded as giving a useful level of immunity from the disease and is now not widely available. Yellow fever and rubella (German measles) vaccinations are produced from live, inactivated viruses and should not be administered during pregnancy.

Q CAN I TAKE SOME UNITS OF MY OWN BLOOD ON HOLIDAY IN CASE I NEED IT?

A No, on a practical level this would never work. Statistically, the tiny likelihood that you would use it means that it would almost certainly not be worth the effort, even were it possible. If you were to need a blood transfusion, you will probably need more blood than you could possibly have "banked" in the previous months without making you anaemic. Furthermore, blood has a limited shelf-life, even when kept in controlled, chilled conditions.

Q SHOULD I TAKE MY HOSPITAL RECORDS WITH ME ON HOLIDAY?

A Yes. Whether abroad or at home, you should carry the details of your care with you, so that if you need medical care, the key points can be established rapidly. Even if you're visiting a country where a different language is spoken, certain facts, such as your blood group and ultrasound scans records, would make your notes extremely valuable to any professional staff caring for you.

Q I GET VERY TRAVEL SICK. CAN I TAKE MY NORMAL TABLETS WHILE I'M PREGNANT?

A This depends entirely on which tablets you take. Some anti-sickness tablets or suppositories are considered safe in pregnancy, and in fact are used to treat morning sickness early in pregnancy. Others aren't. Your doctor or pharmacist will be able to advise you.

Q IF I GET ILL OR HAVE A COMPLICATION ABROAD, WILL I BE FLOWN BACK?

A Not always. If you are in an emergency condition, no doctor would advise travelling. Depending on what stage of pregnancy you are at, if you develop a complication you might not be able to come home, in some cases, until after the baby's birth.

Q WHAT IS THE RISK TO MY PREGNANCY OF GETTING BAD GASTROENTERITIS?

A The most obvious problem is of you becoming dehydrated, which can affect your strength, how your kidneys work, etc. Any infection with a high temperature and dehydration stands a risk of causing preterm labour or even miscarriage. So, diarrhoea and vomiting in pregnancy must be taken seriously, and you may need a day or two in hospital, if only to be rehydrated.

Q CAN I TAKE ANTI-DIARRHOEA TABLETS WHILE I'M PREGNANT?

A Any tablets are best avoided in the first trimester of pregnancy (up to 14 weeks). However, some anti-diarrhoeals can be used in later pregnancy. Consult your pharmacist or doctor for advice. If you have diarrhoea while on holiday, drink plenty of electrolyte solutions in clean, bottled water, or even fizzy sugary drinks from cans. You need sugar, fluid, sodium, and potassium, so pure water on its own is not the answer.

Q I'M TRAVELLING TO A MALARIA ZONE. CAN I TAKE ANTI-MALARIAL DRUGS?

A The risk of you getting malaria in pregnancy is one that must be minimized, as malaria can cause miscarriage and premature delivery. Try to avoid travelling to a malaria zone in the first trimester of pregnancy. It is important to check which drugs you need for the particular strains of malaria prevalent in the area you are visiting. Many anti-malarials can be taken with caution in pregnancy whereas others shouldn't be taken at all. Chloroquine and proguanil are regarded as relatively safe to use. Do note that preventing malaria involves more than just taking tablets. To avoid getting bitten, expose as little bare skin as possible and use mosquito nets and coils.

Q SHOULD I TAKE ANTIBIOTICS ON MY TROPICAL HOLIDAY IN CASE I GET ILL?

A Unless you are medically trained, you are unlikely to know which infection you have picked up, and no antibiotic covers all infections. You can potentially cause problems by taking the wrong or inappropriate antibiotic. The best advice is to find out in advance the name of a good local doctor or clinic before you travel.

Q CAN I STILL RECEIVE FREE ANTENATAL CARE ABROAD?

A For EU citizens travelling within European Union countries, there is a reciprocal arrangement for emergency medical care. You should obtain form E111 from your post office before you travel. Most other countries do not provide free health care, so you will need to take out holiday medical insurance. Even if travelling within Europe, it is advisable to take out holiday medical insurance in any event in case your care turns out to involve more than you are eligible for; this would normally include cover for repatriation to your home country.

KEEPING FIT AND HEALTHY

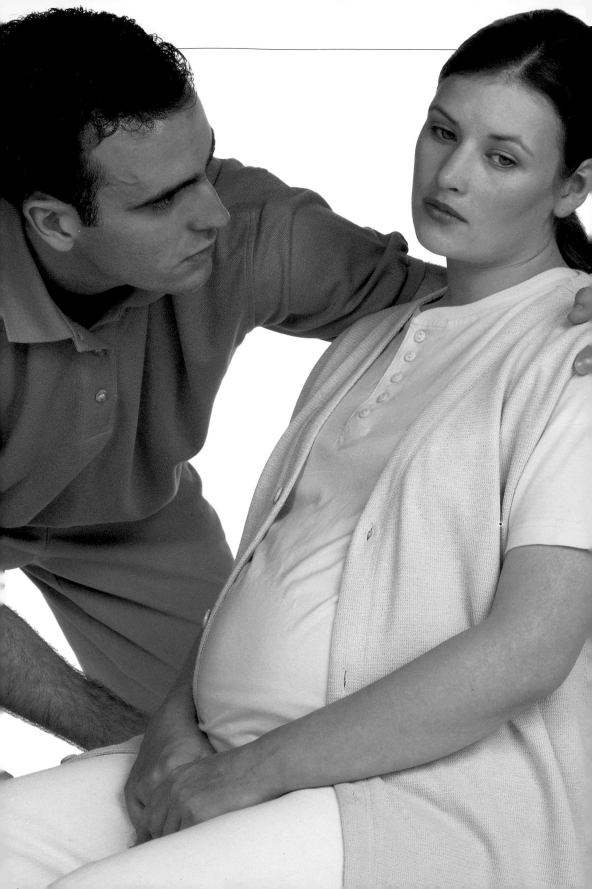

PROBLEMS
IN
PREGNANCY

Few pregnancies run their course without some problem or ailment occurring – most are minor but a few are more significant. Like many couples, you and your partner may find even minor complaints worrying, however, most can usually be dealt with relatively quickly; only very rarely are there indications of a serious condition. This chapter shows you what to look out for during pregnancy, which problems are common and need no further treatment, and which need to be brought to the attention of your doctor or midwife. By understanding what is happening, you will be able to cope more easily with any unexpected developments.

COMMON DISORDERS

Q WHICH PROBLEMS DO I NEED TO CONSULT MY DOCTOR ABOUT?

A The numerous changes your body undergoes throughout pregnancy can cause many problems. Most of these are normal and will not need special medical attention. However, there are sometimes more serious developments in pregnancy, such as infections (see opposite), or diabetes (see p. 136), which need particular attention from an obstetrician, midwife or other specialist. Always mention anything that is troubling you to your doctor or midwife so that they can reassure you or take further action as necessary.

Q WHAT IS CAUSING MY ABDOMINAL ACHES AND PAINS?

A Pregnancy will invariably cause various twinges in your abdomen. The main offenders are the ligaments of your womb, which are stretching, those of your pelvis, and those supporting sacroiliac joints, which are loosening. These pains often lessen if you change position, for instance, or lie down for a while; or you may find that gentle exercises or swimming will help.

Q MY LOWER ABDOMEN ACHES AND I FEEL SICK, WHAT IS WRONG?

A Not every pain is simply due to your pregnancy. If you have stomach pain with other symptoms such as nausea or vomiting, it may be caused by indigestion, food poisoning (gastroenteritis), cystitis (a urinary tract infection, see opposite), or even appendicitis, all of which can occur in pregnancy. Pregnancy can also mask symptoms and exaggerate others; some conditions, cystitis for example, have slightly different symptoms during pregnancy; talk to your doctor if you suspect that anything is wrong.

Q I SUFFER FROM MIGRAINES. WILL THESE GET WORSE IN PREGNANCY?

A Some women suffer more, others find that their migraines completely disappear. Migraines may be linked to blood flow to the brain, which is affected by high oestrogen levels. Some of the symptoms of migraine are similar to those of pre-eclampsia; should you experience a headache with blurred vision or spots in front of your eyes, you should see your doctor.

Q WHAT IS A FIBROID AND CAN IT AFFECT MY PREGNANCY?

A A fibroid is a benign growth of muscle inside your womb, and is normally noticed when you have a scan or an internal examination. Fibroids rarely develop during pregnancy, but if you already have one, the high levels of oestrogen produced by your body in pregnancy can cause it to grow larger. If a fibroid degenerates, it may cause pain in your abdomen. Although unpleasant, this is not usually serious. It is unusual for a fibroid to affect your baby or your labour unless it grows very large or obstructs your cervix. A fibroid may also increase the risk of heavy bleeding after the birth (see p. 190).

Q IS URINE LEAKAGE A COMMON PROBLEM DURING PREGNANCY?

A Leaking urine when you cough, sneeze, laugh, or run around is exceptionally common from mid-pregnancy onwards. This is known as stress incontinence, and you may wish to wear a sanitary pad if it happens frequently. You can help alleviate the problem by practising pelvic floor exercises (see p. 111), and by cutting down your intake of tea, coffee, and alcohol. Cystitis is often a cause of stress incontinence, or it makes the problem worse if you already have it. If you were suffering from incontinence before you became pregnant, and it gets much worse during your pregnancy, you may need to have your bladder examined at a centre specializing in these problems.

Q WHY, WHEN I STAND UP, DO I FEEL PAIN AND WEAKNESS IN MY PELVIS AND LEGS?

A As you approach 37 weeks, your baby's head moves down towards your pelvis and presses against the pelvic bones, causing the ligaments to stretch and making your pelvic area feel extremely uncomfortable. The baby's head may also press hard against your sciatic nerves – those nerves responsible for movement, pain, and sensation in your legs, and this can cause numbness, tingling, weakness, and pain down one or both legs. Known as sciatica, this is fairly common. If it is severe, however, you should see your doctor to eliminate other possible causes, such as a slipped disc (see p. 87).

Infections in Pregnancy

Infections are caused by viruses or bacteria. Chickenpox, rubella (German measles), and herpes are caused by viruses. They cannot be treated by antibiotics. Bacteria are live organisms that can infect your body by multiplying in tissue and in the bloodstream. Serious bacterial infections include toxoplasmosis and listeriosis. Unlike viruses, these can be treated with antibiotics. Although it is unusual for bacteria or viruses to cross the placenta and affect the baby, the exceptions to this rule are rubella, toxoplasmosis, and listeriosis. The baby may also be indirectly affected by an infection (for example, a kidney infection) that causes premature labour.

Urinary tract infections (UTIs)

A urinary tract infection can affect any part of the urinary tract, including the bladder and kidneys. Symptoms include a constant need to urinate, irritation, or a burning sensation when urinating, low abdominal pain and, if untreated, blood in the urine, and fever. If you have any of these symptoms, you will need antibiotics. Delay in treatment may result in a kidney infection, causing severe illness and possibly miscarriage or premature labour.

Thrush

This is a common and usually harmless vaginal infection caused by a fungus. Its main symptoms are vaginal soreness and itching, and a white discharge. Treatment in pregnancy involves a course of cream, and vaginal suppositories.

Toxoplasmosis

If you think you have been in contact with this infection (see p. 106), your blood will be tested for antibodies, which your body produces to fight the infection. If present, your baby may need treatment, and his or her growth will be checked by frequent scans. If the infection is missed, there is a risk of miscarriage or stillbirth, or your baby might be born mentally handicapped or blind.

Listeriosis

This bacterium is found in soft cheeses, pâtés, and pre-cooked foods (see p. 106). If the results of a blood test show that you have been infected, you will be treated with antibiotics and your baby may need to be delivered early. Listeriosis can cause premature labour, miscarriage, or stillbirth. If your baby has to be delivered, he or she may be very ill and will need antibiotics to prevent septicaemia (blood poisoning) and meningitis.

Rubella (German measles)

This virus is now rarely contracted in pregnancy because most young adults have been vaccinated against rubella at school. Rubella can cause your baby heart and brain defects, deafness, and cataracts and, if you are infected with rubella in the first three months, there is a more than 50 per cent chance of your baby being affected; this risk reduces thereafter.

Chickenpox (varicella zoster)

This can cause a severe lung infection or pneumonia in the mother if contracted in pregnancy, but there is only a very small chance that this will harm your baby. If you have been in contact with anyone with chickenpox and are not immune, you will be injected with immunoglobulins to reduce any risk.

Herpes

This virus can cause painful blisters in and around the vagina. The risk of passing this on to your baby at birth, even with recurrent herpes, is low. However, if your first attack is in pregnancy and you have ulcers at the time of delivery, you may be offered a Caesarean section because there is a risk of your baby being infected, which may cause brain damage.

Cytomegalovirus (CMV)

Cytomegalovirus (CMV) is one of the herpes group of viruses. It is one of the major congenital causes of deafness, blindness, and mental impairment; a fact made even more shocking because so few pregnant women have heard about it. The good news is that many women (40 to 80 per cent in Europe) are immune to it through previous infection. The bad news is that if you're not immune, and catch it in pregnancy, there is a 50/50 chance of passing it to the baby.

How do i know when a complaint needs treatment?

Most of the complaints you will experience during your pregnancy are common and nothing for you to worry about; in fact, they are probably a sign that your pregnancy is progressing normally. However, if any discomfort persists or keeps coming back,

SYMPTOMS	POSSIBLE CAUSES	COMMON/MILD CASES
Headaches with blurred vision	Migraines, pre-eclampsia	May be linked to high levels of the hormone, oestrogen, in pregnancy. Just as some women get headaches with the Pill, which contains oestrogen, pregnancy can have the same effect.
Severe tiredness, lethargy, inability to carry out simple tasks, pale complexion	Anaemia	Anaemia is usually caused by insufficient iron, either in your diet or from the demands of pregnancy. This reduces the haemoglobin in the red blood cells.
Severe vomiting, inability to keep food or even fluids down, thirst	Severe morning sickness Urinary tract infection (UTI)	Morning sickness is common, although its severity varies. If you are expecting more than one baby, this can worsen and prolong morning sickness.
Aching under ribs, shortness of breath	Baby's position	In late pregnancy, your womb presses on internal organs, which press on your ribs.
Abdominal aches	Baby's size	Muscles stretch to accommodate the womb, and ligaments become loose.
Abdominal pain – with vomiting and/or diarrhoea	Food poisoning; cystitis; appendicitis	Cause unrelated to pregnancy.
Low backache	Baby's weight and position	Hormones cause the joints and ligaments of your pelvic area and spine to soften, which places strain on your back; this is made worse by bad posture.
Intense itchiness, usually on stomach and back or in folds of skin (under breasts)	Dry skin; skin rash; liver problems	May be due to dryness from lack of vitamin B; varicose veins cause itchiness; a skin rash (intertrigo), can occur due to being overweight and excess sweating.
Leaking urine when you cough, sneeze, laugh, or run	Baby's weight; cystitis	Your bladder is being squashed by your womb, causing it to leak; this is common from mid-pregnancy onwards.
Numbness, tingling, and weakness in fingers, difficulty in gripping objects, may have shooting pain in wrist and arm	Fluid retention	Swollen tissues in the wrist compress nerves, causing pain and weakness. This is called carpal tunnel syndrome.
Pain in pelvic area, numbness, tingling or weakness down one or both legs	Sciatica; slipped disc	In late pregnancy, your baby's head fills the pelvis, stretching ligaments, and may also press against sciatic nerves.
Swollen ankles, toes, and puffy fingers	Fluid retention (oedema); pre-eclampsia	May be caused by increased blood volume. This condition tends to be worse in hot weather or if you are expecting more than one baby.

mention it to your doctor or midwife, because it may be symptomatic of another underlying and possibly more serious condition. The chart below lists common pregnancy complaints, their symptoms, whether they need treatment, and whether they are signs of a more serious condition. If you have any of the symptoms below, don't try to diagnose yourself, tell your doctor or midwife.

IN SEVERE CASES	TREATMENT
If you have a severe headache, blurred vision and/or spots in front of your eyes after 20 weeks of pregnancy, this may indicate pre-eclampsia (see p. 138), and you should contact your doctor immediately.	Prevention is the best option because, apart from paracetamol, most treatments are not safe in pregnancy. Avoid migraines by not letting yourself get dehydrated or hungry, and avoid triggers like bright light, stress, loud noise, cheese, chocolate, and red wine. If a severe headache is diagnosed as pre-eclampsia, you will be cared for in hospital.
When severe, this reduces your immunity and your ability to cope with the demands of pregnancy.	Eat a balanced, nutritious diet containing iron, folic acid, and vitamins (see p. 104). Your doctor may prescribe iron supplements; you can improve their absorption by taking them with an acidic drink, such as orange juice or a vitamin C drink. If you have a stomach upset, change your tablets.
You may be dehydrated and lacking in energy, especially if it carries on past the first trimester. You may also have a urinary tract infection (UTI) (see p. 127).	Drink plenty of fluids; very severe morning sickness may need hospital treatment to replace the nutrients and fluids you have lost. You may be given injections, or suppositories, of anti-sickness drugs that are considered safe in pregnancy. If you suspect a UTI, consult your doctor.
The baby may be in the breech position or you are expecting more than one baby.	Pain and pressure may be relieved by lying on your side rather than your back; or by resting your head on your raised arms (see p. 117).
This does not usually become a serious problem.	Aches may improve if you change position, or lie down; swimming can help by taking the weight of the womb off the rest of your body.
Indicates food poisoning (gastroenteritis), cystitis, or appendicitis.	If you are vomiting and/or have pain and diarrhoea, see your doctor.
If pain is very severe, this may be caused by strain on your sacro-iliac joint, which can make it difficult to walk (see p. 87).	Be aware of your posture (see p. 114), avoid any twisting movements, don't lift heavy objects, and have a massage (see p. 118). If severe, you may need to be treated by an osteopath experienced in treating pregnant women. Ask your doctor to recommend one.
In rare cases this may indicate a liver problem (cholestasis), but this will normally be accompanied by other symptoms (see p. 133).	Special cream or calamine lotion, from a chemist, can relieve rashes. Your doctor may prescribe antihistamine pills; you could also use talcum powder to keep your skin dry. If a liver problem (cholestasis) is suspected, you will be referred to a specialist immediately.
If this occurs with other symptoms, such as abdominal pain, or blood in the urine, it may be a sign of cystitis (see p. 127).	Practise pelvic floor exercises (see p. 111) and cut down on tea, alcohol, and coffee; wear a sanitary pad if needed. If this persists after pregnancy, you may be referred to a urinary specialist.
This does not usually become a serious problem.	Try not to lift heavy objects, avoid using keyboards, and rest your hands in your lap. If the pain is severe, paracetamol may be taken. If symptoms persist, your doctor may refer you to a physiotherapist.
The sciatic nerves may be trapped. Or if very severe, this may indicate a slipped disc.	Pain should cease or lessen before the birth, when the baby's head has fully engaged (see p. 69).
If severe, may be a sign of excess fluid retention, called oedema. Blood pressure should be monitored to check for pre-eclampsia (see p. 138).	Avoid standing too much; wear support tights. Don't drink less fluid, as this won't relieve the problem and may cause you to become dehydrated.

SPECIAL-CARE PREGNANCIES

Q WHAT ARE SPECIAL-CARE PREGNANCIES – IS MY BABY AT RISK?

A These are pregnancies that warrant close attention because you have an existing medical condition such as asthma, diabetes or epilepsy, or because you develop a serious condition caused by your pregnancy (see p. 132). You will be closely monitored by your doctor, or midwife, and be under the supervision of a consultant obstetrician. With careful management, there is usually no reason why your pregnancy should not proceed normally.

Q I AM ASTHMATIC – HOW WILL THIS AFFECT MY PREGNANCY OR MY BABY?

A Mild asthma should not cause problems during your pregnancy if you normally control the asthma with a bronchodilator or a steroid inhaler. Severe asthma, where you have recently been admitted to hospital and require daily tablets, will be a problem for you and your baby only if your attacks increase and the oxygen supply to your baby becomes dangerously low. Don't stop taking your asthma medication unless your doctor has advised you to.

Q I AM EPILEPTIC. WILL I HAVE A NORMAL PREGNANCY?

A Epilepsy should not stop you having a normal pregnancy. It is not an inherited condition, so you should not pass it on to your baby. Your doctor may change or increase your medication before or during pregnancy to ensure that your fits are controlled.

Q SHOULD I STOP TAKING MY EPILEPSY MEDICATION DURING MY PREGNANCY?

A No. Your epilepsy may get worse in pregnancy, so you must take the medication that controls your fits. If you do have a fit, your baby may be harmed if you fall on your bump or if the oxygen getting to your baby is reduced during the fit.

Q I HAVE THYROID PROBLEMS – WILL THIS AFFECT MY BABY?

A If you have an existing thyroid condition, your thyroid function will be regularly checked by blood tests. Your medication should not affect your baby's development, but your baby's thyroid function may be affected and will be checked after birth.

CAN HIV AFFECT MY PREGNANCY?

If you know you're HIV positive but are otherwise healthy, your pregnancy should not be affected, and there is no evidence to suggest that pregnancy increases the risk of developing full-blown AIDS. Any infections should be treated at once, and by taking iron and folic acid you can reduce the chance of becoming anaemic. You should also make sure that you've had a cervical smear and appropriate treament if necessary.

What is the risk to the baby?
If you received no treatment, had a normal delivery, and breastfed your baby, the risk of passing on the infection would be about 20 per cent. By reducing the amount of virus in your bloodstream while you are pregnant, having a Caesarean delivery, and not breastfeeding, the risk is certainly less than five per cent and possibly as low as one per cent. New effective drug combinations (the most common is known as "triple therapy") reduce the amount of virus in the body and seem to be safe in pregnancy.

What care will I receive?
Most large hospitals have special arrangements for HIV positive pregnant women. Your care is likely be shared between an obstetrician, specialist midwives, and an HIV/genito-urinary physician.

When do I know if the baby is OK?
Tests in the first few months are not accurate, as the baby will probably have HIV antibodies in its blood that have come from you and crossed the placenta. An antibody test can be done after a year.

Q CAN SICKLE CELL ANAEMIA HARM MY BABY OR MYSELF DURING PREGNANCY?

A Sickle cell anaemia is a condition that affects red blood cells, and can cause chronic anaemia; it is most likely to affect black Africans and people of Mediterranean origin (see p. 34). If you carry the trait for this condition, but do not suffer from it, you may already be anaemic, which can worsen in pregnancy. You may need iron and folic acid supplements or a blood transfusion if you have severe anaemia. You will also need specialist antenatal care. Sickle-cell anaemia in you can cause premature birth and a low birthweight baby. If your baby has sickle-cell disease, he or she will not be affected while in your womb because symptoms only develop in the first months of life. Your baby will be tested for the disease after the birth.

Q I HAVE A "RISK" PREGNANCY. SHOULD I STAY IN HOSPITAL UNTIL THE BIRTH?

A This is a difficult one. If your doctors are worried about you, then they will almost certainly arrange for you to be looked after in hospital. But unless you or the baby need extra monitoring or specific treatment, there is little point spending weeks in hospital. It is usually better for you, both physically and psychologically, to get around and carry on with your life until you actually need to be admitted.

Q IF I HAVE A "RISK" PREGNANCY, DO I NEED TO STOP WORKING COMPLETELY?

A No, unless you are advised to by your doctor or midwife, or your visits and tests are taking up so much time that it is impractical to continue with work. Work on its own is unlikely to harm your pregnancy, as long as you adopt sensible routines with your employers, and are not over-stressed! Some women, if they are used to being very active, find it more stressful to stay at home.

Q WILL I AUTOMATICALLY NEED TO HAVE A CAESAREAN?

A Not necessarily. However, if your pregnancy has the "special care" label, certainly the odds are that much higher. If you were hoping for a normal delivery but have to have a Caesarean, then it is important that you don't see this as a failure on your part. Instead, try to stay focused on the fact that, while a Caesarean may not be what you would have chosen ideally, the whole point of your pregnancy care is for you to be safely delivered of a healthy baby.

Q MY PREGNANCY MAY BE COMPLICATED. CAN I STILL HAVE A HOME BIRTH?

A If the experts say there could be complications, it may not be advisable for you to consider a home birth. It would be wise to listen to their advice and benefit from their expertise and hospital-based medical care.

Q I HAVE THALASSAEMIA. HOW WILL IT AFFECT MY BABY?

A Thalassaemia is an inherited blood disorder that affects the red blood cells, and causes anaemia, and which appears in two forms. The minor variety of thalassaemia often goes unnoticed and does little harm. Major thalassaemia, however, can seriously restrict growth and damage major organs. Affected children only start to show symptoms of thalassaemia within three or four months of birth, so antenatal screening is used to detect the disease (see p. 34). In very serious cases, where an affected fetus is unlikely to live, the parents may be offered the choice of a termination. A baby born with the more serious type of thalassaemia may be given a blood transfusion after the birth.

Q CAN I HAVE MY BABY LOCALLY IF I'VE BEEN REFERRED TO THE REGIONAL HOSPITAL?

A The reason that you've been referred to the regional unit is almost certainly because they have the expertise to deal with you and your baby, so see this as a positive, not a negative, move. It may well mean, however, that you have to travel further and be more inconvenienced. In certain situations, once the initial tests and treatments are performed, you can be looked after both by your local hospital and by the regional one.

Q I HAVE HAD A KIDNEY TRANSPLANT. WHAT WILL THIS MEAN FOR MY PREGNANCY?

A This puts you into the "special-care pregnancy" category. However, if your kidney is working well, your blood pressure is controlled, and you are suffering no medical problems, the outlook for a healthy baby and a healthy you is good, although you may end up delivering early. Throughout your pregnancy, you should be looked after by a renal physician and a specialist obstetrician, who will regularly check your blood pressure and do blood tests to check that your kidney function is not deteriorating. Before trying for a baby, however, you should discuss taking an anti-rejection drug with your doctor.

PROBLEMS IN PREGNANCY

CONDITIONS OF CONCERN

Q CAN I DEVELOP SERIOUS CONDITIONS BECAUSE OF MY PREGNANCY?

A Yes, there are conditions that may arise because of your pregnancy and if they do develop you will require special treatment. These conditions include pre-eclampsia (see p. 138), thrombosis (see p. 141) and, more rarely, liver diseases (see right). The purpose of antenatal care is to detect these and other conditions, to monitor them, and to deal with them before they become serious. However, without becoming unnecessarily anxious, it is useful to be aware yourself of some of the potential problems that can occur during pregnancy, so that you can alert your doctor or midwife if you suspect that something is wrong.

Q WHAT IS HELLP SYNDROME?

A HELLP syndrome is a severe variant form of pre-eclampsia (see pp. 138–139) . The "H" stands for haemolysis (damage and break up of red blood cells), "EL" for elevated liver enzymes, and "LP" for low platelet levels. It may occur after delivery, and needs to be treated in a specialist unit where complications can be dealt with. While in most cases the condition gets better on its own or after delivery, some mothers with this condition are at risk of kidney and liver damage, or even death. Although it is impossible to predict, luckily it is very rare. If identified early, HELLP syndrome stands a good chance of being treated successfully.

IS IT COMMON TO FEEL VERY DEPRESSED DURING PREGNANCY?

Many women become significantly depressed during pregnancy. This is thought to be caused by hormonal changes during the first trimester, and often eases off without needing treatment. Depression is also more likely if you felt low at the start of your pregnancy, or if you have suffered from depression before becoming pregnant. You are likely to experience depression if you are having problems with your partner, if your baby was unexpected, or if you are not sure if you really want to have a baby now.

Symptoms of depression
Early signs of depression are: you feel irritable and anxious, especially about your baby; you feel continually tired; you have no energy, and find it difficult to enjoy yourself; it is difficult to get to sleep because you are feeling so anxious about things, or you wake up in the early hours of the morning feeling stressed or despondent.

Relieving depression
Mild depression in pregnancy is often easily helped by reassurance and support from your partner, family, or friends. If your depression is very severe and you feel desperate, do not keep it to yourself, consult your midwife or doctor. You may benefit from professional counselling, or your doctor may recommend some medication. There are drugs that are very effective in treating depression, and are also safe for you and your baby during pregnancy, although ideally these should be avoided in the first trimester.

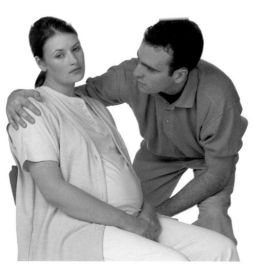

PROLONGED DEPRESSION
The hormonal changes that accompany the onset of pregnancy (see p. 77) can cause depression; if it continues after the first trimester, consult your doctor.

WHAT IS CHOLESTASIS?

Cholestasis is a relatively rare condition of pregnancy, caused by the liver not working as efficiently as normal. The first sign is usually itching all over your body; this is most severe on the arms, legs, abdomen, and back. It is not usual to have a rash. If the condition gets worse, you may feel unwell and pass pale stools and dark urine. You may be prescribed tablets to reduce the itching (urso-deoxycholic acid, UDCA) and vitamin K for two to four weeks before the expected date of delivery to make sure that the liver problem does not affect your blood's ability to clot.

Can itchy skin be serious?
Yes. This may be an indication of cholestasis, which may cause premature delivery or stillbirth. The symptoms are: very itchy and yellowish skin; dark urine; and feeling generally unwell. If you have these symptoms, consult your doctor immediately.

Is cholestasis dangerous for me?
No, almost invariably not. It does not cause more serious problems with your liver, and always gets better after you've had the baby.

Can cholestasis affect the baby?
Yes, in rare cases the baby may come early, stop growing, or become distressed in the womb. If this is overlooked, then there is a rare possibility of stillbirth. This is why your doctor or hospital will want to monitor you and your baby closely if you have the condition.

What are the chances of cholestasis occurring again in a future pregnancy?
Cholestasis has a high risk of recurring in a future pregnancy, so the odds are that it will happen again in your next pregnancy.

How can I relieve the itching?
UDCA tablets are probably the best way of helping the itching. Antihistamines do not tend to work particularly well, and unfortunately neither do soothing creams. Some relief can be obtained from cool baths, but there's a limit to how many of these you can have!

What tests will I have?
Your liver function will be checked at regular intervals, and you may also have a special test to measure the levels of bile acids. Bile acids come from the liver, and in cholestasis they accumulate in your body. These acids are thought to be responsible for the intense itching that is commonly one of the first symptoms you notice. Just occasionally, the diagnosis is not cholestasis, but some other liver condition. So, normally, blood tests will also be taken to check for hepatitis and other conditions that may affect your liver.

Will I get a skin rash?
No, a rash is not usual. If you have a rash, then it may not be cholestasis but some other condition; possibly a viral infection or an allergy.

How will my baby be monitored?
Usually with regular scans to check baby's growth and heart rate traces using cardiotocograph (CTG) or non stress test (NST). But one of the most important ways that you can assess your baby is by monitoring the baby's movements: if you feel that they have decreased over a 12 or 24 hour period, you should contact your doctor or midwife so that they can check you out.

Will my baby get liver damage?
No, the condition only affects your liver and does not affect the baby's liver at all.

Will I need a Caesarean?
Not necessarily. It depends how advanced your pregnancy is when you develop cholestasis, and whether it is affecting you and/or the baby badly enough to warrant delivery. If you do need to have your baby, it is often quite possible for your labour to be induced, especially if the baby is cephalic (head down) and you are at or near term, and there are no other complications.

Can hepatitis cause cholestasis?
No, but if you think that you might be at risk of hepatitis, then you must tell your doctors. Risk factors for hepatitis would include travel to an endemic area, having a prolonged food poisoning type illness with diarrhoea, a recent blood transfusion, or intravenous drug abuse.

BEING UNDER- OR OVERWEIGHT

Q I AM TOLD THAT I'M UNDERWEIGHT. IS MY BABY GOING TO BE SMALL?

A Generally, the baby's size is linked to how big you are, your own birthweight, and that of your partner. If you are underweight, then there is a higher chance that your baby will not grow to its full potential in your womb, and also a higher chance of delivering early. For this reason, you may be offered extra scans to monitor the baby's growth.

Q I HAD ANOREXIA WHEN I WAS YOUNGER. WILL I BE ABLE TO BREASTFEED?

A Even women diagnosed as starving, such as the victims of famine, manage to breastfeed. The fact that your anorexia is now history and you are eating normally, coupled with the fact you were able to get pregnant, suggests that your body has probably recovered and you will be as able as the next woman to feed your baby.

Q DOES BEING OVERWEIGHT INCREASE MY RISKS IF I HAVE A CAESAREAN?

A The short answer is yes, and the degree depends on how overweight you are. If you are over 100kg (220lb), then this is generally considered overweight. The operation itself is made more difficult, and your baby is likely to be bigger than had you not been overweight. There is a higher risk that your Caesarean wound may become infected, and of a chest infection (especially if you have a general anaesthetic). It is really important to be up and moving as soon as possible after the Caesarean: if you lie in bed immobile then there is a risk of you having a deep vein thrombosis (DVT). To counter this risk, most doctors would suggest that you wear special compression stockings and you may well be given daily injections of heparin or a similar drug to reduce the chance of clots forming in your veins.

WHAT SHOULD YOU WEIGH?

To find out if you are a healthy weight, find your weight on the vertical axis, then run your finger across to your height to see which of the zones you fall into. (See below for zone definitions.) Another way is to work out your body mass index (BMI) (see below), which provides a guideline based on height and weight.

Calculating your BMI
To calculate your body mass index (BMI), divide your weight in kilograms by your height in metres, squared. A body mass of less than 20 (zone A) is considered underweight. If your BMI is 20–25 (zone B), you are a healthy weight for your height. A BMI of 25–27 (zone C) is considered slightly overweight. A BMI of above 27 (zone D) is considered obese, and there is an increased risk of many diseases including diabetes and heart disease.

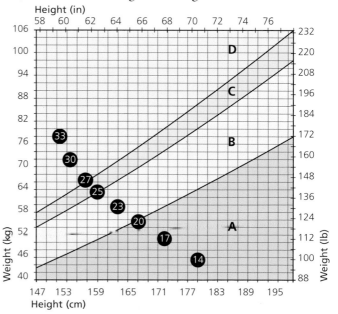

PROBLEMS IN PREGNANCY

IF YOU ARE OVER 40

Q WHAT ARE THE RISKS FOR ME IN PREGNANCY AS I'M OVER 40?

A These include a greater risk of Down's syndrome, greater medical intervention, and, depending on your pre-pregnancy fitness and health, your body may feel the physical effects of pregnancy more than a teenager might. However, this does not automatically mean that you will have a tougher pregnancy or delivery, solely based on your age.

Q WILL I BE REFUSED A HOME DELIVERY BECAUSE OF MY AGE?

A No, you cannot be refused a home birth. If the professionals caring for you feel that there is a medical or practical reason why you should not consider it, they will discuss it with you. The decision should not be based on your age, but on factors concerning you and your baby's well being.

Q WILL I HAVE TO STAY IN HOSPITAL LONGER AS I'M AN OLDER MOTHER?

A Not necessarily. If you are an older first time mother, and feel you could benefit from staying in hospital to gain confidence and new skills, that will be your decision. Usually, the staff caring for you will discuss this and the conclusion will be worked out between you.

Q WILL I HAVE TO HAVE A CAESAREAN BECAUSE OF MY AGE?

A No, age is not an important part of the equation when deciding on a Caesarean. The decision whether or not to have a Caesarean will be based on medical issues. That's not to say you will not end up having one, but if you do then age should not be the major determining factor.

Q I AM OVER 40. WHAT CAN I DO TO REDUCE THE RISK OF DOWN'S SYNDROME?

A You can have prenatal screening (usually based on blood tests or the nuchal thickness measurement of the baby) to establish your risk. You can then decide whether to have "invasive" tests such as amniocentesis or CVS (chorion villus sampling). These do carry a risk of miscarriage, but they will tell you if your baby has Down's syndrome or another chromosomal abnormality. If this were the case, you would then have the option to continue your pregnancy or, where this option legally exists, to terminate your pregnancy.

Q I'M 43. AM I MORE LIKELY TO HAVE A BABY WITH ABNORMALITIES?

A The only increased risk for your baby because of your age is of trisomy; this is where the baby has an extra chromosome. The commonest trisomy is Down's (chromosome 21); much less common are Edward's syndrome (trisomy 18) and Patau's (trisomy 13). The last two are invariably lethal for the baby. There is no evidence of other abnormalities; for example, cleft palate, spina bifida, and heart defects are no more common than if you were 20 years old.

Q DOES MY AGE INCREASE THE CHANCES OF GETTING A MEDICAL CONDITION?

A Most people are still very fit in their 40s. However, you do have a higher risk of chronic conditions such as raised blood pressure, diabetes, heart and kidney conditions, and thromboses (see below). It is important for these to be identified and treated before you get pregnant, so a general check-up with your doctor before trying for a baby is a good idea.

Q AM I MORE AT RISK OF DEVELOPING A THROMBOSIS?

A The risks of getting deep vein thrombosis (DVT) and pulmonary embolus are much higher in the over 40s, and even higher just after delivery, particularly if you have a Caesarean. After delivery, to combat this risk, you will be kept well hydrated, the doctors and midwives will advise you to get up and walk around as soon as possible, and you may need to wear compression stockings on your legs. Many women will be given small doses of heparin or similar drugs, as an injection, for a few days after the birth until fully mobile.

Q IS IT TRUE THAT I WILL BE MORE ABLE TO COPE EMOTIONALLY?

A Women over 40 generally cope very well emotionally with pregnancy, possibly because they have had the time to develop supportive networks, are more established in a job, and may have been with a partner for a long time. Of course, this is not necessarily true for all over 40s. After the baby is born, you will be more tired than if you were 20 years younger, although you are likely to have family and friends to help out and be realistic when it comes to going back to work!

DIABETES IN PREGNANCY

Q WHAT EXACTLY IS DIABETES?

A Diabetes is a condition caused by the pancreas producing too little insulin. Insulin is a hormone that ensures that, when you eat a meal, the sugar is stored in your body for use at a later date. Lack of insulin means that your blood sugar levels can climb dangerously high; in the short term this can make you dehydrated, and in the longer term can affect your kidneys, heart, and blood vessels. It also means that there may be insufficient carbohydrate stores in your body to call on when you need energy. If diabetes remains undiagnosed, you may be very thirsty, feel generally unwell, and lose weight.

Q I HAVE SUGAR IN MY URINE. DOES THIS MEAN THAT I'M DIABETIC?

A Probably not. In pregnancy, kidneys leak sugar out of your bloodstream and into your urine, in what is known as a "reduced renal threshold" for glucose. So it is quite common for pregnant women to leak some glucose, especially after a big meal or a sweet drink, and for this to be picked up by urine tests. However, if the urine tests show persistent large amounts of glucose leaking, and/or you feel lethargic, unwell, thirsty, and are losing weight, then your doctor or midwife should carry out a blood test to check for diabetes.

HOW WILL DIABETES AFFECT MY PREGNANCY?

There are two types of diabetes in pregnancy, pre-existing diabetes mellitus and gestational diabetes. Diabetes should be well controlled to reduce any dangers to you and the baby.

Pre-existing diabetes mellitus
You and your baby will be monitored closely throughout your pregnancy, usually jointly by an obstetrician and a physician at the hospital. Pregnancy doesn't necessarily make diabetes worse, but your insulin requirements and your blood sugar regulation will change; you will also be more susceptible to developing high blood pressure (pre-eclampsia) or having a premature labour.

Diabetes that develops as a result of pregnancy
If you develop diabetes in pregnancy, this is known as gestational diabetes and tends to be less serious than normal diabetes. Your blood sugar levels can either be controlled through your diet, or insulin may be required. This type of diabetes improves after you have had your baby.

How gestational diabetes is diagnosed
Normally, the signs of diabetes are thirst, passing urine frequently, feeling weak, and losing weight. However, in pregnancy, these classic symptoms may not occur because of other metabolic changes taking place; diabetes is often diagnosed only through routine testing of your blood and urine.

Controlling your diabetes
To ensure that your pregnancy progresses smoothly, your diet must be strictly controlled, and normal blood sugar levels maintained. Your doctor will discuss your diet with you but, in essence, you need lots of carbohydrates such as pasta and potatoes, plenty of fibre, and a limited intake of fats and sugar. Eat little and often and do not miss meals. You may be given insulin injections if you are unable to control your blood sugar through your diet. Contact your doctor if you suddenly feel unwell, drowsy, or feverish, or if you cannot feel your baby moving significantly.

Diabetes and your baby
Good blood sugar control during the first few weeks of pregnancy reduces your baby's chances of developing a congenital abnormality, such as a cleft palate. Babies of diabetic mothers can grow very large or have restricted growth. With the care you will receive and careful control of your diet, your baby should develop well and be healthy at birth.

Antenatal care with diabetes
Your doctor can monitor your blood sugar control, and your insulin dose may have to be increased. Your blood pressure and urine will also be checked. You will be offered scans every two to four weeks after 20 weeks to monitor your baby's growth. If your baby seems to be too large, your obstetrician may want to deliver you earlier, at around 37 weeks.

Q IF I'M ON INSULIN, DOES THIS MEAN MY BABY IS MORE LIKELY TO GET DIABETES?

A No. Your insulin-dependent diabetes does not mean your baby is any more likely to develop the condition. It just means that the baby may be exposed to higher levels of glucose crossing the placenta from you. There is, however, a weak link in families for adult onset diabetes.

Q WHY DO SOME WOMEN DEVELOP DIABETES IN PREGNANCY?

A The extra strain on your metabolism means that the pancreas needs to produce extra insulin. This is partially because of the extra energy needs of the baby, and also because the placenta produces hormones that can prevent insulin working properly. In some women, this extra insulin is not produced, leading to gestational diabetes (see box opposite). This almost always gets better afterwards; if you take insulin for the first time during pregnancy, it is highly likely you will be able to stop this immediately after the birth.

Q ARE BABIES OF DIABETIC MOTHERS ALWAYS LARGE?

A No, babies of diabetic mums may be large, medium, or small at delivery. There is a higher chance of large babies weighing more than 4.5kg (10lb) in gestational diabetes, but most babies are of average size. A proportion are small, because in established insulin dependent diabetes, the placenta may not function as well as it should.

Q CAN I USE TABLETS TO CONTROL MY DIABETES IN PREGNANCY?

A The tablets used to treat diabetes should not be used in pregnancy: it is safer and better to change over to insulin injections. The effects of these tablets could become unpredictable in pregnancy, and because they are often very long lasting, difficult to reverse. They may also cross to the baby, affecting its blood sugar levels.

Q I HAVE GESTATIONAL DIABETES AND DON'T NEED INSULIN. CAN I EAT WHAT I WANT?

A Well, you can, but if you do, you will find that your blood sugar levels will rise because of your low insulin levels, and the baby will probably grow bigger and bigger on a diet of fizzy drinks, chocolate, and cakes. This means that there is a higher risk of problems delivering your baby, a higher risk of Caesarean, and a higher risk of the baby needing special care after delivery.

Q ARE DIABETIC BABIES MORE LIKELY TO GET STUCK DURING DELIVERY?

A Most diabetic women are able to have a normal vaginal delivery. However, very large babies may get their shoulders stuck under the pelvic bones at delivery. This is known as "shoulder dystocia" and can be dangerous for the baby, leading to damaged nerve fibres in the shoulder and arm, broken bones, and, rarely, death of the baby. If a baby is thought to be very large before delivery, a Caesarean section may be advised.

Q I HAVE DIABETES MELLITUS. WILL I BE INDUCED EARLY OR NEED A CAESAREAN?

A There are very few absolute rules in obstetrics, but it is fair to say that most obstetricians would suggest that your baby is delivered between 37–39 weeks, to minimize the risk of placental problems. Whether this is done by inducing your labour or by Caesarean section depends on individual circumstances. If you had a Caesarean last time, then this would make a planned Caesarean more likely this time around. If, however, the baby is normal size, you have had a baby normally before, or this is your first pregnancy and there are no other problems, a normal labour and delivery might be planned.

Q I HAVE A URINE INFECTION. WHY ARE MY BLOOD SUGAR LEVELS OUT OF CONTROL?

A Any infection can throw your blood sugar control way out, usually sending levels high. If you have diabetes, an infection in pregnancy is potentially dangerous. You must see your doctor if you suspect anything, and you'll need antibiotics if it is a presumed or confirmed urine infection. If you feel really unwell, you may be admitted to the hospital for frequent blood sugar monitoring, an IV drip, and adjustment of your insulin doses.

Q I KEEP HAVING "HYPOS" ON MY NEW INSULIN REGIME. IS THIS NORMAL?

A No, although it is best for your blood sugar levels to be tightly controlled within a narrow range in pregnancy, this should not mean you getting frequent "hypos" (hypoglycaemic attacks). Your insulin levels may need to be adjusted, along with your diet. Your diabetic physician or specialist nurse will help you with this. Always carry a dextrose drink, fruit, and some sweets with you. Remember: your baby and the placenta are acting as a separate "fuel burning unit" in your body, using your own sugar!

PRE-ECLAMPSIA

Q WHAT IS PRE-ECLAMPSIA?

A Pre-eclampsia is a condition that can only develop in pregnancy, and its symptoms include: high blood pressure; protein in the urine; swollen legs, ankles, and fingers, headaches; nausea and vomiting; blurred or disturbed vision; abdominal pain; and excessive weight gain.

Q HOW IS THE BABY AFFECTED BY PRE-ECLAMPSIA?

A Your baby may be affected by a poorly functioning placenta ("placental insufficiency"). This can cause your baby's growth in the womb to be restricted, which may require early delivery.

Q IS IMMEDIATE DELIVERY THE ONLY CURE FOR SEVERE PRE-ECLAMPSIA?

A If your blood pressure, kidney function, or baby's health become critical, there is no time to wait, irrespective of prematurity. Pre-eclampsia is dangerous for you and your baby if uncontrolled. This condition always improves after delivery.

Q HOW COMMON IS PRE-ECLAMPSIA?

A Around seven per cent of women develop pre-eclampsia with their first pregnancy, but it is much less common in subsequent pregnancies. If you suffer from high blood pressure, diabetes mellitus, or a kidney disease, pre-eclampsia is more likely. The risks of developing pre-eclampsia are also increased if you are over 35, have already had pre-eclampsia, or are having a multiple pregnancy.

Q AM I MORE AT RISK FROM DEVELOPING PRE-ECLAMPSIA IF I SMOKE?

A Smoking increases your chance of bleeding from the placenta and having a small baby. Strangely, if you smoke before conceiving, and stop when pregnant, the risk is actually reduced, but this is no reason to take up smoking!

Q DOES PRE-ECLAMPSIA GET BETTER WITH BED REST?

A Probably not, but resting in the home or hospital away from the stress of work and/or family may delay it getting worse. Strict bed rest is generally a bad idea because immobility increases your risk of deep vein thrombosis (DVT).

Q WHAT IS ECLAMPSIA?

A Eclampsia describes the generalized fitting and loss of consciousness that occurs in severe pre-eclampsia, usually as a result of very high blood pressure and the protein component of your blood leaking out into brain and other tissues through damaged blood vessels. Although the fits themselves are not commonly fatal, extremely high blood pressure may cause a stroke or heart damage. This condition is mercifully rare but needs emergency treatment if it does occur, usually using intravenous blood pressure drugs and anti-convulsants.

Q WHEN DOES PRE-ECLAMPSIA TURN INTO ECLAMPSIA?

A Eclampsia can occur if pre-eclampsia is not carefully supervised and treated. It occurs in the later stages of pre-eclampsia, before, during, or after delivery, and may be fatal for the baby and/or the mother. Thankfully, eclampsia is now extremely rare because doctors have learnt to treat pre-eclampsia before it becomes eclampsia.

Q CAN PRE-ECLAMPSIA BE PREVENTED?

A As the cause of pre-eclampsia is not yet known, prevention cannot be guaranteed; doctors and midwives are familiar with the symptoms, so you should attend all your antenatal check-ups to ensure that your blood pressure is monitored and early signs of the condition are recognized. Low doses of aspirin may be given to pregnant women who are at high risk after 12 to 14 weeks, as aspirin may reduce the severity of pre-eclampsia if it occurs. Your blood pressure will be checked every one to two weeks.

Q MY FACE HAS BECOME QUITE SWOLLEN AND ROUND. IS THIS NORMAL?

A Yes, it is normal. Your face becomes swollen because of the extra fluid that collects under the skin during pregnancy (oedema). In addition to this, the fat distribution of your body changes somewhat because of the influence of oestrogen and another steroid hormone, cortisol, that is produced by your adrenal glands. Just occasionally, if you suffer from pre-eclampsia, you can get generalized and marked swelling of your legs, arms, and face.

Q WHY DO I NEED DRUGS TO TREAT PRE-ECLAMPSIA AND ARE THEY SAFE?

A If you have pre-eclampsia, you may need to take drugs that reduce your blood pressure (anti-hypertensives). These do not actually stop you getting pre-eclampsia, but reduce the dangerous effects of high blood pressure on you. There are several types of drug used in pregnancy for this and all are safe for you and the baby. The most commonly used drug is methyldopa, but others are also used.

Q WILL MY BLOOD PRESSURE GO BACK TO NORMAL AFTER MY BABY IS BORN?

A Pre-eclampsia is a condition caused by pregnancy, so when you've had the baby, the symptoms go away and your blood pressure should return to normal again. This can sometimes take a few weeks, and you may still need to be on tablets and have your blood pressure checked in the meantime. It is very unusual for you to have permanent blood pressure problems as a result of pre-eclampsia.

Q CAN VITAMINS REDUCE MY CHANCE OF PRE-ECLAMPSIA?

A There is a promising area of research involving the use of vitamins to prevent injury to your blood vessels in pregnancy, reducing the risk of pre-eclampsia. It may be that vitamins C and E are the most useful; however, several studies have shown them to be of no value in established pre-eclampsia; one study suggests possible value if given as supplements early in pregnancy. Until further, larger studies have been done, we do not know for sure whether vitamins can help prevent pre-eclampsia.

Q I HAD PRE-ECLAMPSIA IN MY FIRST PREGNANCY. WILL I HAVE IT AGAIN?

A Your chances of developing pre-eclampsia are lower in your second pregnancy, as long as you did not suffer from it in your first pregnancy. However, a minority of women who have had severe pre-eclampsia in their first pregnancy do, for an unknown reason, develop it in subsequent pregnancies.

HOW CAN A DOPPLER SCAN HELP TO DETECT PRE-ECLAMPSIA?

Doppler ultrasound enables doctors to assess how good the quality of the blood flow is from you to the placenta (uterine artery Doppler) and in the baby (fetal Doppler).

Uterine artery Doppler
Uterine artery Doppler scans are most commonly performed at 20–24 weeks. The uterine artery takes oxygenated blood from you to the placenta, and abnormal flow is characterized by high resistance Doppler waveforms. If this is the case, you may need more regular scans and blood pressure checks, as there is a risk of you developing pre-eclampsia or having a small baby.

Fetal Doppler
Doppler scanning of the umbilical artery (from baby to the placenta) and other fetal blood vessels gives valuable insight into blood flow in the baby to the placenta. If the baby's oxygen levels are reducing, the baby diverts blood towards the brain. This does not mean that the brain is damaged but that the baby is adapting to slightly lower oxygen levels, as can happen if the placenta is not working very well.

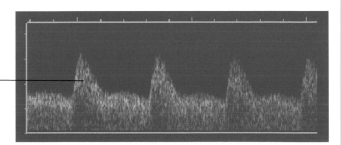

UTERINE ARTERY DOPPLER
A uterine artery Doppler at 23 weeks, showing normal blood flow from mother to placenta.

Normal uterine artery Doppler waveform with low resistance flow, making future pre-eclampsia very unlikely

BLEEDING IN PREGNANCY

Q IS VAGINAL BLEEDING A SERIOUS PROBLEM IN PREGNANCY?

A Vaginal bleeding at any stage of pregnancy should be taken seriously, and should be brought to the attention of your doctor. Severe bleeding in the early weeks may be a sign of miscarriage or, after 24 weeks, of placental bleeding, and you must seek medical advice at once.

Q CAN THRUSH CAUSE BLEEDING?

A Thrush can make your vagina sore and itchy, which may cause a raw area that bleeds, especially after intercourse. This condition can be treated with vaginal suppositories and cream, although it commonly recurs during pregnancy.

Q WHERE IS THE BLEEDING COMING FROM – ME OR MY BABY?

A Apart from a threatened miscarriage, the most common sources of bleeding are your cervix (the neck of the womb) and the placenta (see below). It is very unusual for any blood to come from your baby.

Q SHOULD I BE WORRIED ABOUT BLEEDING FROM MY CERVIX?

A During pregnancy, the rise in oestrogen can cause the cervix to become slightly reddened, causing an "erosion". This usually clears up after the birth. Occasionally, there may be light bleeding from your cervix, especially after intercourse. If you have had abnormal smears, the bleeding may be more significant and you should see your doctor.

WHAT HAPPENS IF I HAVE BLEEDING FROM THE PLACENTA?

Bleeding after 24 weeks may be one of the first signs of a low-lying placenta, known as placenta praevia or abruption of the placenta. Both of these conditions are potentially serious, and require hospital investigations.

What a low placenta means

Early in your pregnancy you will have a scan to check the placenta's position. If the placenta is low, you will have regular scans to see if it has moved upwards away from the cervix as the womb expands. If it does, you will be able to have a normal delivery. Also, if the placenta is very near the cervix, but not actually in the way of the baby's head, a normal delivery may be possible. However, if the placenta completely obstructs the cervix, the baby will have to be delivered by a Caesarean section.

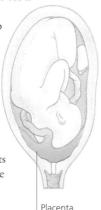

Placenta

PLACENTA PRAEVIA
When the placenta is positioned directly over the cervix, it is called a major praevia. This prevents a normal vaginal delivery and you will need a Caesarean if the placenta is in this position.

What placental abruption means

If the bleeding is fresh (bright red) and you have abdominal pain, the baby is not moving normally, and your womb feels tense and tight, contact your doctor or go to hospital at once. You may have placental abruption – the placenta has partially come away from the womb wall. This is serious and means that your baby may have to be delivered as soon as possible, even if you are not at term.

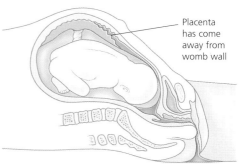

Placenta has come away from womb wall

PLACENTAL ABRUPTION
When the placenta separates prematurely from the womb wall, it is termed abruption. This is serious and may necessitate an immediate delivery.

BLOOD CONDITIONS

Q AM I LIKELY TO GET A BLOOD CLOT DURING PREGNANCY?

A A blood clot, or thrombosis, is more likely to occur in pregnancy because of the changes in the way your blood clots. It is not a common condition, but some factors increase the risk: being overweight or inactive for long periods, smoking, having a personal or family history of deep vein thrombosis or pulmonary embolus. The older you are, the more likely you are to have a thrombosis.

Q HOW DO I KNOW IF I'VE GOT A BLOOD CLOT AND IF IT'S SERIOUS?

A A pain in your calf or thigh, perhaps with slight swelling and redness, is a sign of a blood clot. Your leg may also be painful to walk on and tender to touch. The danger with a blood clot is that part of it may break off and pass to your lungs. This is called a pulmonary embolus and, although not common, it is potentially very serious, if not fatal.

Q HOW WOULD I KNOW IF I HAVE A PULMONARY EMBOLUS?

A You will be short of breath and have chest pain, especially when inhaling. If you develop either of these symptoms, inform your doctor as soon as possible. You will need to have a special lung scan and an X-ray test called a venogram, or a Doppler scan (see p. 38), to look at the veins in your legs.

Q WHAT IS ANTI-PHOSPHOLIPID (HUGHES') SYNDROME (APS)?

A This unusual condition causes the blood to clot a little more easily, and produce antibodies in your bloodstream directed against the membrane (coating) of the body's own cells. APS may cause blood clots and may also be linked to some cases of pre-eclampsia and recurrent miscarriages. It may also stop the baby growing properly in the womb. Taking low dose aspirin from conception onwards may help, perhaps combined with blood thinning injections, though this is not proven yet.

WHAT IS RHESUS DISEASE?

Each person's blood has a Rhesus (Rh) factor, which is positive or negative. This is a problem only when an Rh negative woman has a partner who is Rh positive – this may result in a Rh positive baby. If the mother's and the baby's blood come into contact during the birth or through often unnoticed bleeding in pregnancy, her body produces antibodies against the baby's blood.

How does this affect my baby?
Your blood is tested every few weeks to check if you are making antibodies. If you are, the present baby won't be affected but a subsequent baby may become severely anaemic because your antibodies will cross the placenta and destroy the baby's red blood cells. This is now rare, however, because women in this situation are given injections of anti-D, which coats the baby's Rh positive blood cells and prevents the manufacture of antibodies from your bloodstream.

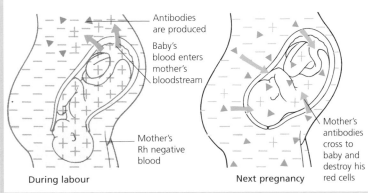

During labour

Next pregnancy

Antibodies are produced

Baby's blood enters mother's bloodstream

Mother's Rh negative blood

Mother's antibodies cross to baby and destroy his red cells

RHESUS DISEASE
Antibodies produced against Rhesus positive blood by the mother during delivery (far left), cross the placenta in later pregnancies (left) to cause severe anaemia in the next baby, and may even cause a miscarriage.

– Rhesus negative blood

+ Rhesus positive blood

▲ Mother's antibodies

PROBLEMS IN A MULTIPLE PREGNANCY

Q HOW WILL MY PREGNANCY BE AFFECTED IF THERE IS MORE THAN ONE BABY?

A If you are pregnant with more than one baby your pregnancy is automatically classed as high risk. As well as all the normal problems of pregnancy, you have a greater chance of developing a potentially serious condition such as pre-eclampsia (see p. 138). Your pregnancy will be more closely monitored by your doctor and midwife, and you will have experienced staff on hand to supervise the birth. It is also unlikely that you will carry your babies to 40 weeks.

Q WHY AM I MORE LIKELY TO GET PRE-ECLAMPSIA IF I AM EXPECTING TWINS?

A Multiple pregnancies place extra strain on your body's resources at an earlier stage in the pregnancy, so you are slightly more likely to suffer from high blood pressure and excessive weight gain, two of the possible symptoms of pre-eclampsia.

Q WILL I HAVE MORE ANTENATAL CHECK-UPS IF I'M EXPECTING TWINS?

A Yes, you will have more frequent antenatal check-ups to monitor your babies' growth rates, and your blood pressure and urine will be tested more frequently.

Q ONE OF MY TWINS IS LARGER THAN THE OTHER, IS THIS A PROBLEM?

A It is relatively common for twins to grow at a different rate in the womb. If there is a big size difference, your babies may have to be delivered early. Size difference also needs to be investigated to eliminate a rare condition called twin-to-twin transfusion syndrome (see opposite); this only occurs if your twins are identical and share a placenta.

Q AM I LIKELY TO HAVE A PREMATURE LABOUR?

A Yes, it is very likely that your babies will be born early. With twins, you can probably expect to go into labour between 34 and 38 weeks, and with triplets between 32 and 36 weeks. This is partly because of the increased weight that you are carrying, and because the extra amniotic fluid stretches your womb and puts extra pressure on your cervix. If your babies are born before term, they will probably be smaller than full-term babies and may need to spend some time in a special care baby unit (see p. 228).

Q MY TWINS ARE IDENTICAL, WILL THIS AFFECT THE DELIVERY?

A It is very important, not least for the delivery, to determine whether the twins are identical or not and, if they are identical, whether they are in separate placental sacs. Identical twins are more likely to be born by a Caesarean delivery, as they usually share a placenta, and are occasionally in the same amniotic sac. These factors can make a vaginal delivery difficult and dangerous. Provided that at least one of them is head down (cephalic), non-identical twins can often be delivered vaginally.

Q AM I MORE LIKELY TO HAVE A CAESAREAN DELIVERY?

A Yes, twin or multiple deliveries are more likely to be by Caesarean, especially if the first baby is not head down, or if there are other complicating factors. The Caesarean will usually be a planned procedure involving a team of professionals, with an obstetrician, a midwife, an anaesthetist, and a paediatrician for each baby.

Q CAN I INSIST ON A TRIAL VAGINAL DELIVERY?

A For the reasons given above, twin vaginal deliveries are considered to be higher risk than the delivery of one baby. Ask your doctors exactly why they are suggesting a Caesarean section. It is unlikely that they are proposing this simply as a standard procedure; there is probably a specific reason for avoiding a vaginal delivery. However, you do always have the right to refuse their advice if you feel strongly about this.

Q IF ONE TWIN DIES IN THE WOMB, CAN THE OTHER CONTINUE TO DEVELOP?

A Yes, if one twin dies and even miscarries early on in the pregnancy, the healthy baby may continue to develop in the womb. This does not usually cause serious problems for the surviving baby and the dead twin may even be absorbed into the placenta. However, if one baby dies during or after the second trimester, the placenta of the miscarried twin can remain in the womb and may act as a focus for infection. During the third trimester, the death of one twin is more likely to cause premature labour; or the dead twin may simply remain in the womb while the other twin continues to grow.

Q WILL I BE ABLE TO TELL IF ONE TWIN IS NOT MOVING?

A Usually, after about 24 weeks, the babies stay on one side and you can tell what position they are in. Most women can feel their babies moving separately and are even able to tell when one is sleeping. If you notice that one twin's movements have significantly changed, or a twin has stopped moving, inform your doctor or midwife immediately.

Q WHY DO I FEEL GUILTY ABOUT LOVING MY SURVIVING TWIN?

A It will obviously be distressing for you and your partner if a twin dies. Even though you still have one baby to cherish, you will feel the loss of your other baby. However, it is important to realize that you can be overjoyed by the arrival of your healthy baby, and at the same time grieve deeply for the one who died.

Q WILL THE LOSS OF ONE TWIN AFFECT THE SURVIVING BABY?

A You may worry that the death of one twin will affect the emotional well-being of the surviving one, but there is no evidence of this. The living twin has every chance of being healthy and happy.

QUESTIONS TO ASK

Are my twins identical?

Will I have regular scans to check the babies' growth?

Will I be seen by a professional experienced in dealing with multiple pregnancies?

Do I need to come to hospital for my antenatal care?

TWIN-TO-TWIN TRANSFUSION SYNDROME

This is a rare condition that occurs only in identical twins with a shared placenta. It is caused by an abnormal blood vessel in the placenta that connects one baby directly to the other. As a result, one baby (the donor) uses most of its energy pumping blood not only around its own body but around the other baby's body (the recipient). This means that the donor twin does not grow properly, and the amniotic fluid is reduced. The recipient twin grows much bigger and an excessive amount of amniotic fluid accumulates rapidly over hours or days.

What are the symptoms?
The rapid increase in amniotic fluid may cause swelling and pain in the abdomen, and premature labour may begin.

What is the outlook for the babies?
This depends on how severe the condition is and how early it is discovered. There have been attempts to treat this condition using lasers to destroy the abnormal blood vessel and by draining the amniotic fluid from the sac around the larger twin. Neither technique is ideal and the risk of premature labour and stillbirth in severe cases is high.

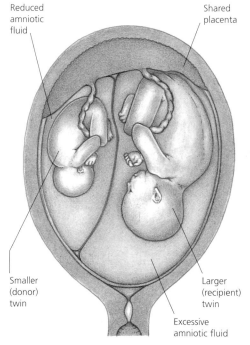

Reduced amniotic fluid

Shared placenta

Smaller (donor) twin

Larger (recipient) twin

Excessive amniotic fluid

WHY THE WOMB SWELLS
The larger "recipient" twin receives more blood than the smaller one and therefore excretes more fluid into the surrounding amniotic fluid. This swells the womb and causes the mother to experience increasing pain.

PROBLEMS IN PREGNANCY

IF SOMETHING IS WRONG

Q WHAT TYPES OF ABNORMALITIES CAN OCCUR IN MY BABY?

A Different abnormalities can occur: congenital abnormalities, that is, physical defects that are present at birth for no reason, such as hare lip, cleft palate or club foot; these do not endanger the baby's life. Chromosomal abnormalities occur when there is a problem in the baby's genetic make-up; these include conditions such as Down's syndrome (see opposite). Genetic defects, such as cystic fibrosis, can be inherited from the parents (see p. 39).

Q ARE FETAL ABNORMALITIES COMMON?

A Up to two per cent of babies are born with what is called a congenital abnormality, but often this is something relatively minor, such as an extra digit, or a heart murmur. More rarely, a baby is born with a serious abnormality, such as a heart defect, or spina bifida. Chromosomal abnormalities, such as Down's syndrome, are relatively rare.

Q WHEN ARE ABNORMALITIES USUALLY DISCOVERED?

A Since the widespread introduction of ultrasound scans, many major abnormalities are picked up at an early stage in pregnancies (around 18 to 22 weeks). Some of the less obvious abnormalities may sometimes be missed, even by experienced scanners, and in this situation you may not find out until your baby is given a post-natal check after the delivery.

Q WHAT SUPPORT WILL I BE GIVEN IF MY BABY IS FOUND TO HAVE A PROBLEM?

A If an abnormality is discovered or suspected during an antenatal scan, you will usually be referred to an obstetrician who specializes in fetal medicine. Ask the doctor or sonographer (or both) to explain everything seen on the scan; ask what the outlook is (see opposite), and whether you will need further scans or invasive tests (see p. 40). You will be given time to think about the situation, obtain further information, talk to your family or your own doctor, and be invited to come back with questions.

Q WHAT IS THE NEXT STEP ONCE AN ABNORMALITY IS DISCOVERED?

A With major abnormalities, such as cardiac defects, where an operation is needed that may endanger your baby's life or where your baby may have a permanent disability, ask to see the paediatric surgeon and obstetrician to discuss this. Only then can you make an informed choice about whether to continue the pregnancy. With minor abnormalities that won't endanger your baby's life, or need only a small operation, the situation is less serious but should still be discussed with the paediatric surgeon.

Q COULD I HAVE DONE ANYTHING TO PREVENT MY BABY'S ABNORMALITY?

A No reason can be found for the majority of abnormalities. Only rarely are abnormalities caused by factors such as diabetes, infections, anti-epilepsy drugs, or alcohol. It may be difficult but it is most important that you should not feel guilty about what has happened.

Q WHAT IS THE DIFFERENCE BETWEEN A MAJOR AND A MINOR DEFECT?

A Parents are invariably shocked and upset if a defect is found in their baby, no matter how small, but doctors divide abnormalities into minor and major ones. Minor defects such as cleft palate, hare lip, or blemishes, will not endanger your baby's life and require no treatment or just a small operation, or physiotherapy, to correct. Major abnormalities, such as serious heart defects, can endanger the baby's life and require major surgery and the baby may have a permanent disability.

QUESTIONS TO ASK

What does the scan show?

Would you advise a second opinion?

How serious is the condition?

Will my baby need surgery after birth?

Is it likely that my baby will have a normal life?

What are the options in continuing with the pregnancy?

WHAT IS THE OUTLOOK IF MY BABY HAS AN ABNORMALITY?

The outlook for your baby depends on how severe the abnormality is. It also depends on whether you have access to paediatric surgeons who can carry out corrective surgery. It is usually very hard for the parents to come to terms with their baby's abnormality, no matter how minor, even though many conditions can be treated successfully in the first few months of life.

Disfiguring blemishes
Marks on the baby's face from labour, bruising from forceps, and even acne, are fairly common at birth; most are not serious or permanent and usually disappear within days.

Cleft palate/hare lip
Babies with these defects have a palate and/or lips that do not join properly in the middle, leaving a gap. Once the baby is born, depending on the severity, plastic surgery can be carried out (often successfully); sometimes there may be several operations over a number of years.

Club foot
A baby born with a club foot usually has one foot twisted at the ankle so that it doesn't point in the normal direction. Physiotherapy or corrective surgery (involving several operations for severe cases) can correct the problem after the birth.

Extra or absent fingers and toes
Often an hereditary defect, extra digits are quite easily removed by surgery after the birth. Absent digits are very rare and usually not correctable.

Water on the kidney (hydronephrosis)
This is a swollen kidney as a result of a blockage lower down in the urinary tract that stops the flow of urine. Minor cases often get better spontaneously at or before delivery. More severe cases, however, can eventually cause kidney damage, and surgery will be needed after the birth to remove the obstruction, or even the damaged kidney itself.

Heart (cardiac) defects
These are relatively common, varying from a small hole in the heart that often closes naturally, to more serious conditions of the heart and arteries, which may need major surgery once the baby is born.

Diaphragmatic hernia
This is a condition where the baby's abdominal contents (bowels and sometimes liver) push up through a hole in the diaphragm into the chest cavity, compressing the lungs and stopping them from developing properly. Major diaphragmatic hernias can also compress the heart, pushing it to one side. This condition must be operated on within a few days of birth. The outlook depends on how big the hernia is and whether the lungs and heart have been damaged.

Spina bifida
This defect occurs when the bones, usually at the bottom of the spine, don't join properly so that the spinal cord, which contains vital nerves supplying the lower part of the body, is exposed. It is only after the birth that the true extent of the nerve damage becomes obvious. Severely affected babies can suffer from disabilities including paralysis of the legs, and bladder problems. Spina bifida often occurs in conjunction with hydrocephalus (water on the brain), which can cause mental retardation. Minor degrees of spina bifida, in which the spinal defect can only be detected by an X-ray, can also occur; successful corrective surgery after the birth is possible. With the advent of invasive testing and scanning, this condition is more easily diagnosed. The condition is becoming rare; the incidence of spina bifida is known to reduce if mothers take supplements of folic acid in early pregnancy.

Down's syndrome
Although dreaded by most parents, Down's syndrome is quite rare, affecting about one in every 650 fetuses. Caused by the presence of an extra chromosome, Down's syndrome may be detected on a Nuchal scan at 11 to 14 weeks (see p. 38), by Triple or Bart's test screening, or by ultrasound scanning at 18 to 22 weeks (see p. 36); but diagnosis can only be confirmed by an invasive test (see p. 40). Most Down's syndrome children have some physical abnormalities; the face and features tend to be small, while the hands are short and broad; there are also varying degrees of mental disability. Medical and surgical advances, together with enhanced long-term care facilities, have greatly improved the outlook for Down's children, who can make the most of their capabilities with constant educational and environmental stimulation.

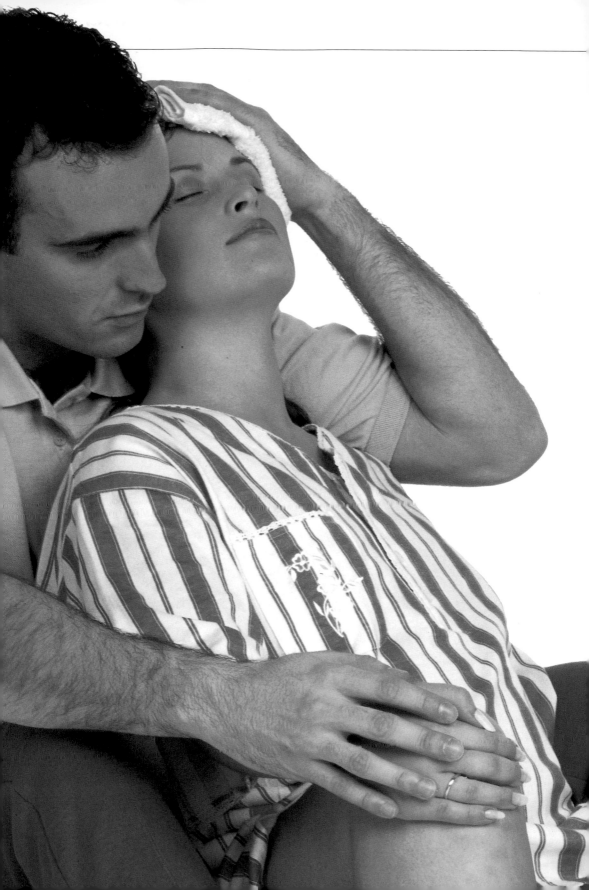

LABOUR
AND
BIRTH

Few other events in life can compare with the
anticipation and excitement of the birth of a
baby; soon you will meet the tiny human being
you have carried and nurtured for so long – and
you will treasure the moment forever. You may
have fears about what will happen during the
delivery, and you may be concerned about how
you will react to the physical exertion of labour.
This chapter explains the types of delivery,
your choices of pain relief and their relative
effectiveness, and what happens during the
three stages of labour. With this information,
you can feel really positive
about what is to come.

PREPARING FOR LABOUR

Q HOW WILL MY LABOUR BE INFLUENCED BY HOSPITAL POLICIES?

A Hospitals have policies on all aspects of labour, birth, and post natal care, so it's worth discussing these with your midwife or doctor. However, these are usually only guidelines and, if you have a request that conflicts with hospital procedure, you can often negotiate.

Q WHAT ASPECTS OF MY LABOUR CAN I NOT DECIDE ON?

A You can be involved in all aspects of the planning of your labour, but when it comes to the actual delivery, it's important to listen to the professionals. They will guide you in the choices available to you, based on the immediate needs of yourself and your baby. If any medical intervention is necessary, there is usually a good reason for it.

Q HOW CAN I LET THE HOSPITAL KNOW WHAT KIND OF LABOUR I WANT?

A One way is to outline your ideas in a birth plan (see opposite). A birth plan is a document that tells hospital staff how you would like your labour and delivery to progress. It can cover the type of delivery you want, who you would like with you, and your preference for pain relief. However, certain requests depend on the facilities available, such as whether or not there is a birthing pool.

Q WHY IS WRITING A BIRTH PLAN A GOOD IDEA?

A Even jotting down a few lines is an excellent way to focus your mind on the choices that are available to you during labour; it can also make you feel more confident and more in control. Also, there will probably be periods during your labour when you won't feel like answering lots of questions: if you have prepared a birth plan, the staff will look at this when you start your labour and will be aware of your preferences.

Q WHO SHOULD I TALK TO ABOUT MY BIRTH PLAN?

A Discuss your birth plan with your midwife and doctor at the hospital at around 32 to 36 weeks. They will be familiar with the hospital's policies and facilities, and will know whether your plan is feasible.

Q HOW LIKELY AM I TO GET WHAT I REQUEST IN MY BIRTH PLAN?

A Most labour wards will try to accommodate your wishes, but be flexible and open-minded: your labour may not go as expected, so try not to be disappointed if something happens that means that you have to abandon all or part of your birth plan. Be positive and emphasize the things you are looking forward to, such as breastfeeding your baby afterwards, or your partner cutting the cord.

Q CAN I SAY THAT I DON'T WANT STUDENTS PRESENT DURING LABOUR?

A Yes, you can, but the students are not only there to learn about birth, they can also provide useful support to the main medical team and to you, and are always closely supervised.

Q DO I HAVE TO WRITE A BIRTH PLAN?

A You don't have to. In fact, many women choose not to, especially if they have had a baby before, but if you have particular likes or dislikes, fears and requests, a birth plan is the place to state these. However, during labour, the medical team will always consult you before carrying out any treatment.

Q CAN I CHANGE MY BIRTH PLAN?

A What you put in your birth plan is not written in stone; keep a copy of it with your hospital notes so that you can change it at any time if, on further reflection, your original thoughts don't seem like such a good idea.

QUESTIONS TO ASK

Is it this hospital's policy to follow birth plans as closely as possible?

If there is a change of staff, will my new midwife be told of my birth plan?

Does the hospital have the facilities to comply with my requests?

Are all the medical staff open to discussion about procedures?

WRITING A BIRTH PLAN

There is no set format for a birth plan; it can consist of a few simple instructions, or detailed notes. It is important to include those issues that most concern you, and to list your preferences, but try not to sound too confrontational. Discuss the plan with your doctor or midwife, and ask them to sign and date it. You need two copies, one for yourself and one to attach to your hospital notes.

WHAT IT MIGHT COVER	WHAT YOU SHOULD CONSIDER
Who you want to have present as a birth partner	■ Who will be your birth partner: your partner, a friend, or a relative? Can you have more than one person with you? If you need to have a Caesarean delivery or stitches, would you prefer your birth partner to leave?
THE FIRST STAGE	■ How do you feel about being induced if you go past your due date? ■ Do you want to be as active as possible during labour? ■ How do you feel about fetal monitoring, which could confine your movements? ■ How do you feel about your labour being artificially speeded up, either by having your waters broken or by a hormone drip (see p. 170)? ■ Have you practised certain breathing or relaxation techniques, and would you like to be coached in these during labour to relieve the pain? ■ If you are giving birth in a teaching hospital, do you object to medical students or student midwives being present?
Pain relief	■ Do you want to be offered pain relief or do you want the medical team to wait until you ask for it? ■ Do you have preferences for certain kinds of pain relief – TENS, gas and air, pethidine, or epidural (see p. 164)? ■ If you have an epidural, would you prefer it to be timed so that it wears off when you are ready to push?
THE SECOND STAGE	■ In what position would you prefer to deliver your baby (see p. 178)? ■ Would you prefer to be allowed to tear naturally or would you prefer a cut made to the perineum (an episiotomy) to make room for your baby's head on delivery? ■ Would you like to see your baby's head being delivered? ■ Would you like your birth partner to cut the umbilical cord?
When your baby is born	■ Would you like your baby to be delivered straight on to your abdomen? ■ Does the hospital routinely suction the baby's air passages after birth? ■ Do you want a midwife to help you breastfeed? ■ Would you and your partner prefer to be left alone with your baby in the delivery room?
THE THIRD STAGE	■ Does the hospital routinely use the drug syntometrine to speed up the delivery of the placenta? Would you prefer to deliver it naturally? ■ If you need stitches to your perineum, would you prefer an experienced midwife to do them rather than a student? Would you object to having a local anaesthetic for this? ■ Providing all goes well, how soon would you like to leave the hospital?

LABOUR AND BIRTH

HAVING YOUR BABY IN HOSPITAL

Q WHAT PLANS SHOULD I MAKE BEFORE MY LABOUR IN HOSPITAL?

A There are a number of arrangements that need to be made well in advance of your labour so that everything runs smoothly when you have to go into hospital. Make a list of relevant contact numbers, keep them by the telephone, and tell another person where they are in the event of an emergency. This list should include your midwife's contact number, or the number of the labour ward and your labour partner's daytime telephone number. Keep your hospital notes handy.

Q WHAT OTHER ARRANGEMENTS SHOULD I MAKE?

A Work out your travel arrangements in advance because once your contractions start, you should not attempt to drive yourself to the hospital. If no one else is available to drive you to the hospital, call a taxi or, in an emergency, call an ambulance. If you have children, you should make arrangements for someone to come over at short notice to look after them. They should be prepared to come even if you go into labour in the middle of the night.

GETTING READY FOR YOUR HOSPITAL BIRTH

Plan what you will need to pack in your hospital bag, and make sure that it is ready at least three weeks before your baby is due.

If you leave the packing until you go into labour, you are more than likely to forget something in the excitement.

WHAT YOU NEED

In most hospitals you will need the basic essentials shown here, but you can take other things for relaxation and massage.

Socks

A big T-shirt or nightdress for labour

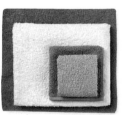
Flannels and towels

Slippers

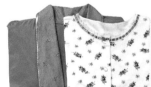
A dressing gown and nightdress for afterwards

Extra items

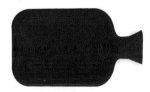
A hot water bottle for backache

A natural sponge, lip salve, water spray, and massage oil and equipment

Essentials for your labour
- A nightdress or big T-shirt ✓
- Socks ✓
- Face flannels and towels ✓
- Slippers ✓
- Dressing gown and fresh nightdress ✓
- Sponge bag with toiletries ✓

Extra items
- Hot water bottle
- Natural sponge to suck on and lip salve
- Water spray bottle
- Massage equipment
- Music for relaxation
- A hand-held mirror

After delivery for you
- Nursing bras and breast pads
- Disposable briefs
- Sanitary pads ✓
- Food and drink to snack on

Q WHAT DO I NEED TO TAKE TO HOSPITAL FOR MY LABOUR?

A You will need to pack a bag of basic essentials (see below). Before you begin to pack, however, ask your midwife for a list of basics the hospital provides in the way of toiletries and bulkier items such as cushions. Assemble the things you'll want for your comfort during the delivery, such as a cooling face spray and a natural sponge to suck on when your mouth feels dry, as well as your usual toiletries for washing and freshening up. You can usually wear your own clothes, such as a large T-shirt or short-sleeved nightdress, during labour. For later in the post-natal ward, you will need a dressing gown as well as fresh nightdresses (front-opening if you intend to breastfeed). Don't forget to pack your sanitary towels, maternity bras, and breast pads.

Q APART FROM ESSENTIALS, ﹖ BRING ANYTHING ELSE?

A You may both be glad to have ﹖ to distract you during what c﹖ prolonged early labour, so your p﹖ arrange to bring in tapes and a ca﹖ games, or playing cards. Remember to bring your favourite massage oils and equipment if you are using them. If you want to record the birth of your baby, pack a camera or video camera. Change or a phone card for the hospital telephone is essential, as mobile phones – which can interfere with equipment – are not allowed. You might consider refreshments for your partner during a long labour, because few hospitals provide food during the night. A change of clothes for your partner is also useful.

WHAT YOUR BABY NEEDS

You need to provide a set of clothing for when your baby is born. The following list is very basic, but should cover your baby's immediate needs after the birth. You will buy more clothing as your baby grows over the coming months (see p. 210).

(see p. 210)

Essentials
- Two to three stretchsuits or nightdresses, and vests ✓
- Scratch mittens ✓
- A shawl or baby blanket ✓
- Cream, such as zinc and castor oil or petroleum jelly, for baby's bottom
- Disposable nappies ✓
- Cotton wool ✓

Afterwards for taking your baby home
- An extra layer of outdoor clothes or blankets
- A carry cot, pram, or car seat
- A hat

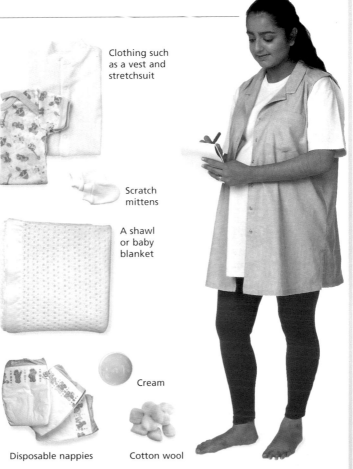

Clothing such as a vest and stretchsuit

Scratch mittens

A shawl or baby blanket

Cream

Disposable nappies

Cotton wool

THE DELIVERY ROOM

A hospital environment can seem frightening to an outsider but if you understand exactly what is going on when you have your baby, you can be more relaxed. Your hospital will invite you to tour their Maternity Unit as part of your antenatal preparation. It is a good idea to go along to see the delivery rooms and post-natal wards, and to ask any questions you might have about the hospital's procedures and equipment.

WHAT IS THE EQUIPMENT FOR?

The labour room is full of equipment, some of which can look quite worrying to prospective parents. Below is a guide to the most important items you will see:

■ **Baby's cot** This is where your baby is laid when being checked over by the midwife or doctor.

■ **Delivery bed** Although high, the delivery bed is practical: for delivery it can be raised and lowered, and the end can be removed to facilitate the delivery and stitching.

■ **The resuscitation trolley** This trolley is equipped with oxygen for your baby, and suction apparatus to extract any mucus from your baby's lungs. There is also a heater for the newborn. This equipment is always prepared and available in the event of a problem.

■ **Sphygmomanometer** This instrument measures your blood pressure.

■ **Oxygen** Piped oxygen, if you need it for pain relief, reaches you through a mask.

■ **Gas and air** This is a mixture of oxygen and nitrous oxide that you can inhale to help take the edge off your pain.

■ **CTG (cardiotocograph)** This records your contractions and your baby's heartbeat, and shows them on a continuous print-out.

■ **Extra comforts** Some hospitals supply aids, such as a bean bag, birthing chair or stool, or a rocking chair, for a more active birth.

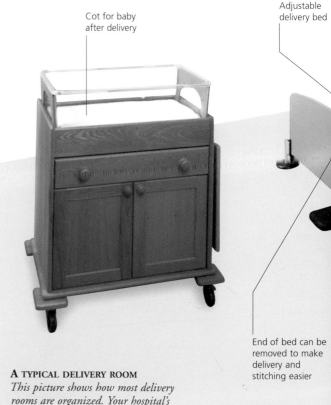

Cot for baby after delivery

Adjustable delivery bed

End of bed can be removed to make delivery and stitching easier

A TYPICAL DELIVERY ROOM
This picture shows how most delivery rooms are organized. Your hospital's delivery room may not look exactly like this one but most modern hospitals provide the equipment shown here. Some also offer private bathroom facilities, and there may be a birthing pool.

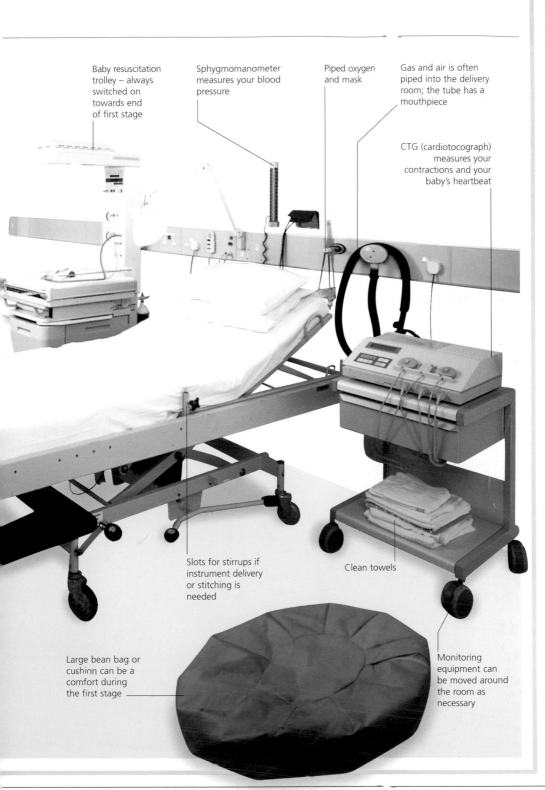

Baby resuscitation trolley – always switched on towards end of first stage

Sphygmomanometer measures your blood pressure

Piped oxygen and mask

Gas and air is often piped into the delivery room; the tube has a mouthpiece

CTG (cardiotocograph) measures your contractions and your baby's heartbeat

Slots for stirrups if instrument delivery or stitching is needed

Clean towels

Large bean bag or cushion can be a comfort during the first stage

Monitoring equipment can be moved around the room as necessary

LABOUR AND BIRTH

PREPARING FOR A HOME BIRTH

Q WHAT ARE THE ADVANTAGES OF HAVING MY BABY AT HOME?

A There are many positive aspects, the most important being familiarity with your surroundings; you and your partner will not have to travel anywhere when you go into labour, and you may both feel more relaxed about participating fully in the event. You will also have more freedom to move around, and to give birth in whatever position feels natural and comfortable. You can create a soothing atmosphere with music and candles, and your labour can be as private – or as social – an event as you wish, yet you will have the reassurance of a professional presence in your midwife. If you have other children, they can come in immediately afterwards.

Q IS A HOME BIRTH AS SAFE AS A HOSPITAL BIRTH?

A If your pregnancy and labour are considered to be straightforward, there is no evidence to suggest that a home birth is less safe than a hospital one. You may feel more reassured if you talk to your midwife to find out exactly which situations she can deal with.

Q WHAT DO I NEED TO DO IN PREPARATION?

A When you midwife visits you, ask her about what equipment you should provide for her in preparation for labour; she will probably supply a list of essential and optional items. You also need to prepare the room or areas in which you intend to give birth (see p. 156).

QUESTIONS TO ASK

Are there any medical reasons why I should not consider having a home birth?

What are my options if labour does not proceed normally?

How can I find a midwife who will be sympathetic to my ideas about home birth?

What kind of pain relief can the midwife offer me during a home birth?

Q WHAT KIND OF ROOM IS BEST FOR A HOME BIRTH?

A It can be anywhere in your home but it should be warm (with extra warmth available for the baby when he or she arrives), quiet (where you are not likely to be interrupted by other members of the household), and ideally near a bathroom. If you intend to have an active or water birth, the room must be spacious enough for you to clear a birthing area and cover it with plastic sheets for protection, with space for pillows or bean bags if you wish. You'll also need a clear table top that can be used as a work area for the midwife's equipment, as well as somewhere to put all your comfort aids. Your midwife will inspect your room beforehand to check that there are no problems.

Q CAN I ASK MY FAVOURITE MIDWIFE TO ATTEND MY LABOUR?

A Midwives usually work within a small team, and you should have the chance to meet most of your team during the antenatal period. If you have a favourite midwife, ask her if she minds putting herself on "extra" call to look after you, but there is a chance that she might not be able to.

Q WHAT HAPPENS WHEN LABOUR STARTS?

A Call your midwife and your birth partner as soon as you feel that your labour has begun (see p. 166). Your midwife will give you her paging number at the hospital, or a mobile phone number if she has one. Keep the relevant numbers to hand as your estimated date of delivery approaches.

Q WHAT SHOULD WE DO WHILE WE WAIT FOR THE MIDWIFE TO ARRIVE?

A You will be relaxing and breathing through your contractions. If you have not already done so, your birth partner can prepare the room by clearing away furniture, laying out plastic sheets, setting up the birthing pool if you are using one, and creating a comfortable atmosphere with heating, lighting, and relaxing music. He or she can also organize care for any of your other children, and prepare drinks and snacks for everyone to have later.

Q WHAT WILL MY MIDWIFE DO DURING MY HOME BIRTH?

A When your midwife arrives, she will ask questions about your progress. She will probably give you an internal examination to confirm the stage of labour and the position of your baby, and she will record the strength and frequency of your contractions. She will check your blood pressure, temperature, and pulse to ensure that there are no problems, and will regularly monitor your baby's heartbeat (usually with a hand-held Doppler sonicaid device), to check that your baby is not in distress. Your midwife will deliver your baby and the placenta and, if necessary, stitch any tears or cuts after the birth.

Q WHAT IF PROBLEMS DEVELOP DURING THE BIRTH?

A Your midwife is trained to spot potential problems, and if any develop, she will call an ambulance to take you to hospital. She will then accompany you to the hospital, stay with you, and deliver the baby with the appropriate medical back-up. This may be disappointing if you've had your heart set on a home birth, but it is important to keep an open mind about transferring to hospital. Remember that the safe delivery of your baby will always be your midwife's priority, whether you are giving birth at home or in a hospital.

Q IS IT REALLY NECESSARY TO BOIL WATER FOR A BIRTH – OR IS THIS A MYTH?

A Midwives used to have to sterilize their equipment in boiled water, but this is no longer necessary. Some warm water will be needed to clean your baby after he or she is born.

Q CAN MY CHILDREN WATCH THE BIRTH?

A Only you can gauge how your child or children will react, but if he or she is likely to be frightened by seeing you in pain, it may not be a good idea. Also, you may lose your partner's support while he or she tends the child or children elsewhere in the home. The child or children could perhaps be there to meet the new arrival immediately after the birth.

Q WHAT WILL HAPPEN IN THE FIRST FEW HOURS AFTER MY BABY IS BORN?

A Once delivered, you will be able to give him or her a cuddle; your baby will then be cleaned, examined, and weighed (see p. 187). The midwife will need warm water, cotton wool, and a nappy ready. This is a time for you and your partner to bond with your baby; the home is ideal for undisturbed contact. The midwife stays long enough to check that all is well. She will usually return to check you both later in the day.

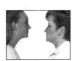

DISCUSSION POINT

DECIDING ON A HOME BIRTH

Some women feel more secure if their labour is managed by doctors in a hospital, others relish the chance to have their babies without medical intervention. If you are self-confident enough to ask, you can get the kind of birth you want.

The medical reaction

Because they cannot predict how your labour may progress, doctors generally are not keen on first babies being delivered at home, so you may find that your doctor prefers you to have had at least one normal delivery in hospital before agreeing to a home birth. However, if you are really set on a home birth, and there are no medical objections (see p. 26), talk to your midwife about it.

Pain relief

You may choose a home birth because your goal is a more natural approach, and you particularly want to avoid medical intervention such as an epidural anaesthesia and electronic fetal monitoring. This is fine, but however determined you are to keep the birth as natural as possible, you may change your mind and perhaps require pain relief once the labour begins. Your midwife can offer you gas and air or injections of drugs such as pethidine; she cannot give you an epidural.

Organization

Organizing a home birth is perhaps not as easy as booking into a hospital, but most women who do manage it find that having their baby at home is a very satisfying experience.

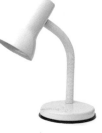

What do I need for a home birth?

Because you have chosen to give birth in your own home, you and your partner are in control of your birth environment and can provide the atmosphere you prefer. There are, however, certain essentials you should provide; ask your midwife for a list.

What you will need

The midwife attending your delivery will bring with her all the necessary medical equipment (see panel, right). Decide where you would like to have your baby; the only requirements are warmth and cleanliness. In addition to some items of equipment you will be required to provide, consider the optional items shown below.

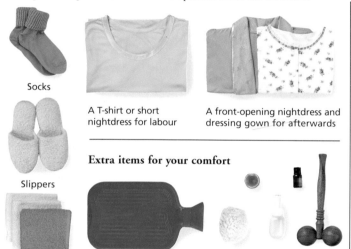

Socks

A T-shirt or short nightdress for labour

A front-opening nightdress and dressing gown for afterwards

Slippers

Extra items for your comfort

Flannels

Hot water bottle

A sponge, lip balm, water spray, massage oil and equipment

Essentials for you
- Something comfortable to wear (a large T-shirt or short nightdress)
- Socks, flannels

Extra items for your comfort
- Small natural sponge to suck on
- Ice chips or cubes
- Hot water bottle
- Water spray bottle
- Lip balm; massager, oil

Items you will need afterwards
- A fresh nightdress
- Slippers and dressing gown
- Nursing bra and breast pads
- Disposable knickers
- Sanitary pads
- Towels

Equipment you will need to provide

Your house probably already contains most of the things you need, but you may want to provide extra cushions so that you have several alternatives for changing positions when coping with contractions. Dim lights may help you to relax during labour, but your midwife will need a bright light for stitching.

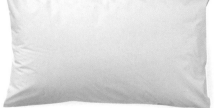

Extra pillows or large cushions

Clean towels

Lamp

FOR YOUR BABY

About three weeks before your baby is due, start assembling all the basic items that will be necessary for your new baby. The main requirements are nappies, warm clothing, and somewhere to sleep.

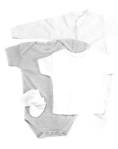

Stretchsuits, vests, and scratch mittens

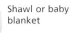

Plenty of nappies, baby cream, and cotton wool

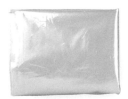

Shawl or baby blanket

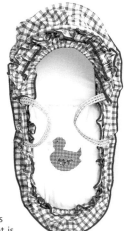

A portable Moses basket or carrycot is best for a newborn baby

Essentials
- Soft, clean towels and sheets
- Nappies (disposable or towelling as preferred)
- Clothing such as two to three stretchsuits, vests, or nightdresses
- Scratch mittens
- Shawl or baby blanket
- Cotton wool
- Zinc and castor oil cream or petroleum jelly
- Moses basket or carrycot
- Changing mat (optional)

THE MIDWIFE'S PACK

Your midwife arrives with a delivery pack containing essential medicines and sterile instruments for the safe delivery of your baby.

Basic labour kit
- Antiseptic solutions
- Blood pressure monitor
- Thermometer; stethoscope
- Doppler sonicaid
- Syringes
- Urine testing sticks
- Oxygen
- Equipment for stitching
- Gloves, scissors

For pain relief
- Gas and air
- Opiate-type drugs such as pethidine (your midwife may ask you to get this on prescription from your doctor beforehand)
- Local anaesthetic

In case of emergency
- Resuscitation equipment for your baby
- A drip in case of haemorrhage

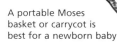

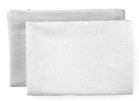

Plastic sheeting

Clean sheets

Checklist for the labour
- Clean sheets for your bed in case you use it, and/or waterproof cover for the mattress
- Plastic sheeting for the floor
- Lamp or bright torch for stitching, if necessary
- Pillows or cushions
- Hot water, soap, and clean towels
- Energy snacks and drinks for you, your partner, and the midwife

For afterwards
- Bags for rubbish disposal
- Clean sheets for your bed

Optional extras
- Bean bag(s) or large floor cushions
- Hand-held or portable fan
- Portable electric heater if the room needs extra warmth
- Music, candles, and/or scented oils to create a relaxed atmosphere
- Camera or video camera loaded with film
- A low stool
- Hand-held mirror
- Birthing pool – you must order this in advance, if wanted

LABOUR AND BIRTH

YOUR CHOICES IN CHILDBIRTH

Q WHAT ARE MY CHOICES IN TYPES OF CHILDBIRTH?

A You can choose between a natural, or alternative birth, an active birth or an actively (medically) managed birth – or even a combination of these.

Q WHAT DOES A NATURAL BIRTH INVOLVE?

A A natural birth avoids the use of drugs for pain relief, encourages active labour positions; it also favours the use of natural or complementary types of pain relief (see below).

Q WHAT ARE THE BENEFITS OF NATURAL OR COMPLEMENTARY PAIN RELIEF?

A Stress in labour increases tension and reduces your capacity to deal with pain. Natural methods of pain relief (see below) or distractional stimuli, such as massage, stimulate your body to release endorphins, its own natural painkillers; these help you to cope with the pain, which reduces stress and enables you to feel more in control of your labour. Whether you go for a completely natural childbirth, or combine natural with medical pain relief, be prepared for your plans to alter.

WHAT NATURAL PAIN RELIEF METHODS ARE AVAILABLE TO ME?

Natural pain-relieving methods soothe and relax you, but will not entirely stop all pain; however, by easing tension, they increase your capacity to deal with pain. You will need to organize, practise, and familiarize yourself with these methods before the birth. Most methods can be used with medical types of pain relief (see p. 164). Most midwives and doctors accept these approaches and are open to their use during labour, but if you decide to have a natural birth, discuss this before labour.

ALONE OR WITH YOUR PARTNER

■ **Heat and cold** Applying heat or cold is soothing in labour and can ease tension; in itself it will not get rid of pain but it can make pain easier to cope with. A hot water bottle alternated with a flannel soaked in cold water can reduce backache or cramp. Some women find that a cold flannel on the face can ease tension.

■ **Movement** Keeping mobile improves your circulation and can help to reduce backache, as well as act as a distraction to the pain. Try different positions in labour, using cushions, bean bags or chairs for support, until you find a position that suits you best.

■ **Massage** This relieves tension in your shoulders, neck, face, and back, as well as relaxing you and improving circulation, thereby reducing the intensity of labour pains. You and your partner can practise this together before labour (see p. 118).

■ **Aromatherapy** This technique involves essential oils combined with massage, which helps to reduce tension, and can relieve, but not eliminate pain, particularly in early labour. You can also place oils in vapourizers in the room to help soothe you.

WITH AN EXPERT

If you are considering using any of the following methods you will need to arrange for a qualified practitioner to be with you throughout labour to ensure that everything is done correctly.

■ **Acupuncture** Fine needles inserted into specific body points (see p. 108) relieve pain by releasing the body's own painkillers, endorphins.

■ **Reflexology** Applying pressure to specific points on your feet can relieve pain and muscular problems in other parts of the body (see p. 108). Gentle foot massage can also be very relaxing.

■ **Hypnosis** This works by suggestion: if you believe that you can control the pain, you may be less disturbed by it. Try hypnosis only if you have tested it before labour.

Q WHAT DOES AN ACTIVE CHILDBIRTH MEAN?

A An active childbirth means that you move around during the early part of labour, and give birth in any position other than the traditional one of lying on a bed on your back. You can sit, stand, squat or kneel on all-fours; you will, however, need assistance from your birth partner, midwife or hospital staff. An active childbirth should not be confused with the "active management of labour". This is a medical phrase that originated in the 1960s from a group of obstetricians in Dublin who believed in the close supervision of labour and, if necessary, early intervention in the labour process with the labour-inducing drug, syntocinon, or by artificially rupturing the membranes (see p. 170).

Q WHAT ARE THE BENEFITS OF AN ACTIVE BIRTH?

A Active positions may help your labour to progress through the use of gravity; they can make your contractions more effective in the first stage of labour, increase your stamina, and help your cervix to open up more easily. In the second stage of labour, an upright rather than a supine position means that you won't feel as if you are pushing uphill, which can help progress.

Q HOW DO I PREPARE FOR AN ACTIVE CHILDBIRTH?

A The principles of this type of birth are usually covered in independent antenatal classes; you will be taught to trust your body and your instincts, as well as to strengthen your body by exercise.

GIVING BIRTH IN WATER

Immersion in water was originally used just for pain relief during the first stage of labour, and it was not intended that the actual birth take place under water. Recently, actual water births have become popular, however, the safety of births under water is now being investigated.

The benefits of water
Sitting in water and/or giving birth in water is often used as a form of pain relief in labour and can be very enjoyable. Water supports the body and might also speed up a slow labour. A water birth may reduce your chances of tearing during labour because it helps you to relax.

Arranging a water birth
Some hospitals now have the facilities available for water births. If your hospital does not provide this, you may be able to hire a birthing pool to take into the hospital. Or you could use one at home. Discuss this with your doctor and/or midwife.

Assistance during a water birth
Not all midwives are experienced in supervising water births. If you would like one, check with the hospital or midwife beforehand to ensure that you will have the assistance of a midwife experienced in the supervision of this type of birth.

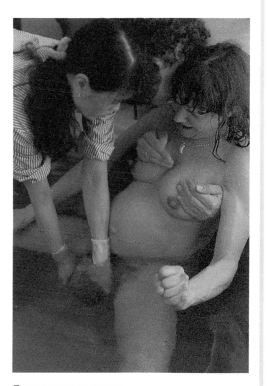

GIVING BIRTH IN WATER
While the mother and her partner watch, a midwife guides the head of the baby out into the water during this water birth. Many women stay in the water only for the first stage of labour, and get out to deliver their babies; this may be safer for the baby.

LABOUR AND BIRTH

Coping With Pain in Labour

Q DO MOST WOMEN USE SOME TYPE OF PAIN RELIEF DURING LABOUR?

A Although many women think that they would like to go without pain relief in labour, it is quite common to have some kind of help, whether it is self-administered or given by a midwife or doctor. A minority of women need no assistance, while some women use every method of pain relief available. The majority of women, however, fall between these two extremes. Remember, giving birth isn't a race or an endurance test and you shouldn't feel that you are a failure if you ask for a pain-relieving drug.

Q WHAT IS THE PAIN OF LABOUR GOING TO BE LIKE?

A As you will probably have experienced degrees of pain before in your life, you will have some idea of your particular pain threshold. The pain of labour is, however, quite unlike any other, inasmuch as it is not a warning that something is wrong. Also, unlike most other pains, labour contractions come and go, giving you intervals of respite. Some women say they are like strong period pains; others say that they seem to overwhelm the whole body and are so excruciating that they are hard to bear.

What are the Main Methods of Pain Relief?

The three main medical types of pain relief used in childbirth are entonox (gas and air), pethidine (or other opiate drug), and epidural anaesthesia (see p. 162). Non-medical methods include breathing techniques, and the TENS machine which, although they may not completely eradicate the pain, can take the edge off it. Some women combine other non-medical pain relief methods (see p. 158) with drugs and anaesthesia.

Entonox (gas and air)

Entonox, which is nitrous oxide, a mixture of gas and oxygen, has been used during labour since the middle of the last century and is considered a very safe form of pain relief.

How does it work?
You inhale it, slowly and deeply, through a special mask or mouthpiece. It helps to ease your perception of pain but does not remove the pain entirely. Its effect is not immediate; if inhaled at the start of a contraction, it takes effect by the time the contraction is at its peak.

Why choose this method?
Nitrous oxide is particularly useful in early labour, but can be used at any time, and in combination with other methods of pain relief. It is impossible to overdose on gas and air, so you can have as much as you want, and it won't affect your baby.

What are the drawbacks?
Some women find that it is not really strong enough if contractions are very severe. It can also make you feel "out of it" and nauseous.

Pethidine (or other opiate drug)

Pethidine is a synthetic analgesic drug that is similar to morphine. This type of pain relief is administered by an injection into the muscle of your buttock or thigh about every three to four hours.

How does it work?
Pethidine relieves pain by stimulating specific "opiate" receptors in your brain and spinal cord that are also the target of endorphins, your body's own painkillers.

Why choose this method?
Pethidine can be an effective pain reliever; it is particularly useful when you can't have, or don't want, other forms of pain relief, such as epidural anaesthesia.

What are the drawbacks?
Reactions to this drug include nausea, vomiting, blurred vision, sleepiness, and mood changes. If you are given pethidine within the two hours prior to your baby's birth, it can make your baby sleepy and affect his or her ability to breathe and move spontaneously or to respond to stimuli. For these reasons, pethidine should not be given too late in labour.

Q WHAT IF I CAN'T COPE WITH THE PAIN OF LABOUR?

A Remember that labour pains are simply a sign that your body is working hard to open up your cervix and move the baby down the birth canal. No one can predict how you will cope with the pain of your first labour; and subsequent labours often do not follow the same pattern, so try not to panic or feel disappointed if you need help.

Q WHAT FACTORS MIGHT AFFECT HOW I DEAL WITH PAIN DURING LABOUR?

A How you cope during labour will depend primarily on the intensity of the pain. Certain factors can also affect your capacity to deal with the pain, such as when you last ate and slept, how long your labour lasts, how your baby is lying, and how comfortable and relaxed you are. A birth partner can really help to make you feel relaxed by being supportive, talking you through the contractions, and distracting you.

Q HOW CAN I PLAN MY PAIN RELIEF BEFORE I START LABOUR?

A It is a good idea to think about the method of pain relief you might prefer and to find out which methods are available, their benefits, and possible side-effects. It is also important to find out whether or not you have to practise or organize them before the onset of labour. Keep an open mind about this, however, because labours do not always go to plan.

USING A TENS MACHINE

TENS (Transcutaneous Electrical Nerve Stimulation) is a battery-operated device with wires that are attached to your body by adhesive pads.

How does it work?
A tiny electrical current passes through your skin, reducing pain messages to your brain and at the same time stimulating the production of endorphins, the body's natural painkillers.

Why choose this method?
By using a handset, you are in control of the machine and the intensity of the current. You can walk about and stay upright; it can also be used with relaxation and other self-help methods.

What are the drawbacks?
Most hospitals do not supply the machine; if you decide to try it, you will have to hire your own set beforehand and take it with you when you first go into labour (see p. 256).

USING TENS
Press a button on the handset at the start of a contraction. Electric impulses give a mild tingling sensation that blocks the pain.

BREATHING TECHNIQUES

Special breathing techniques help you to relax and reduce your reaction to the pain; they can be used with other types of pain relief (see p. 164).

How do they work?
Known as psychoprophylaxis, this method involves the use of practised levels of breathing during contractions. Concentration on breathing distracts you from the pain and also relaxes your muscles so that tension, which heightens pain, is eased. To be effective, you should go to antental classes to learn about and practise these techniques. Take your partner so that he or she can help during labour.

Why choose this method?
It is a natural method that does not involve drugs or medical supervision; you are in control.

What are the drawbacks?
This method is not always successful because it depends on how your reaction to your labour pains, which cannot be predicted, and on your ability to concentrate on something other than the pain.

Two pairs of pads are taped to your lower back

LABOUR AND BIRTH

HAVING AN EPIDURAL

Q WHY SHOULD I CONSIDER AN EPIDURAL?

A An epidural should be considered when you, or your obstetrician or midwife feel that the pain is more than you can cope with. You are more likely to need epidural pain relief if your baby is in the posterior position, and intensive contractions result in little progress (see p. 172). You might have an epidural if you need a Caesarean delivery, or with a forceps or ventouse delivery. An epidural may also be necessary with a multiple birth or if your baby is in the breech position. Your doctor or midwife will tell you if they think you need an epidural, but the final decision will be yours.

Q HOW WILL AN EPIDURAL AFFECT ME?

A An epidural should act as a total pain block, numbing all sensation in your abdomen. However, it can also affect the nerves that control the movement in your legs and bladder, which means that your legs may feel quite heavy and difficult to move, and you may not be able to feel when you need to pass urine. When an epidural is inserted, you will be encouraged to lie down, and a small plastic tube (catheter) will usually be passed into your bladder to prevent it from becoming too full; an overly full bladder could impede the progress of your baby or cause bladder problems.

HOW DOES AN EPIDURAL WORK?

An epidural anaesthetic works by numbing the nerves in your spine that lead to your abdomen. A small amount of local anaesthetic is injected into the lower part of your back to numb the area before the main anaesthetic is injected. This procedure usually takes around 20 to 40 minutes, and the effect should last for several hours. The anaesthetic can then be topped up every few hours through the end of the catheter where a filter valve is attached in order to prevent bacteria from entering your body.

THE PROCEDURE

■ To stop your blood pressure dropping suddenly, you will be connected to a drip. You will be asked to lie very still on your side or to sit up, and your lower back is then made sterile.

■ The anaesthetist will give you a local anaesthetic.

■ The anaesthetist will carefully place a fine, hollow needle between two vertebrae in the lumbar region of your lower back.

■ To check that the needle is in the right place, a small amount of anaesthetic is given through the needle. If this numbs your abdomen satisfactorily, a catheter is inserted through the needle, and a full dose of anaesthetic injected.

CONNECTING THE CATHETER
The catheter or tube is taped into position along your back so that you will then be able to move around if you wish and be "topped up" later, if necessary.

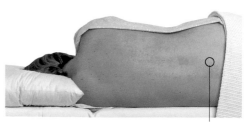

Position for an epidural   Insertion point

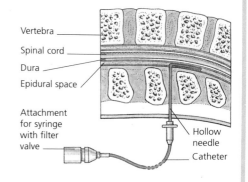

Vertebra

Spinal cord

Dura

Epidural space

Attachment for syringe with filter valve

Hollow needle

Catheter

Q WHO WILL GIVE ME AN EPIDURAL – AND WHEN SHOULD I ASK FOR ONE?

A Epidurals are normally given by trained anaesthetists. The vast majority of delivery units have such anaesthetists available around the clock; however, it would be wise to check this with your local hospital to avoid disappointment. When you are in labour it might be a good idea to request an epidural sooner rather than later, just in case the anaesthetist is not available immediately; if you leave it too late, you may find that your labour is too advanced to have an epidural because the baby is descending into the birth canal and you need to push.

Q WILL I STILL BE ABLE TO PUSH MY BABY OUT IF I HAVE AN EPIDURAL?

A It is commonly believed that you cannot push with an epidural in because you cannot feel your contractions. You can push, but your midwife will need to put her hand on your abdomen to feel for contractions, and then tell you when to push. It is not as easy to push without the strong urge that comes with normal second stage contractions, but it is possible. Alternatively, your midwife may wait for the epidural to wear off slightly so that you can feel the contractions and push for yourself.

Q IS THERE A RISK OF BACKACHE WITH AN EPIDURAL?

A There has been a lot of research in recent years into whether women who have had an epidural experience more backache after delivery than those who haven't. However, there is no evidence to link chronic post-natal backache with epidurals. Many women experience backache for some time after the birth, but this could be due to a long, difficult labour rather than the epidural.

Q CAN I HAVE A CAESAREAN DELIVERY UNDER AN EPIDURAL?

A With the improvements in Caesarean operations, an epidural anaesthetic is preferable to a general anaesthetic; this type of anaesthetic will also enable you to see and to hold your baby as soon as he or she is born (see p. 196). More importantly, an epidural anaesthetic is safer for you than a general anaesthetic. Having an epidural anaesthetic also means that you won't be sleepy or have to spend as much time recovering after the operation as you would after a general anaesthetic.

Q WILL I BE CONFINED TO BED WITH AN EPIDURAL?

A You will find it easier to remain on a bed because it will probably be difficult for you to move your legs. Some maternity units offer "mobile epidurals", which use a type of anaesthetic drug that blocks the pain and still allows you to walk around and empty your bladder. However, these are not available everywhere, and not all anaesthetists are familiar with them.

Q HOW DOES A MOBILE EPIDURAL WORK?

A A mobile epidural is so-called because a different, and "lighter", combination of drugs is used compared to a conventional epidural. So, instead of your legs being numbed, and needing a catheter to pass urine, you can theoretically walk around and urinate as normal.

Q WHAT IS A SPINAL ANAESTHETIC?

A With a spinal anaesthetic the needle is inserted into your spinal canal, a small shot of anaesthetic is given, and the needle is removed. This takes effect more rapidly than an epidural, but only lasts one to two hours, and cannot be topped up.

Q CAN AN EPIDURAL GO WRONG?

A As with any medical procedure, there is a risk attached, but it is virtually impossible for an epidural to injure or paralyse you. The only problem that can arise is if the epidural anaesthetizes only half your abdomen. In this case, the anaesthetist will be called back to get the epidural working properly. He or she does this by gently moving the tube in your back to allow the anaesthetic to reach all the relevant nerves. It should not hurt. Occasionally, the epidural needle needs to be repositioned completely, which takes a few minutes.

QUESTIONS TO ASK

Is there an obstetric anaesthetist available at the maternity unit at all times?

How long will the tube be left in my bladder after the epidural?

Do my previous back problems mean that I won't be able to have an epidural?

Which type of pain relief is best for me?

	BREATHING	AROMATHERAPY	REFLEXOLOGY/ HYPNOTHERAPY/ ACUPUNCTURE	MASSAGE
Do I need to organize or practise this in advance, or is it supplied?	You need to learn how breathing techniques work, and to practise them, before going into labour.	You need the oils and vaporizer or burner and, if combined with massage, to have a person present who can massage you.	You should have contacted a therapist and tried these prior to labour, then organized for the therapist to be with you during labour.	Your partner should practise massaging you before labour (see p. 118), or your midwife may be happy to do this if she is free.
How will it affect me?	Deep, controlled, slow breathing distracts you from pain by making you focus on something else; it also reduces nausea and dizziness.	It relaxes you and can reduce stress and tension; only use oils that are suitable during pregnancy (see p. 118).	These all help to relax you and to reduce pain, or to distract you from pain during labour (see p. 108).	It will help you to relax by relieving stress and tension, and by helping to sooth aching and tense muscles.
How will it affect my baby?	It will not affect your baby. This helps you to relax, so your labour should progress better.	It will not affect your baby and, if relaxed, your labour may progress better.	These will not affect your baby.	It will not affect your baby.
How quickly does it work if I decide to use it?	Immediately	If you have the essential and base oils with you in labour, aromatherapy can begin to work immediately.	Once the therapist begins using the treatment, you should feel the benefits within 15–30 minutes.	Immediately, but make sure someone is present who knows how to massage you (see below).
How long will it last?	As long as you control your breathing.	Whether used intermittently or continuously, you should feel the benefits throughout the labour.	The effects vary, depending on which therapy is used and for which symptom; all can be made to last the entire labour.	If done properly, the effects of massage can last for a considerable time.
Can I combine it with other methods of pain relief?	Yes, you can use this technique in conjunction with any other types of pain relief.	Yes, it is commonly combined with massage (see p. 118) and other types of pain relief.	Yes, you may find that these do not provide adequate pain relief on their own.	Yes, you can combine this with any other method of pain relief.
Can I use it in a home birth?	Yes	Yes	Yes	Yes
Can I use it before I come into hospital?	Yes	Yes	Yes	Yes

WATER BUOYANCY	TENS	GAS AND AIR (nitrous oxide and oxygen mixture)	PETHIDINE OR OTHER OPIATE DRUG	EPIDURAL/SPINAL ANAESTHETIC
The labour ward may have a bath that you can use in early labour, or a birthing pool; you may have to book the pool in advance.	You may be able to rent a TENS machine from the hospital. If not, you can rent or buy one from a specialist company.	This will be supplied in hospital, and by the midwife at a home birth.	This is supplied in all labour wards, and brought to a home delivery by your midwife (see below).	It will be supplied by the hospital and is not something you can organize in advance, although you should enquire about availability.
This relieves tension by supporting you; you may have to leave the water for your baby to be monitored (see p. 168).	It makes pain less intense by reducing the pain stimuli reaching the brain, and by stimulating the body's natural painkillers, endorphins.	This takes the edge off contraction pains, but may make you feel light-headed, sleepy, and sometimes nauseous (see p. 160).	This relieves pain, but can cause light-headedness and nausea; you may need an anti-sickness injection with it (see p. 160).	This should numb your stomach, back passage, and vagina, stopping all feeling; your blood pressure may fall slightly (see p. 162).
It will not affect your baby	It will not affect your baby.	It will not affect your baby.	If given late in labour, it can make your baby sleepy and affect his or her breathing; some oxygen will be given to wake your baby.	It won't affect your baby unless your blood pressure drops and the blood flow to the placenta is reduced.
Provided you have arranged this in advance, it will begin to work as soon as you get into the water.	After switching on the machine and adjusting the output to the correct strength, the effects can be felt immediately.	Provided in hospital or at a home birth if your midwife has brought it, the effect should be immediate.	This can take 10–20 minutes; an internal check will be carried out to ensure that you are not about to give birth imminently.	This can take 30–45 minutes; an internal check ensures that you are not just about to give birth, and an anaesthetist is called.
The effect will last if you stay in the water, but you may find it less effective as labour becomes more painful.	It may be less effective in more painful labour.	The effect wears off in a few seconds, but you can use it consistently throughout labour.	It takes 20 minutes to take effect and should last for about three hours.	This depends on the type of epidural (see p. 163), but it can be topped up, giving pain relief throughout labour.
Yes, within limits. You can have gas and air, or even pethidine, but it is impossible to have an epidural while lying in water.	Yes, except in water.	Yes, you can use this with all other methods of pain relief.	Yes, you could try, massage, breathing techniques, gas and air or even an epidural with it.	This should totally block the pain and you shouldn't need anything else. If really necessary, you can use gas and air.
Yes	TENS is ideal for use in a home birth.	Yes, your midwife will bring a supply with her.	Yes, your midwife can bring this; it may have to be prescribed and collected from a pharmacy in advance.	No, because it must be administered by an anaesthetist. You and your baby will need monitoring.
Yes	Yes, practise using it before labour. The start of labour is the most effective time to use it.	No, it can only be used under medical supervision.	No, you will have to come in to hospital for this.	No, this must be administered in hospital by an anaesthetist.

THE FIRST SIGNS OF LABOUR

Q WHAT ARE THE SIGNS THAT LABOUR HAS BEGUN?

A There are several signs that indicate whether or not you may be starting the first of three stages of labour. These signs can be divided into two groups: those that are possible indicators of labour, and those that are absolute signs of labour (see chart, opposite). There may be certain signs, such as a "show" (see below) several days or even weeks before you actually start labour, which can lead you to think that labour has begun. In fact, the only true sign that labour is underway is the occurrence of frequent and regular contractions that are causing your cervix to dilate (open).

Q WHAT DOES HAVING A "SHOW" MEAN?

A During pregnancy, a plug of jelly-like mucus seals the lower end of your cervix to prevent infection getting into your womb. This plug comes away towards the end of your pregnancy, and although it may mean that labour is going to start soon, it can dislodge (with no harm to the baby) up to six weeks before your labour starts.

Q WHAT SHOULD I DO IF I HAVE A SHOW?

A Try not to panic if you see a small amount of blood. It's normal for a show to contain either fresh red blood or old dark blood (like at the end of your period) as part of the clear or cloudy mucus of the plug. Unless you have other symptoms, such as strong, regular contractions, a show is not an absolute sign that labour is starting now, but it is best to ring your midwife or doctor for advice.

Q HOW DO I KNOW IF I'M JUST IN FALSE LABOUR?

A You will be experiencing regular Braxton-Hicks' contractions (see p. 85), which can often be mistaken for the real thing – particularly if they are especially strong and if this is your first baby and you don't know what to expect. The difference between these "practice contractions" and labour pains is that they occur irregularly, perhaps one or two an hour, then fade away, whereas labour pains usually begin slowly and build in intensity and frequency.

Q I AM HAVING REGULAR UNCOMFORTABLE CONTRACTIONS, WHAT SHOULD I DO?

A Time your contractions from the beginning of one to the beginning of the next, also how often they occur. There are no hard and fast rules, but as a rough guide: if they are regular (less than 30 minutes apart), and painful (you have to stop what you are doing until they pass), you should contact your midwife, doctor, or labour ward.

Q WHAT DOES "BREAKING OF WATERS" MEAN, AND WHEN SHOULD MINE BREAK?

A The "waters" are the aminiotic fluid (contained in membranes) that surround and protect your baby in the womb (see p. 58). The membranes usually break as your cervix opens, once labour is actually in progress. The contractions that are opening your cervix may cause the baby to press down, creating pressure that bursts the membranes. If they don't break spontaneously, they may be broken artificially by your midwife or doctor to speed up your progress (see p. 176).

Q HOW DO I KNOW IF MY WATERS HAVE BROKEN, AND WHAT DO I DO?

A This question can be worrying, especially as any slight leakage could be of urine. If there is quite a large amount of fluid, you will be in no doubt about what has happened. But if the waters break, and produce a trickle, and you are still in doubt, put on a sanitary pad and examine the pad. Urine will look and smell different to amniotic fluid. Waters are normally clear or a light straw colour, with no odour, and trickle beyond your control. If you think your waters have broken, contact your midwife, doctor, or labour ward; what happens next will depend on whether or not you are in labour.

Q WHAT IF MY WATERS BREAK BEFORE I AM IN LABOUR?

A If you are between 37 and 42 weeks pregnant, and your waters break without contractions having begun (see opposite), it is quite likely that you will go into labour within 24 hours; within 48 hours, over 90 per cent of women will have gone into labour. In certain situations, you may be induced to help labour get started (see p. 170).

Q HOW WILL I KNOW IF THERE'S ANYTHING TO BE CONCERNED ABOUT?

A If you see a dark green fluid when your waters break, it means your waters contain meconium, the substance in your baby's digestive system (see p. 66) that is usually passed in the first bowel movements after birth; if passed earlier, it can mean that your baby is distressed, and you should contact your midwife immediately. If you have a lot of blood mixed with the fluid, or bright, fresh bleeding that continues after your waters have broken, this needs to be checked out straight away.

Q WHAT SHOULD I DO IF I THINK I AM IN LABOUR?

A True labour contractions occur very regularly, and grow stronger and more frequent. If you think you are in labour, contact your midwife or labour ward for advice. Your midwife will probably come to see you, or you will be asked to go to your hospital to check if labour has indeed started. Remember to take your hospital notes and your labour bag with you. It is important to try not to panic; you have prepared for this moment, and should have plenty of time.

HOW CAN I TELL IF I AM IN LABOUR?

The only true sign that you are in the early first stage of labour is that you are experiencing regular contractions that are causing your cervix to open; whether or not this is happening needs to be confirmed by an internal examination. However, if you are in any doubt, check your symptoms on the chart below and contact your midwife, doctor, or labour ward for information and reassurance.

YOU ARE HAVING	IF...	WHAT TO DO	BUT IF...	WHAT TO DO
Contractions	1 or 2 contractions per hour	Wait, labour has not begun	Contractions 5–10 minutes apart	Call your midwife or labour ward
Baby's movements have become less frequent	With or without contractions	Contact your midwife or labour ward for advice	All movements have stopped	Go to hospital immediately
Strong contractions	Less than 5 minutes apart	Contact the labour ward and get to hospital immediately	Some contractions are weak and irregular	Contact your midwife or hospital
Waters broken	⟶	Contact your midwife or labour ward for advice	With dark green stains (meconium)	Go to hospital immediately
Had a show	⟶	Contact your midwife or labour ward for advice	With lots of blood	Go to hospital
Constant backache	It can be eased by changing position, or by massage	Wait and see	It does not ease and with other signs (see above)	Contact your midwife or labour ward for advice
Diarrhoea	Without other signs (see above)	Wait and see	With other signs (see above)	Contact your midwife or labour ward for advice
Strong urge to push	⟶	Labour is in progress	⟶	Contact your midwife or labour ward/ go to hospital

GOING INTO HOSPITAL

Q WILL I NEED TO INFORM THE HOSPITAL THAT I'M ON MY WAY?

A If you are part of the Domino scheme or have booked a private midwife, she will probably come to your home when your contractions have started, decide when you should go into hospital, and inform the hospital that you are on your way. If you are booked into the hospital or are a part of a Team midwife scheme, try to ring the hospital before you set off so that they can allocate a room for you and organize a midwife to care for you.

Q WHAT HAPPENS WHEN I ARRIVE AT THE HOSPITAL?

A You will be welcomed to the ward, and meet your midwife – unless, of course, she came with you. You can then change into a nightdress or a T-shirt and familiarize yourself with the ward. Your midwife will discuss your symptoms and check the notes and any birthplan you have brought with you.

Q WILL I BE GIVEN MEDICAL CHECKS AT THE HOSPITAL?

A Your temperature, blood pressure, and pulse will be checked, and your urine tested for protein, sugar, and blood. Your midwife will examine your abdomen to check your baby's position, and the strength and frequency of your contractions. Your baby's heartbeat will be checked by a cardiotocograph (CTG) to ensure that he or she is not in distress and that all is well (see below). Continuous monitoring may be needed if there are complications such as a breech baby, twins, a very small or a very large baby, or the presence of meconium.

Q HOW WILL MY MIDWIFE CONFIRM THAT I AM IN LABOUR?

A Your midwife will confirm that you are in labour by giving you an internal examination to see if your cervix has softened sufficiently and is beginning to dilate (see p. 173).

HOW IS MY BABY'S HEARTBEAT MONITORED?

A CTG (cardiotocograph) electronic monitor records your baby's heart rate and your contractions. If your baby's heartbeat is normal and there is nothing else of concern in your labour, you can be disconnected from the CTG so that you can move around. Your midwife will listen to your baby's heartbeat intermittently during the labour.

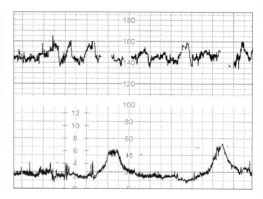

HOW THE CTG WORKS
The CTG monitor is securely attached to your abdomen by two belts. Your baby's heartbeat is detected by ultrasound.

WHAT THE CTG PRINT-OUT SHOWS
The top line of the print-out (above) shows your baby's heartbeat, the lower shows your contractions. These can be interpreted to discover if your baby is distressed.

Q IF I GO INTO LABOUR AND I'M ALONE, SHOULD I DRIVE MYSELF TO HOSPITAL?

A No, this is not a good idea. If you are getting painful contractions, and your waters are about to break (or have broken), driving will not only be very uncomfortable and dangerous for you, it will also make you a hazard on the road. Try to have a contingency plan for this eventuality – for example, a friend or neighbour with a car who you know might be available. If this is not possible, phone for an ambulance.

Q I'M 36 WEEKS NOW. HOW WILL I KNOW WHEN TO GO INTO HOSPITAL?

A You should go to the hospital, or contact your doctor or midwife, if you have regular, painful contractions (more than one every ten minutes), if your waters break, if you have fresh vaginal bleeding, if your womb becomes painful without contractions, or if you feel your baby's movements reduce over a short space of time. If you are not sure, or have other symptoms, call the hospital!

Q WHAT SHOULD I TAKE TO HOSPITAL WITH ME?

A From 36 weeks onwards, you should have packed what you will need for hospital and have everything in a suitcase waiting by the front door (see pp.150–151). Don't forget your notes, some small change, and your diary or personal organizer, and let a friend or your partner know that you're going to the hospital.

Q IF I'M NOT NEAR MY HOSPITAL WHEN I GO INTO LABOUR, WHAT SHOULD I DO?

A You should go to the nearest maternity unit. If an ambulance collects you, it will usually take you to the nearest unit anyway. If you are making your own way there, although it is tempting to drive back to your own hospital, which feels safe and familiar, it is much better to go to the local unit. If everything settles down, they will usually let you go home or transfer you to your own hospital.

Q THE HOSPITAL IS A BIG PLACE. WHERE EXACTLY SHOULD I REPORT TO?

A In most cases, the maternity unit has its own entrance, often open 24 hours a day. It is worth getting to know the exact location of the hospital, maternity unit, and entrances some weeks in advance, so that your mind is at rest when you are on your way there in the middle of the night or in the early hours!

Q WHAT HAPPENS IF I GO TO HOSPITAL BUT MY CONTRACTIONS DIE OUT?

A The midwives and/or doctors will establish whether or not you are in labour. Once you have been thoroughly examined and the baby monitored, and it is confirmed that you are not yet in labour, it is likely you will be advised to return to your home. If you are admitted to the hospital during the night, however, you may be advised to stay for a few hours until the morning.

Q WHAT IF I GO INTO HOSPITAL SEVERAL TIMES WITH FALSE ALARMS?

A There are no set rules as to how often you can come into hospital. You are not supposed to be the expert on labour and birth, especially if this is your first baby. You come to the doctors and midwives in the hospital for their expertise and advice, and together you decide what care you need, depending on your own circumstances.

Q WHAT IF I DON'T WANT TO STAY ONCE I GET TO HOSPITAL?

A The fact that you go in at all suggests that you may well need to be there. If you do need to stay but do not wish to, perhaps it is because you are anxious that your labour may be about to start and you are naturally apprehensive. If you are in labour, you will need to stay in hospital but if not, normally you will have the choice to go home. It would be foolish to return home against the advice of your midwives and doctors. However, if you find yourself in these circumstances, you may be able to negotiate alternatives.

Q CAN I BE MADE TO STAY IN HOSPITAL UNTIL I'VE HAD THE BABY?

A This is a common concern among mothers-to-be – going into hospital and not being allowed to return to your comfortable home for days or weeks until after you've had the baby. Please don't worry! Unless you are in labour, or have a serious condition such as pre-eclampsia, or there is another reason why you have to be kept in for monitoring and/or treatment, the chances are that you will be allowed home soon. If you simply need to be checked out on the delivery unit and you and the baby are fine, you are often allowed to go straight home.

INDUCTION OF LABOUR

Q **AM I MORE LIKELY TO NEED FORCEPS OR A VENTOUSE IF I'M INDUCED?**

A Yes, there is a greater likelihood of requiring an assisted delivery, by forceps or ventouse. There is also a greater likelihood of needing a Caesarean section.

Q **MY WATERS BROKE TWO DAYS AGO. WHY IS MY LABOUR BEING INDUCED?**

A Once your membranes have ruptured, there is a high chance that you will go into labour naturally within 24–48 hours. The longer you wait after this, the stronger the risk of infection getting into your womb and affecting the baby. To reduce this risk, many hospitals will give you the choice of induction of labour straight away, or waiting for a day or two before starting the induction process off.

Q **DO I NEED AN EPIDURAL FOR MY INDUCTION?**

A No, you don't actually "need" an epidural, but if the signs are that your labour is going to be a long process (for example, first baby, big baby, or unfavourable cervix), then an epidural early on will mean that you can be comfortable throughout the labour. And, nowadays, you may be able to have a mobile epidural (see p. 165). With a mobile epidural, you will still have sensation in your legs and you can usually walk around rather than being confined to the bed! But this should not stop you trying out other methods of pain relief and relaxation, which can also be effective: a TENS machine, aromatherapy, and even acupuncture can help create "low tech" pain relief and a relaxed atmosphere early on in labour.

Q **CAN I SAY "NO" TO INDUCTION?**

A You have a perfect right to say no to any intervention. As with all things, if an induction is recommended, there are usually good reasons for it, so it is important to speak to your doctor or midwife and then ask the relevant questions. If the doctor's or midwife's replies satisfy you, then go ahead with the induction on their advice. It is not advisable to say "no" without knowing what the risks are for you and/or your baby if you decline induction.

Q **WHY DOES LABOUR NEED TO BE INDUCED AT 41–42 WEEKS?**

A You may argue "nature will decide" when you'll go into labour, and this is generally true. However, the placenta, which feeds the baby, is operating on lower efficiency from about 38 weeks, and certainly after 41 weeks. This means that, from about 41 weeks onwards, the baby has a progressively higher chance of not being fed oxygen and nutrients. There are no really accurate tests to tell us which placentas are working well, and which aren't. Most doctors, therefore, advise induction of labour between 41–42 weeks. After 42 weeks, the chances are still that you will go into labour at some point and deliver a healthy baby, but the risk of fetal distress in labour, and even stillbirth, climbs steeply. Daily monitoring is not the answer – it tells you how the baby is at the time of monitoring, but not how the baby will be in 10 hours or even 10 minutes.

Q **CAN I HAVE A CAESAREAN INSTEAD OF BEING INDUCED?**

A You must discuss this with your doctor or midwife. The chances of a successful induction (i.e., vaginal delivery) depend mainly on whether you've had a vaginal delivery before, whether your cervix is "favourable" (see p. 177) and the baby's head is engaged, how large the baby is, and how big/tall you are. Overall, there is a 70–80 per cent chance of having a vaginal delivery following induction of labour.

Q **IS AN INDUCED LABOUR LONGER THAN ONE THAT STARTS SPONTANEOUSLY?**

A Usually, yes. This is because the whole labour process must be initiated first: this may take many hours. Usually this is done by breaking your waters (ARM: artificial rupture of membranes) and giving prostaglandin gel or a prostaglandin tablet (by mouth or into the vagina). Once you are in labour, you may also need an intravenous drip with oxytocin (pitressin/syntocinon) to get your contractions coming regularly. Sometimes, especially if you've had babies before, just breaking your waters or giving one dose of prostaglandin is enough to get your labour going on its own, without further outside help.

WHAT IS AN INDUCED LABOUR?

It is sometimes necessary to start labour artificially. This is known as induction of labour or, if your waters have already broken, stimulation of labour. Induction of labour is usually easier if you have had one or more babies before by normal delivery, and if your cervix (neck of your womb) is already ripe.

Why your labour might be induced

■ If you are beyond 41, or in some cases, 42 weeks pregnant (known as "post dates" pregnancy).

■ If your doctors are concerned that your baby's growth has slowed down or stopped; your baby is not moving well; there is a reduced amount of amniotic fluid; or the placenta is no longer nourishing your baby (placental insufficiency).

■ If you have reached 40 weeks and you have a medical condition that means that an early delivery would be in your interest.

■ If you are at 40 weeks, and you have a vital personal reason to have your baby delivered.

■ If your baby has a condition, such as "hole in the heart", that needs surgery, it is in your baby's interests to be delivered during working hours when the necessary expertise is readily available.

■ If you develop pre-eclampsia, your doctors may decide, for your and for your baby's safety, that your labour should be induced. This may be as much as a few weeks before your baby is due.

■ If you have another medical condition, for example, diabetes or kidney disease.

The procedure for inducing labour

Your obstetrician will check that your baby is "head down" in your womb, and has engaged low in your pelvis, then will ascertain if your cervix is ripe. You will be asked to return to the hospital at a certain time to have your labour induced. When you come in, your baby's heartbeat will be monitored for about half an hour on a CTG machine to check that he or she is not in distress. You will then be induced by one of the following methods:

■ **Prostaglandin** (vaginal gel or tablets orally). This substance is found naturally in your womb lining and one of its functions is to stimulate uterine contractions so that labour can begin. If your cervix is firmly closed, your midwife or doctor may put a gel or a tablet containing synthetic prostaglandin into your vagina, which helps to ripen your cervix. This procedure may be repeated several times in one day, or even continued the next day, until you go into labour or your cervix has opened enough for your waters to be broken.

■ **Artificial rupture of the membranes (ARM)**
If your cervix is sufficiently ripe, this can be an effective way of inducing labour. Your doctor or midwife will give you an internal examination, then use a long, thin plastic hook to brush against the delicate membranes, which is usually enough to break them (see p. 176).

■ **Syntocinon** This is a synthetic substance fed into your arm via a drip to increase the strength and regularity of your contractions. It is similar to oxytocin, the hormone produced by the pituitary gland, which causes the womb to contract, stimulating labour. This method is often combined with the artificial rupture of your membranes (see above). It is very safe, but if too much syntocinon is given it can cause your womb to contract too much; it can also make your contractions very painful (and sometimes causes double contractions).

Why inductions are not more common

Although inductions are usually successful, labour is not induced more frequently or on demand because there is a risk that you will not go into labour; if the induction fails, then you will need a Caesarean. You are also more likely to need an assisted delivery with forceps or ventouse (see p. 194). An induced labour is less likely to be successful if your cervix is completely closed and your baby's head has not properly engaged in your pelvis.

What to consider

An induced labour may be more painful and take longer than one that starts naturally. You may need to have an epidural; this means that you will be prepared if you later need a Caesarean, or even an assisted delivery with forceps or a ventouse cup.

THE FIRST STAGE OF LABOUR

Q WHAT ARE THE MAIN STAGES OF LABOUR?

A Labour has three distinct stages: the first starts with regular contractions that open up your cervix, and lasts until the cervix is fully open (about 10cm/4in); the second stage of labour begins when your cervix is fully open, and concludes with the birth of your baby; the third stage is from the birth of your baby until after the delivery of the placenta.

Q HOW LONG DOES EACH STAGE OF LABOUR LAST?

A Every birth is different and the timescale varies, but as a rough guide, doctors expect the first stage of labour to last eight to 14 hours, the second stage one to two hours, and the third stage ten to 60 minutes. If this is your first baby or your labour needs inducing, it can take longer; if this is not your first baby, labour may be quicker.

Q WHEN SHOULD I DISCUSS MY BIRTH PLAN OR PREFERENCES FOR THE BIRTH?

A Once your midwife confirms that you are in labour, you should discuss your birth plan if you haven't done so (see p. 148). Remember, this is to make your feelings clear. If you feel unable to converse because of the contractions, ask your partner to discuss your birth plan with the midwife.

Q WHAT WILL HAPPEN ONCE IT IS ESTABLISHED THAT I AM IN LABOUR?

A Once you are having between two and four contractions every ten minutes, you, your baby, and the progress of your labour will be regularly monitored. Many hospitals use a system whereby the progress of labour is recorded on a graph called a partogram that shows the rate at which your cervix is dilating and acts as a visual guide so that problems can be spotted immediately.

THE POSITION OF YOUR BABY

Your baby's position in the womb will affect your labour. For an easy passage through the birth canal, the best position for your baby is head-down (cephalic) with the back facing your abdomen (anterior position). If your baby's back has turned towards your back (posterior position), your baby presents the widest part of the head (occiput) into the birth canal; this can give you back pain, and also a prolonged labour that may have to be assisted (see p. 194). A breech presentation means that the feet or buttocks are delivered first, and this will also require the assistance of an experienced doctor or midwife.

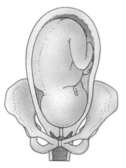

OCCIPUT ANTERIOR
Your baby's head is downwards with his or her back facing your abdomen.

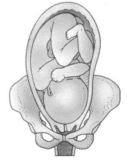

OCCIPUT POSTERIOR
Your baby's head is downwards with his or her back turned towards your spine.

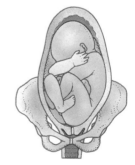

BREECH PRESENTATION
Your baby is presented bottom first, with his or her legs flexed at the knees and hips.

Q HOW WILL I FEEL DURING THE FIRST STAGE OF LABOUR?

A You may feel a range of intense emotions. At one moment you may feel excited and joyful and the next you may feel despondent, afraid, and tired; or you may feel exhilarated throughout. You will probably be stretched to your physical limits, and at times feel that you cannot carry on. Express your emotions and laugh or cry depending on how you feel; this can help you to relax, which can help the labour to progress. You may also be oblivious to your surroundings because your entire being is centred on pushing out and delivering your baby.

Q WILL I FEEL MUCH PAIN DURING THE FIRST STAGE?

A The degree of pain felt varies from woman to woman. The pain usually intensifies towards the end of the first stage of labour when your contractions are becoming stronger and your cervix is almost fully dilated.

Q WILL I NEED PAIN RELIEF IN THE FIRST STAGE?

A This will depend on the intensity of your contractions, also on how your midwife and doctors feel you are coping with the pain; if they become concerned about your progress, they may ask if you want, or suggest that you try, some form of pain relief (see p. 164). If you do need relief, the first stage is usually the best time for this.

Q DOES THE CERVIX START OPENING ONCE CONTRACTIONS BEGIN?

A No, the cervix needs to soften before it can dilate. Labour doesn't always begin when your contractions start. You may have irregular, painful contractions for hours or even a day or two before your cervix dilates, especially if this is your first baby. So you may feel tired, nauseous, and be unable to eat properly while waiting for your cervix to dilate. This is called the "prolonged latent phase".

Q WHAT WILL HAPPEN IF MY CONTRACTIONS STOP DURING THE FIRST STAGE?

A Contractions can sometimes start regularly, but then die away halfway through your labour. If this happens and the progress of your labour comes to a halt for a few hours, your midwife may suggest breaking your waters (if they have not already broken) or artificially stimulating your labour with syntocinon (see pp. 170 and 176).

HOW YOUR CERVIX OPENS

The first stage of labour begins with the onset of regular contractions. This causes the cervix to thin out, known as "effacement". Once the cervix has softened, the contractions cause the cervix to dilate (widen) progressively, so that your baby's head can pass through. Contractions draw the cervix up over the baby's head like a glove, towards the vaginal walls.

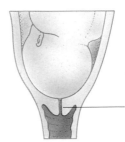

BEFORE LABOUR
The cervix is thick and closed (known as "uneffaced") and your baby's head is engaged.

Cervix is closed

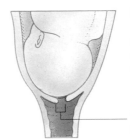

EARLY FIRST STAGE
The cervix thins and softens (effacement) before it can stretch and dilate.

The cervix starts to dilate

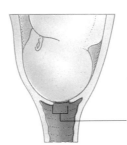

LATE FIRST STAGE
At about 5cm (2in), the cervix is said to be half way towards full dilatation.

Dilatation is proceeding

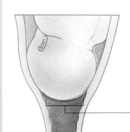

FULLY DILATED
The cervix is fully dilated when its opening measures about 10cm (4in) in diameter.

The cervix is now fully opened

LABOUR AND BIRTH

POSITIONS FOR THE FIRST STAGE

In the first stage of labour, when there is no urge to push yet, you are usually freer to move around and find a comfortable position. Some women instinctively find a position that suits them and stay in this position for the entire first stage. Others prefer to walk around and keep upright as much as possible. Staying upright is beneficial because gravity helps your baby's weight to press down on your cervix which, in turn, helps to open your cervix. If you want to stay mobile, work out a small circuit in the delivery room and place chairs or cushions strategically so that you can stop and concentrate on breathing during a contraction. Try different positions until you find one that you prefer.

STANDING
Stand behind a chair, facing the back, and place your arms on the back for support. This can help you to rest during a contraction if you are moving around during the first stage of labour.

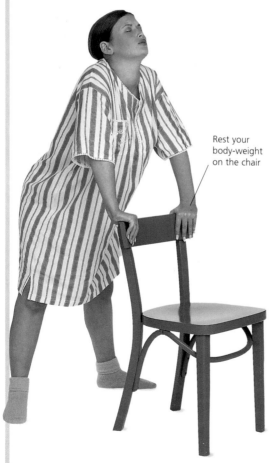

Rest your body-weight on the chair

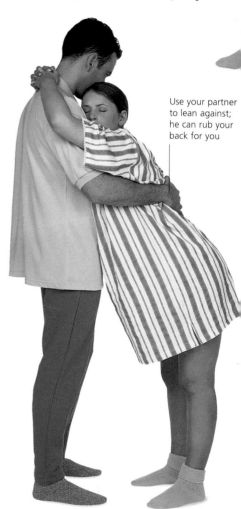

Use your partner to lean against; he can rub your back for you

LEANING
Stand facing your birth partner with your arms around him or her and lean forward so that your body-weight is supported. Ask your birth partner for a low back massage at the same time if this helps.

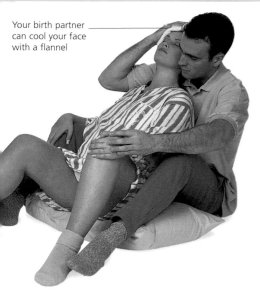

Your birth partner can cool your face with a flannel

SUPPORTED SITTING
Get your partner to sit against a wall or sit on a bean bag or cushion. Sit in front of him or her, allowing your body-weight to be supported. This position can also be used during the second stage.

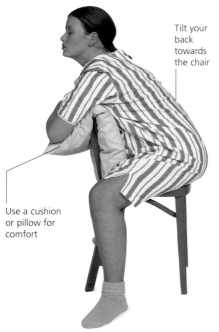

Tilt your back towards the chair

Use a cushion or pillow for comfort

SITTING
Sit on a chair, facing the back, and place your arms over the back for support. Your birth partner can then stand in front of you and sponge your face, or stand behind you and massage your back and shoulders.

THE ROLE OF THE BIRTH PARTNER

Your role as a birth partner is to support your partner both emotionally and physically. Mop her brow or hold her during a contraction; you can also make helpful suggestions, and offer her encouragement and praise. Because she knows you best, the chances are that your partner will take any anxieties or irritations out on you. Be prepared for this to happen, be understanding and try not to take it personally! The following is a list of ideas that you could use to help your partner through her labour:

■ Ask her what you can do to make her more comfortable. She may not know herself, so be ready to make suggestions. Don't get annoyed if she doesn't seem to want to take your advice.
■ Suggest a change of position if you can see that your partner is feeling tired or stressed.
■ Offer to massage her back, feet, or shoulders.
■ Talk her through the contractions and always try to praise her achievement.
■ Remind her how much further on she is than this time yesterday, or a few hours ago.
■ Encourage her to take little drinks every few hours.
■ Remind her to urinate every two hours or so.
■ For distraction, if she is agreeable, read to her, or play a game together.
■ If labour is very long and you are also feeling tired, have some refreshment so that you can recharge your batteries and be of optimum help to your partner.
■ Join your partner in breathing exercises.

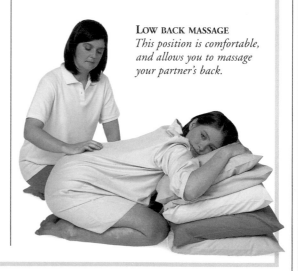

LOW BACK MASSAGE
This position is comfortable, and allows you to massage your partner's back.

As the First Stage Ends

Q WHAT HAPPENS BETWEEN THE FIRST AND SECOND STAGES?

A After the cervix has fully dilated there is often, but not usually, a period before the second stage of labour – with its intense urge to push arrives. You may find this interlude, called transition, one of the most difficult stages of labour.

Q WHY IS THIS A DIFFICULT TIME IN LABOUR?

A Transition can last for a few minutes or for several hours, and can be confusing and hard to cope with for several reasons: your contractions may become more intense and frequent, which can make you nauseous or cause you to vomit; you may also feel shivery, or anxious and out of control. Transition usually occurs after you have already experienced several hours of strong contractions, when your strength is beginning to wane, and you feel tired and irritable, and think that you are getting nowhere. This low point can make some women wish they had never become pregnant in the first place!

Q NOW I'M AT THE END OF THE FIRST STAGE, IS THIS A GOOD SIGN?

A Despite being uncomfortable, the transition stage is a very positive sign that you are making progress – the time to push your baby out is about to begin. While you wait for the next stage to start, you could try: changing your position by sitting up if you have been lying down, or by standing up; walking around the room if you are able to; asking your partner to massage you gently, or sponge your face, or simply to ask you questions that require your concentration; changing partners for a while if you have more than one person with you; making eye contact with your partner.

Q WHAT HAPPENS IF I NEED TO PUSH AND MY CERVIX IS NOT DILATED ENOUGH?

A Your midwife will give you an internal examination to confirm that your cervix is fully dilated, so will not be damaged. If you feel a strong urge to push but your midwife says you are not quite ready, she will ask you to pass this time by distracting yourself through breathing.

What happens if my waters don't break naturally?

Your waters may break spontaneously at any time before labour (see p. 166); this can be a sign that labour may be about to begin. It can also happen as your baby's head descends into the birth canal during the first stage.

Do my waters need to be broken?
Your waters do not need to be artificially broken unless there is a problem such as: a long labour not progressing satisfactorily – artificially breaking your waters could speed things up a little because your baby's head will be able to bear down on the cervix and help it to dilate; signs that your baby is distressed (see p. 188); the need to attach a monitor called a fetal scalp electrode to your baby's head.

How are my waters broken artificially?
Your midwife or doctor will give you an internal examination, then use a long, thin, plastic hook to brush against the delicate membranes, which break, releasing the amniotic fluid.

Can I refuse to have my waters broken?
Yes, but it is very unlikely that your midwife or doctor will suggest breaking your waters unless they have a good reason to do so; if you are unsure about it, discuss it with them. No midwife or doctor should "routinely" break your waters.

Are there reasons why my waters should not be broken?
There are instances when breaking your waters is not a good idea. One reason is if your baby's head is too high and is not yet engaged properly in your pelvis; in this situation, if your waters are broken artificially, there is a risk of the umbilical cord coming down ahead of the baby (cord prolapse). Also, if your baby is very premature, it is better to deliver with the membranes intact, so that your baby has more protection during the birth. If you are carrying twins, your midwife or doctor may be reluctant to break your waters artificially because doing this too early can complicate the delivery of the second twin.

THE SECOND STAGE OF LABOUR

Q WHAT IS THE SECOND STAGE OF LABOUR?

A The second stage begins when your cervix is fully dilated, and is completed with the birth of your baby. This stage averages about one to two hours for a first baby. The second stage means that you can now bear down and push your baby out; this stage may start as soon as full dilatation is confirmed. If the head still has quite a way to come down through your pelvis, you may be discouraged from pushing immediately, so that you do not become exhausted. Therefore, the second stage is often divided into "passive" (you wait for the head to come down on its own) and "active" (you push with each contraction).

Q HOW DO I KNOW WHEN I'M IN THE SECOND STAGE?

A An internal examination by your midwife will confirm full dilatation, but there are other signs that indicate the onset of the second stage, such as a strong urge to push, and involuntary grunting with contractions (you can get this urge before full dilatation). Your back passage may bulge because your baby's head is just behind it; you may feel a need to defecate and may do so. Don't be embarrassed; this is involuntary and your midwife or doctor will have seen it often; in fact, it shows that things are about to happen in earnest.

Q WHAT DETERMINES HOW LONG THE SECOND STAGE LASTS?

A Various factors can influence the length of the second stage: how strong your contractions are; the size and position of your baby's head; and the size of your pelvis. The second stage tends to be shorter with second and subsequent births.

Q ARE THE CONTRACTIONS THE SAME AS BEFORE?

A No, your contractions will change, often becoming less frequent and more intense. You may only have two every ten minutes but they will last longer and allow you more time to make the most of your pushing technique. Also, you will have a strong urge to push now. If your waters have not yet broken, they probably will now, or the midwife may break them for you (see left).

Q AM I LIKELY TO BE TOO TIRED TO PUSH MY BABY OUT?

A If your labour has been long, and without adequate pain relief, you may be exhausted when the time comes to have your baby. However, modern management of your labour by midwives and doctors should prevent this and you should have been able to rest, especially with good pain relief. This active second stage, when you push your baby out, can last up to two hours; if it lasts any longer, you may get tired, and your baby may become distressed.

Q HOW DO I PUSH?

A When you get the urge to push, take a deep breath at the start of the contraction, put your chin on your chest, and push down into your bottom for as long as you can. You can usually take several breaths with each contraction and, as you bear down, your baby will gradually move further through your pelvis. Your partner's or midwife's encouragement can help you to continue pushing for as long as possible with each contraction, even if it seems as if nothing is happening.

Q CAN I PUSH IF I HAVE HAD AN EPIDURAL?

A It is generally thought that you can't do this, but just because you can't feel contractions doesn't mean you can't push. If your epidural is still working in the second stage, the midwife will put her hand on your abdomen, feel for contractions, and tell you when to push. Alternatively, your epidural may be allowed to wear off partially, so that you can feel the contractions, and start pushing.

Q WHO NEEDS TO BE THERE FOR THE BIRTH?

A If everything progresses normally, there should just be you, your partner, and the midwife present. An obstetrician may be there if a problem is anticipated, and a paediatrician (baby specialist) will be called in if, for example, your waters contain meconium, because the paediatrician will need to check if your baby swallowed any, and if you are going to need an assisted delivery.

POSITIONS FOR THE SECOND STAGE

The positions shown here are all suitable for the second stage of your labour. At this stage, when your contractions are lasting longer and you feel quite tired, you might be tempted to lie down – this should be resisted, however, because lying flat is not a beneficial position and does not help your baby to come down the birth canal. The best position is one in which you are upright, so that gravity can assist the process; relaxed, with your pelvis as open as possible; and one in which your weight is supported. Some women stay in one position, others change position as and when they feel they need to.

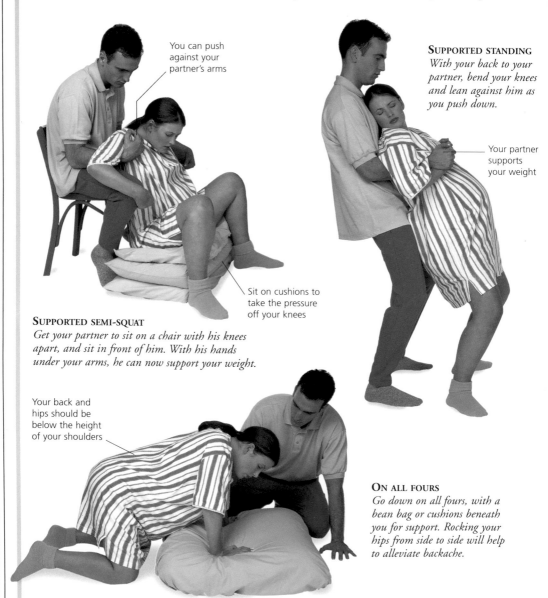

You can push against your partner's arms

Sit on cushions to take the pressure off your knees

SUPPORTED SEMI-SQUAT
Get your partner to sit on a chair with his knees apart, and sit in front of him. With his hands under your arms, he can now support your weight.

SUPPORTED STANDING
With your back to your partner, bend your knees and lean against him as you push down.

Your partner supports your weight

Your back and hips should be below the height of your shoulders

ON ALL FOURS
Go down on all fours, with a bean bag or cushions beneath you for support. Rocking your hips from side to side will help to alleviate backache.

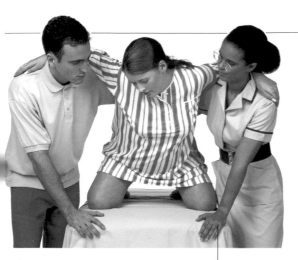

SUPPORTED KNEELING
Kneel on the bed between your birth partner and the midwife. Place your arms around their shoulders for support, and concentrate on pushing down.

The midwife can help to support you

THE ROLE OF THE BIRTH PARTNER

By the second stage your partner will probably be feeling very uncomfortable, very tired, and possibly overwhelmed as the baby begins the descent into the birth canal. As in the first stage, be quietly supportive and encouraging; remind her that she is nearly there, that the baby will be born very soon. You could also try the following:

■ Help her to get into a position in which she is comfortable for the delivery.
■ Talk her through her contractions and pushing; massage her back if required.
■ Spray her face with water or apply cold flannels if she wishes.
■ As the baby is being born, communicate with your partner through touch, rather than trying to talk over the midwife's instructions.
■ Watch for the baby's head as it crowns (see p. 180); if you have brought a mirror, angle it so that she can also see the head.
■ If you wish, you could cut the cord after delivery, and help to lay the baby on your partner's abdomen.
■ Take photographs!

LYING WITH LEG SUPPORT
Place some cushions or a bean bag on the floor, lie on your side, and support your head on another pillow. Get your partner to lift your leg.

Your partner can support your upper leg

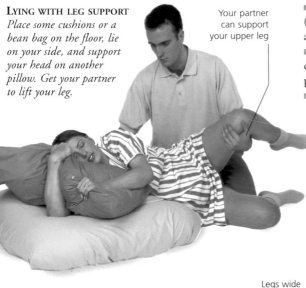

Keep as upright as possible

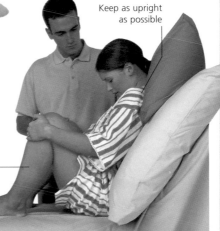

Legs wide apart

SITTING
Sit upright with pillows behind your back for support. Keep your legs apart and push down with contractions.

LABOUR AND BIRTH

THE BIRTH OF YOUR BABY

The final countdown to the most exciting part of your delivery has begun: the actual birth of your baby. However exciting this is, though, you must now concentrate hard during contractions to push your baby out. Your midwife will talk you through the next hour or so, while your partner provides support and comfort. Although you may have read or thought often about this moment, you may be unprepared for how you feel when you see your baby for the first time. Amazed by the completeness of this tiny human being, you will probably be engulfed in a wave of emotion; for most, all the pain and effort will suddenly seem a small price to pay for such a miracle.

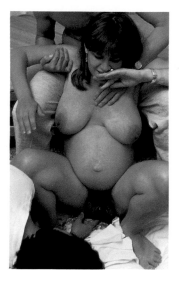
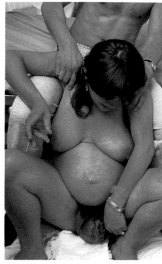
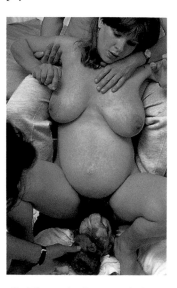

1 Now that the mother has begun to push with each contraction, the baby will move slowly through her pelvis until eventually the top of the baby's head will be visible at the entrance to the vagina. This process may take from a few minutes to two hours.

2 Initially, the baby's head slips back inside the vagina between contractions, but eventually it stays visible; this is called "crowning". The mother can put her hand down and feel the head or see it in a mirror. At this stage, as the tissues stretch, she may feel burning or stinging.

3 The midwife may ask the mother to pant now to slow the head's delivery a little and to give the vaginal area time to stretch rather than tear. As the head appears, the mother may cry out involuntarily. The baby usually emerges face down but will turn to one side at once.

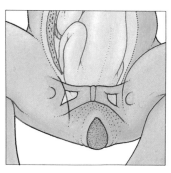
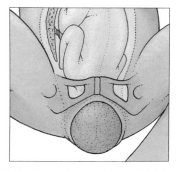
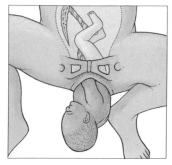

WHAT EFFECT DOES THE BIRTH HAVE ON MY BABY?

During the hardest part of labour your baby is squeezed and pushed down the narrow vaginal canal. This will cause your baby's heartbeat to slow intermittently, but this is not serious. When your baby arrives, it is a wonderful moment, but you may be concerned about the way he or she looks. Your baby will probably be covered in blood or the white greasy cream (vernix) that protected the skin while in the womb. Your baby's face may be bruised from the pressure of the delivery, and may appear blue or bright red from congestion caused during delivery. Although disappointing, remember that these marks are only temporary and will soon disappear. Once you hold your newborn baby, all you will probably feel is an immense tenderness for him or her.

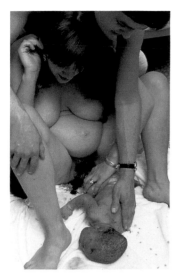

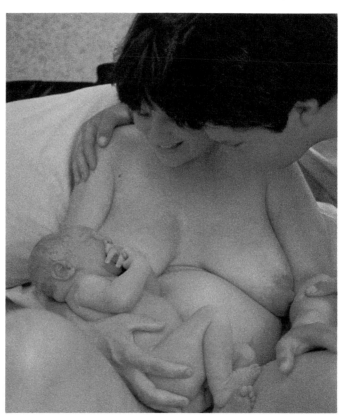

4 The midwife will wipe the baby's eyes, nose, and mouth clear of any mucus; if necessary, any fluid in the air passages will be sucked out through a tube. During the next one or two contractions the baby's shoulders, then body, will usually slide out quickly.

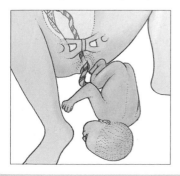

5 The baby may lie quietly or cry lustily straight away. The midwife will check the baby's condition and, provided that all is well, lift him or her on to your abdomen. Instinctively, the mother and her partner will welcome and comfort the baby by stroking or touching. At this stage, the cord will still be pulsating; it will now be clamped and cut, either by the midwife or the mother's partner, if preferred.

As Your Baby is Born

Q WILL I TEAR AS MY BABY'S HEAD COMES OUT?

A Not necessarily. In fact, this can be very difficult to predict, although tearing does tend to be quite common with a first baby. If it seems likely that your baby's head cannot come out easily, or that you might tear badly, your midwife will perform (with your permission) an "episiotomy", which is a small cut made with scissors at the entrance to your vagina (see below).

Q HOW COMMON IS IT TO NEED AN EPISIOTOMY?

A It is more common to need an episiotomy if you are having your first baby, because the vaginal opening may not stretch on its own to accommodate the baby's head. With subsequent babies, the vaginal tissues are more likely to stretch sufficiently.

HOW IS AN EPISIOTOMY DONE?

When your baby's head appears, the midwife gets your permission to make a small cut at the entrance to your vagina, so that it will be easier for you to push your baby out without tearing. Your pelvic floor area will be numbed with an injection of local anaesthetic, and the cut will be made from the bottom of the vagina, at the peak of a contraction. There are two types of episiotomy cut – midline and medio-lateral.

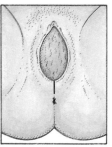
MIDLINE CUT
The cut extends directly backward from the vagina, stopping short of the anus.

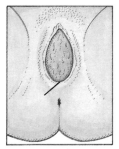
MEDIO-LATERAL CUT
The cut starts off like the midline cut, but goes to one side to avoid the anus.

Q ARE THERE OTHER REASONS FOR HAVING AN EPISIOTOMY?

A There are other complications that may mean it is necessary for an episiotomy to be performed. You will need an episiotomy if;
- There is a risk that you might tear badly and that this is likely to involve your back passage.
- It is anticipated that your baby is very large, and that there may be a problem when delivering him or her.
- Your baby is in the breech position.
- You need to be delivered with the assistance of forceps or a ventouse vacuum cup.

Q IS THERE ANYTHING I CAN DO TO AVOID A TEAR OR AN EPISIOTOMY?

A Unfortunately, there is no certain way to avoid having either a tear or an episiotomy. As your baby's head stretches the outlet of the birth canal, the natural reaction is to tense the muscles of the pelvic floor, when what you really need to do is to relax them. The pelvic floor exercises suggested in Chapter 5 (see p. 111) help you relax the muscles of the pelvic floor during labour. You may find that giving your body time to stretch can help: try to push down for as long as possible, so that the perineal area is encouraged to stretch. However, if you have an epidural, do not push down too hard as the baby's head is delivered. A warm flannel placed on the perineal area between the vagina and the anus during labour can help this area to stretch more easily. Massaging the area during pregnancy with oils or creams (particularly vitamin E creams) may also help it to become more supple.

Q WHAT HAPPENS IF THERE IS A TEAR?

A There are different degrees of tearing; most are not serious. It is more common to tear backwards, towards your back passage. Tearing towards the front is very painful, and is more likely to happen if you deliver in the all-fours position, because the pressure is more towards your labia or clitoris. If you have what is called a second-degree tear, this involves the skin as well as the muscles of the vagina, and those that lie beneath. Rarely, a tear may involve the muscles or lining of the back passage, which is known as a third-degree tear. This will need to be repaired by a senior doctor, sometimes under a general anaesthetic.

Q CAN MY PARTNER HELP TO DELIVER OUR BABY?

A This obviously depends on the circumstances of the birth, and whether or not the midwife or doctor supervising the delivery is happy with this. If the birth is progressing normally, with no complications, there is no reason why your partner cannot assist in lifting the baby out, as long as your midwife or doctor agrees.

Q AT WHAT STAGE IS THE CORD CUT?

A This depends on the methods of the doctor or obstetrician present, but the cord is usually clamped straight away. However, there is also a school of thought that believes that your baby can benefit from the blood and oxygen he or she receives from the placenta during the first ten minutes after the delivery, and that the cord should be left intact until it stops pulsating. The cord is then clamped and you or your partner can enjoy the ritual of cutting the cord if you want to. If you do not wish the cord to be cut immediately, you should state this in your birth plan (see p. 148) and discuss it with your midwife or doctor. Your baby's umbilical cord stump will drop off about ten days after the birth (see p. 210).

Q WHAT HAPPENS IF THE CORD IS WRAPPED AROUND MY BABY'S NECK?

A As soon as your baby's head is born, the midwife will check to see whether the cord is around the neck because this is quite common. If the cord has wound round just once, the midwife can slip it over your baby's head, which can sometimes cause a slightly bloodshot eye. If the cord is wound round more than once, or if it feels tight, the midwife will clamp and cut the cord immediately, to ensure that your baby can come through without restriction, and to prevent the placenta from being pulled away from the wall of the womb.

Q WHAT HAPPENS TO MY BABY ONCE THE CORD IS CUT?

A Immediately after your baby is born, the doctor or midwife will examine your baby and use the Apgar score (see p. 187) to assess his or her condition. If there are no problems, and your baby is breathing properly, he or she will be handed to you at once. However, if your baby is not breathing satisfactorily, he or she will be treated immediately with the resuscitation equipment at hand. A paediatrician will be called to check your baby over, and you and your partner will be kept informed of your baby's condition.

IS IT BETTER TO TEAR NATURALLY OR TO BE CUT?

Tearing is a hazard of giving birth; most tears are minor and heal easily, but if your midwife thinks that tearing will be severe, she may feel that an episiotomy is necessary and ask you for permission to perform one.

Cutting – cruel or kind?
The subject of episiotomy is still controversial. Many women fear that this procedure is still treated as a "routine" aid to getting the baby's head out, rather than as an "emergency" procedure when there are genuine complications. Those in favour of episiotomy argue that it prevents the vaginal entrance from overstretching, and that it is much easier and neater to stitch a cut back together than an uneven tear. However, supporters of natural birth argue that if you are left to tear naturally – and only have a minor tear – then you may not need stitching at all, and that tears heal better and faster.

Can I refuse to have an episiotomy?
Unless there are complications in the labour (see below), you should be able to choose whether or not you are prepared to have an episiotomy. A good midwife will always try to avoid having to perform one unless absolutely necessary – although many first-time mothers will be encouraged to have one if the perineum is not stretching easily. If you are strongly opposed to this, include your wishes in your birth plan (see p. 148), and tell your midwife. If medical staff still insist that an episiotomy is necessary, there is obviously a good reason for one, and it is advisable to follow their advice.

Is an episiotomy ever essential?
Where the baby is in the breech position and where an assisted delivery is necessary, whether by forceps or ventouse vacuum cup, an episiotomy is essential, and will have to to be carried out.

THE THIRD STAGE OF LABOUR

Q WHAT IS THE THIRD STAGE OF LABOUR?

A This stage starts immediately after your baby's birth and concludes with the delivery of the placenta, it can take as little as 15 minutes or last an hour or more.

Q WHAT HAPPENS DURING THE THIRD STAGE?

A A few minutes after the birth of your baby you will begin to have mild contractions, which you may hardly notice. Your midwife will ask you to give a little push to deliver the placenta while she pulls gently on the cord (see below).

Q IS IT NECESSARY TO ASSIST THE DELIVERY OF THE PLACENTA?

A With your consent, your midwife will inject syntometrine into your thigh during a contraction immediately after birth to speed up the delivery of the placenta; this is known as an "active" third stage (see below). It also reduces the risk of postpartum haemorrhage (see p. 190).

Q WHAT IS SYNTOMETRINE?

A This is a combination of the drug ergometrine, and the hormone oxytocin, which is used to induce labour (see p. 170). Oxytocin causes the womb to contract rapidly, and ergometrine prolongs the contraction. Syntometrine is usually safe, although it can make you feel nauseous because it causes the muscles of the womb to contract. You will be advised by your doctor to avoid having this injection if you have high blood pressure because it can aggravate your condition.

Q CAN THE PLACENTA BE DELIVERED NATURALLY?

A If you do not want to be injected with drugs to assist the delivery of the placenta, you can tell the midwife that you would like to have a natural third stage. This does mean, however, that the delivery of the placenta can take considerably longer than with an active delivery – sometimes up to an hour or more.

HOW IS THE PLACENTA DELIVERED?

It is usual for your midwife to deliver the placenta (see right). This will not cause you any pain, because the placenta is soft and comes away easily with a contraction.

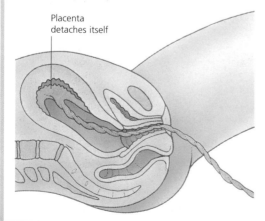

Placenta detaches itself

Speeding up the process

As soon as your baby is born, you are given an injection of a synthetic hormone called syntometrine in your thigh, which encourages the womb to contract and the placenta to detach itself from the womb wall; this can also reduce the risk of a haemorrhage occurring. When the womb has contracted to the size of a small melon and the placenta has peeled away, your midwife will place one hand on your abdomen and gently pull on the cord to ease the placenta out; you may be asked to give a little push at the same time. Your midwife will then feel your abdomen to ensure that your womb has contracted tightly into a ball.

WHEN THE PLACENTA HAS SEPARATED

A small gush of blood, and a lengthening of the cord between your legs indicates to your midwife that the placenta has separated from your womb wall.

Q HOW DO I SPEED UP THE THIRD STAGE WITHOUT USING DRUGS?

A You can try to speed up the process by getting your baby to suckle at your breast. This sucking action stimulates the release of oxytocin, the hormone in your body that causes your womb to contract, thereby encouraging the placenta to shear away from the womb wall. If you prefer, or if your baby doesn't suckle immediately, you can roll your nipples between your thumb and forefinger, which should have the same effect.

Q WHAT ARE THE RISKS OF DELIVERING THE PLACENTA WITHOUT DRUGS?

A There is a greater risk of you having a haemorrhage during a natural third stage because part of the placenta may remain in the womb, or the placenta may not separate from the womb wall. In these situations you will probably be given a general, epidural, or spinal anaesthetic and the placenta, or what remains of it will be removed. Occasionally, this happens in an active third stage of labour.

Q CAN COMPLICATIONS ARISE DURING THE DELIVERY OF THE PLACENTA?

A There are certain factors that can make the delivery of the placenta difficult, for example, a full bladder. This is usually solved by passing a catheter into your bladder to drain the urine. A more serious, but rare, problem is the presence of large fibroids obstructing the placenta. In this situation, you would probably be taken to the operating theatre to have the placenta removed under a general anaesthetic.

Q WHAT HAPPENS TO MY PLACENTA?

A Once your placenta has been delivered, your midwife will check it to make sure that it looks healthy, and that none of it is missing and has remained inside your womb. If there is no need to keep it for tests – and you do not wish to keep it for any reason – it will be disposed of by the hospital.

Q HOW MIGHT THE THIRD STAGE AFFECT ME?

A You will probably feel quite shaky after the birth of your baby and the delivery of the placenta. However, this is the point at which you can finally relax – you and your partner should be able to spend some quiet time together with the new addition to your family.

WHY MIGHT I NEED STITCHES?

Small tears, or cuts that only involve the skin of the vagina, will heal naturally and do not therefore require stitches. However, larger tears, especially those affecting the muscles around the vagina, will be stitched to ensure that they heal properly, and to prevent haemorrhage.

When will I be stitched?
If you are bleeding, you will be stitched as soon as the placenta is delivered, otherwise your midwife may leave you and your baby to rest first. Stitches are less painful if done straight after the delivery of the placenta; the longer you wait, the more painful the procedure can be; also, pain relief used in the delivery will be wearing off.

What is the procedure for stitching?
The tear or cut is repaired in layers: first, the vaginal skin is stitched, then the underlying muscle, and finally the perineal (external) skin. You will be given a local anaesthetic to numb the area; or your epidural will be topped up; you can also use gas and air. You will probably need to rest your legs in stirrups, however ungainly this may seem, because your legs will be very shaky after the delivery. It will take about half an hour to be stitched.

Will I need a catheter if I have stitches?
If the tear has affected your urethra, this can make it difficult to pass urine and you may therefore need a catheter. If you had an epidural, a catheter may be left in overnight or until feeling has returned to your bladder.

How long will the stitches take to heal?
Nowadays stitches that dissolve and fall out as you heal, are used. The area around your vagina has an excellent blood supply, so provided that no infections develop, the cut or tear should heal rapidly, leaving no scar.

How many stitches are normally used?
It is very difficult to be precise because the number of stitches depends on the length of the tear or cut. Technically, you will only have one stitch because they are made with one continuous length of material.

LABOUR AND BIRTH

AFTER YOUR DELIVERY

Q HOW WILL THE BIRTH OF MY BABY AFFECT ME?

A At last, the moment has arrived when you can greet the little stranger that you've carried around inside you for the past nine months. You may feel a sense of instant recognition; when you look at your baby in those first euphoric seconds, you may find yourself saying, "Oh, there you are!". Not everyone feels an immediate bond though; some women feel slightly detached at first, particularly after an exhausting and prolonged labour. This is also quite normal. You'll probably feel different after a rest or a good sleep.

Q WHAT HAPPENS IMMEDIATELY AFTER THE DELIVERY?

A You and your partner should be left alone for a short spell so that you can enjoy some precious time holding and getting to know your baby before he or she is weighed and checked. This is an ideal time to begin the bonding process (see below).

Q HOW LONG WILL I HAVE TO STAY ON THE LABOUR WARD?

A You will probably remain on the labour ward a few hours after the birth; if you need to have stitches, these will be done and, if possible, you can have a bath; you will then be moved to another ward. If you are only staying in hospital for a few hours, the paediatrician will check your baby.

Q WHAT WILL MY BABY LOOK LIKE AFTER THE BIRTH?

A Most babies look quite normal, but don't be surprised if your baby looks blotchy and wrinkled. Some babies have bluish fingers and toes as a result of initial circulation changes, but this is not serious. If your baby's head took a while to come through, it may look pointed, and the face can look blue and engorged; if the delivery was assisted, there may be marks on the face and head. With a breech birth, the bottom may be swollen or bruised. These marks will lessen in a few days.

ENJOYING THOSE FIRST MOMENTS

As soon as your baby is born, you and your partner will probably want to spend some quiet, private time to greet and to bond with your new arrival because your baby is already alert and responsive to your voices, smell, and touch.

The origins of bonding

"Bonding" was a revolutionary idea in the 1970s; research discovered that the most sensitive period for establishing contact with your baby is during the first hour of life. But if you are unable do this, remember that bonding is not some magical process that guarantees a lifetime of closeness. Indeed, before the idea was invented, generations of parents formed perfectly loving relationships with their children.

EVERYDAY CONTACT

As important as early bonding is the long-term daily contact of caring for, feeding, and loving your baby.

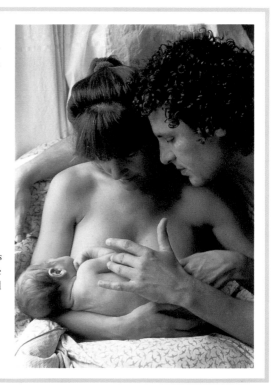

Q WHO CHECKS MY BABY?

A Your midwife and possibly a paediatrician will check your baby after the birth. The check is usually swift but thorough and it is carried out to establish that your baby is normal and to detect anything that is unusual or abnormal (see p. 204). Your baby will be weighed and his or her length measured. While doing this, the midwife will also observe your baby's colour, breathing, heart rate, muscle tone, and any delivery mark.

Q WILL I NEED ANY CHECKS OR TREATMENT IMMEDIATELY AFTERWARDS?

A Common problems in this early stage after giving birth include feeling dizzy, faint, and sick. Your blood pressure, temperature, and pulse rate will be recorded, and special attention will be paid to your bleeding, which will probably be very heavy. The midwife will feel your stomach to check that your womb is contracting well because a relaxed womb can lead to postpartum haemorrhage (see p. 190). You will be encouraged to pass some water in the first few hours, because a full bladder can also prevent your womb from contracting properly.

Q CAN I PUT MY BABY TO THE BREAST?

A Yes, you can. It may only be for a short while until you need to be stitched up but it is worth getting your baby to suckle as soon as possible; this helps you and your baby to bond, and also helps to stimulate the womb to contract down and expel the placenta. Feeding is not immediately possible if your baby needs to be given oxygen to help with breathing, or is taken to neonatal intensive care, or if you're still feeling sleepy after an anaesthetic.

Q HOW LONG WILL MY PARTNER BE ALLOWED TO STAY WITH ME?

A Your partner can stay with you while you're in the labour ward, but once you've been transferred to a post-natal ward, overnight visits aren't usually allowed. You should, in any event, encourage your partner to go home and get some rest, as he'll be feeling emotionally drained; this will also give you a chance to rest. You should also remember when considering visits from friends and family that you will be very tired and so don't be afraid to limit visits to a brief period, or perhaps ask people to wait until you are at home before they come to see you and your baby.

WHAT DOES AN APGAR SCORE ASSESS?

Within one minute of birth, a baby's well-being is assessed by five simple tests recorded by the doctor or midwife (see below). Called the Apgar score, this system evaluates a newborn's condition. Scores are given out of ten. An Apgar score of seven or over indicates a baby in good condition; a low score (between four and six) may mean that a baby needs help with breathing or resuscitation; under four means he or she could need lifesaving techniques. The tests are repeated five minutes later, when a score of seven or more indicates a good outlook. If the score is low, the baby needs monitoring.

INSTANT APPRAISAL

The Apgar score was developed by an American doctor, Virginia Apgar, for short-term diagnosis of a baby's physical condition straight after the birth. It is of little significance in terms of assessing a baby's long-term development, so don't worry if your baby had low scores but recovered within the next few minutes; he or she will almost certainly turn out to be normal and healthy.

SIGN	0	1	2
Heart rate	absent	slow	more than 100/minute
Breathing	absent	slow	good; crying
Muscle tone	limp	some tone	active motion
Response to stimulus	none	some response	sneezes or coughs
Colour of body	pale/blue	blue/pink	pink all over

WHAT CAN GO WRONG

Q WHAT PROBLEMS CAN OCCUR IN LABOUR?

A It should be said that most labours are quite straightforward but at any stage there may be complications – minor or major – that mean you or your baby require some form of medical help. Complications include a prolonged labour, unexpected bleeding during labour, premature labour or your baby becoming distressed.

Q CAN LABOUR TAKE TOO LONG?

A There are wide variations in the length of time labour takes; in fact, there is really no such thing as a "normal" length of time for labour. If it's your first labour it can last anything up to 20 hours (although this is unusual). If you are tired, the labour may be speeded up. There are also time limits for each stage to indicate when it seems necessary to lend a helping hand (see p. 172).

Q DOES LABOUR TAKE LONGER IF IT IS MY FIRST BABY?

A Yes, first labours are usually slower than subsequent ones. After you have been through one labour your womb muscles tend to be more co-ordinated, and your cervix dilates more rapidly. There is no known scientific explanation for this.

Q WHY DO SOME LABOURS TAKE LONGER THAN OTHERS?

A Labour can be slow for various reasons. The baby may be quite big, or his or her head may be in the wrong position (its back to your back, "OP" position, or sideways "OT" position, see p. 172). Your contractions may not be strong or co-ordinated enough to make labour progress efficiently, or it may be a combination of all these.

Q CAN ANYTHING BE DONE TO SPEED UP LABOUR IF IT IS GOING TOO SLOWLY?

A If your contractions are not powerful or regular enough, your midwife may rupture the membranes around your baby (see p. 176) to speed up contractions. If this doesn't work, you may be given a drip containing syntocinon (see p. 171). The drip is regulated according to the rate of your contractions.

Q HOW EFFECTIVE IS SYNTOCINON?

A Syntocinon simply performs the task of the hormone oxytocin, which regulates womb contractions, so as long as it is given carefully, it is considered very effective and safe.

Q IS IT USUAL TO BLEED DURING LABOUR?

A It is quite common to have a small amount of bleeding from your vagina during labour. As your cervix opens up (dilates), it bleeds slightly and as the membranes come away from the wall of your womb, this causes a small amount of bleeding. Too much bleeding, however, may suggest that there is a problem and will always be taken seriously by your midwife and obstetrician (see below).

Q CAN BLEEDING IN LABOUR BE SERIOUS?

A If there is severe bleeding in labour, this is called an antepartum haemorrhage and it may be coming from your placenta. If the placenta is "low" (near the cervix, known as placenta praevia, see p. 140) and you go into labour, it can cause heavy bleeding. (If it is so low that your baby can't pass it on the way down the birth canal, you may need a Caesarean delivery. You will have been told that this is a possibility when you had a scan.) Another cause of bleeding is when part of your placenta separates from the wall of your womb, known as placental abruption, which produces pain and bright red bleeding (see p. 140). This is also potentially dangerous and may mean that your baby needs to be delivered imminently, or that you need an emergency Caesarean delivery. Whatever the cause, the bleeding is coming from you, not from your baby.

Q WHAT IS MEANT BY FETAL DISTRESS?

A Fetal distress usually occurs when the blood flow from the placenta to your baby is reduced, so that your baby is not receiving enough oxygen. This may mean your baby will need to be delivered quickly. If it is severe, your obstetrician may decide to deliver your baby by a Caesarean.

Q HOW WILL THE DOCTORS KNOW THAT MY BABY IS IN DISTRESS?

A Your baby's heartbeat is monitored regularly during labour by using a CTG (see p. 168) and any changes in the rhythm will be picked up. If there are irregularities, or your baby's heart beats persistently fast or very slowly, it can mean that your baby is short of oxygen. Another common sign of distress is if your baby passes dark green "meconium"; this drains out of your vagina if your waters have broken (see p. 66). Serious signs of distress indicate that your baby must be delivered quickly and treated if necessary.

Q WILL MY BABY BE AFFECTED IF HE OR SHE BECOMES DISTRESSED?

A Many babies show some signs of distress in labour because the baby's body endures high levels of stress and pressure, but usually the baby's heart rate returns to normal or you give birth to your baby before serious problems develop. Very rarely, a severe lack of oxygen to the baby can result in brain damage; in extreme situations, oxygen deprivation can be fatal. However, your midwife and doctor are trained to identify the signs of fetal distress and to minimize the risk of any complications developing.

WHAT HAPPENS IF I GO INTO PREMATURE LABOUR?

In about five per cent of pregnancies, labour starts before 37 weeks of pregnancy. If your baby is born between 34 and 37 weeks of pregnancy, he or she should be fine and will probably not need special care after the birth. However, if you go into labour before 30 weeks of pregnancy, your baby is likely to be very immature and will need to be cared for in a neonatal intensive care unit or special care baby unit (see p. 228).

Why might labour start early?
Premature labour is more likely to happen if you have had a premature baby before, if you have an infection that is giving you a high temperature, if you are having a multiple birth, or if you are suffering from an infection in your womb.

Is the start of premature labour the same as normal labour?
Yes, often the signs are the same (see p. 166). However, if you are very early (24 to 28 weeks), it is possible that you will only feel low back pain and not experience proper contractions. If you do think your labour is starting early, contact your midwife or doctor immediately.

What can be done to stop premature labour?
Nothing can actually stop your labour once it is underway but your contractions can be temporarily slowed down with drugs called tocolytics. These are not very effective in the long term, and some have unpleasant side-effects, so in general they are not given to you for longer than 48 hours.

What else can the doctors do?
If there is any hint of infection, for example you have a high fever, they can give you antibiotics; if you are feeling very nervous, you may be given a mild dose of a pain reliever such as pethidine. If you become dehydrated, they might also put you on a drip. Often these measures alone can calm your contractions down.

Will the hospital be able to cope if my baby is born prematurely?
If your hospital's special care unit is unable to cope, either because there is no more room or because it does not have the proper facilities to look after premature babies, you and your baby will be transferred to a nearby hospital that has the necessary resources.

Will my premature labour be any different from a normal full-term delivery?
Yes, in general, a premature labour is faster than a full-term labour, because the baby is smaller.

Is there anything that can help to prepare my baby for premature birth?
As immature lungs cause the most problems for premature babies, you will be given a course of steroids 24 to 48 hours before delivery to improve your baby's chances. Steroids can be given to you via an injection or orally; these cross the placenta to your baby and help your baby's lungs to develop more rapidly. If doctors know that you have a high risk of delivering early, you may be given steroids every couple of weeks or so during pregnancy; this is perfectly safe for you and your baby.

BLEEDING AFTER BABY IS BORN

Q WHAT CAUSES SEVERE BLEEDING AFTER DELIVERY?

A Severe vaginal bleeding after a delivery (called post partum haemorrhage) occurs when your womb has not emptied completely and so cannot contract down tightly enough to stop the bleeding. It usually occurs because a small fragment of the placenta has been retained by the womb, or because the womb muscles are too tired to contract.

Q HOW COMMON IS POST PARTUM HAEMORRHAGE?

A Post partum haemorrhage is quite rare because your womb has a self-protecting device to stop it from bleeding. Once your baby has been born and the placenta has been expelled, your empty womb contracts down to the size of a grapefruit, quickly closing the uterine arteries so that they cannot bleed excessively.

Q WHAT CAN BE DONE IF I HAVE A HAEMORRHAGE?

A You will be given an injection that will help to expel the placenta and make your womb contract down tightly. If even after the injection the bleeding does not stop quickly enough, you may need an operation to clean out your womb under either a general or an epidural anaesthetic; you may also need a blood transfusion.

Q HOW LIKELY IS IT THAT I WILL NEED A BLOOD TRANSFUSION?

A Your chances of needing a blood transfusion are very low indeed, and an obstetrician will only suggest this if it is absolutely necessary – if you lose a lot of blood and your circulation is suffering, your blood pressure is dropping, and your pulse rate is increasing. In certain situations, a transfusion of blood can save your life, so it is unwise to refuse one.

HAEMOCHORIAL PLACENTATION

The design of the human placenta is unique, and is known as haemochorial placentation. The placenta is attached, like a pancake, to the inside of your womb (see below). Little fingers project out from the baby's side of the placenta (see inset diagram) with lots of branching blood vessels, containing baby's blood. These little fingers (known as villi) are bathed in blood from you. This blood circulates between the placenta and the inside wall of your womb. This allows waste products from the baby to pass into your circulation for removal, and nutrients and oxygen to pass from you to the baby, without your blood and the baby's ever mixing.

When the baby is born, your uterus will contract down and the placenta should shear off the wall of the womb and come out naturally. If the womb doesn't contract down, and/or the placenta does not detach properly, then there is a large raw surface in your womb. This is how the majority of post partum haemorrhages (PPHs) occur. There will be continued bleeding until the blood vessels are eventually "turned off" like taps by the muscle of the womb squeezing down making it into a ball.

THE AREA OF ATTACHMENT
A network of blood vessels connects the wall of the womb to the placenta, and consequently, if the placenta fails to detach completely or the maternal blood vessels do not close, there is a risk of bleeding.

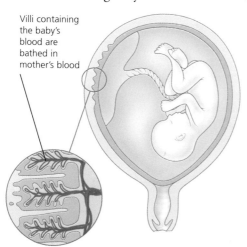

Villi containing the baby's blood are bathed in mother's blood

RARE COMPLICATIONS AT DELIVERY

Q CAN MY BABY'S SHOULDERS GET STUCK AT DELIVERY?

A This situation is, thankfully, very rare. Called shoulder dystocia, it occurs when the baby's head is delivered, but his shoulders get stuck behind your pelvic bones. It is more common with large babies, but some smaller babies also get stuck. The midwives and doctors will move quickly if this occurs and, in most cases, a few simple manoeuvres will allow your baby to be born. There is a potential risk of damage to the baby's bones or nerve fibres if these attempts at delivery are not successful.

Q I'VE HEARD THAT CLOTS IN THE LUNG CAN OCCUR AT DELIVERY. IS THIS TRUE?

A Being pregnant increases the risk of deep vein thrombosis (DVT) and pulmonary emboli (PEs). This risk is increased if you are overweight, smoke, have a Caesarean, or have prolonged bed rest. This is why you may be given compression stockings to wear after you've had the baby; these reduce the chance of blood clots developing in your calves. In some cases, low dose injections of blood thinning drugs such as heparin are given for a few days after your delivery; these reduce the risk of DVTs and blood clots travelling to the lungs (pulmonary emboli). Blood clots may occur at any time in pregnancy or afterwards, but the risk is probably greatest at delivery or within days of delivering your baby. So any calf pain, tenderness, or redness, especially if only on one side, should be reported to your doctor or midwife straight away.

Q HOW DO I KNOW IF I DEVELOP A CLOT IN MY LUNG (A PULMONARY EMBOLUS)?

A You would generally feel chest pain, usually one side or the other and worse when you breathe in, you may be a little short of breath and feel unwell. In extreme circumstances, your heart rate increases, you may become faint and unconscious, and you would need emergency treatment (oxygen and blood thinning drugs) and special tests (lung scans) to confirm the diagnosis.

Q WHAT IS AMNIOTIC FLUID EMBOLUS (AFE)?

A Amniotic fluid embolus (AFE) is an extremely rare condition that may occur in advanced labour or at the time of birth. It may be caused by amniotic fluid leaking into your bloodstream, causing an allergic reaction, making breathing difficult and upsetting your blood clotting system. It is very unpredictable and dangerous, but, thankfully, highly unlikely to occur.

Q I'VE HAD A CAESAREAN BEFORE – CAN MY SCAR RUPTURE AT NEXT DELIVERY?

A If you have a normal delivery following a Caesarean, then there is a small risk of the Caesarean scar rupturing. If it occurs before the baby is born, it will normally be recognized, because the baby's heart rate trace becomes abnormal. After the birth, heavy bleeding (post partum haemorrhage) and severe abdominal pain would warrant immediate investigation.

CAN BEING HIV POSITIVE AFFECT HOW MY BABY IS BORN?

There is good evidence that the combination of anti-HIV drugs in pregnancy, Caesarean birth, and not breastfeeding reduce the risk of your baby being affected to less than 5 per cent. Your baby has less chance of catching HIV if delivered by a Caesarean rather than vaginally because, as the baby makes its way down the birth canal, there is contact with your blood and fluids that may contain the virus. Therefore, any procedures that can cause contamination, such as fetal blood sampling in labour, are best avoided.

Physical contact
While you can cuddle and kiss your baby as much as you wish, it is important not to allow any of your blood to come into contact with him or her. Unfortunately, the HIV virus can also be transmitted by other body fluids, including breast milk, so you should not breastfeed.

Confidentiality
If you request it, the fact that you're HIV positive will not be written on your hospital notes and only those midwives and doctors specifically looking after you need to know that you are HIV positive.

WHAT IF MY BABY DIES?

Q HOW WOULD I KNOW IF SOMETHING IS WRONG WITH MY BABY?

A You may have obvious signs that something is not right, such as vaginal bleeding, cramps, an infection, abdominal pain, and reduced or absence of movements. If you feel that the baby's movements suddenly stop, or reduce, and then become absent for more than 12 hours, you should be checked out by your doctor. The indications that something is amiss will depend on how advanced your pregnancy is, but these signs cover a multitude of minor and major problems and do not automatically mean that something is seriously wrong with your baby.

Q HOW IS THE DIAGNOSIS OF STILLBIRTH MADE?

A Initially, the doctor or midwife will probably use a hand held Doppler device to listen for the baby's heart (this makes a "whooshing sound") to see if the baby's heart has stopped beating. If your doctor or midwife is unable to hear the baby's heart, normally the heart is checked again using an ultrasound scan.

Q IF I THINK SOMETHING IS NOT RIGHT, WHAT SHOULD I DO?

A Contact your doctor or midwife for advice. If you are less than 24 weeks, it is quite common not to feel movements all the time, and, because the baby is too premature to survive, delivery would not be an option. However, much of what you feel to be "wrong" may actually just be different and connected to normal pregnancy.

Q WHY DO BABIES DIE?

A There is no simple answer to this. Pregnancies that end in the first trimester may be nature's way of dealing with abnormality in the baby's chromosomes or development. This does not mean that future pregnancies will end the same way. There are many reasons for stillbirth later in pregnancy, but, unfortunately, sometimes no reason is found. Sadly, too many couples blame themselves when no medical answer can be found. Try not to go down this path – it is self-destructive, and will not help you to recover from your tragedy.

Q MY BABY IS DEAD. WHY DO I HAVE TO GO THROUGH A LABOUR?

A Your first thought may be "I want my baby to be delivered by Caesarean". Well, this is not recommended for two reasons. Firstly, there are always risks with an anaesthetic and any surgery. On top of the pain of losing your baby, you will have to cope with recovery from major surgery. Secondly, you need to go through the labour – your delivery is the start of the grieving process.

Q WHAT TESTS ARE DONE TO FIND OUT THE CAUSE OF STILLBIRTH?

A This varies from hospital to hospital, and country to country. Basic tests include blood tests to check whether you are diabetic, whether the baby's blood cells have entered your circulation, and to check for auto-antibodies that may have affected the baby or placenta. Swabs are taken to check for infection in you, the baby, or placenta, and chromosome tests may be taken from the baby. A post-mortem examination of the baby (autopsy) may give valuable information about whether there was anything wrong with the baby.

Q DOES OUR BABY HAVE TO HAVE A POST-MORTEM?

A You will most likely be offered this if your baby dies after 20 weeks. Do remember, however, that the post-mortem may be inconclusive, so try and be prepared for this eventuality. Your choices about exactly what happens at post-mortem, whether baby's organs are examined and/or retained, will be discussed with you. If a post-mortem is carried out, you may well be given the opportunity to see your obstetrician within weeks of the event to discuss the findings and tests that were done on you.

Q WHAT WILL HELP US TO COPE AT THIS DIFFICULT TIME?

A Your partner, relatives, and friends will be the mainstay. If you find that you can't talk to friends and family, there are organizations that offer support from others who have already been through a similar experience (see p. 256).

Q WHEN WILL WE GET OVER THE DEATH OF OUR BABY?

A Never. You will remember this baby for the rest of your life. The pain will ease, the anger fade, and eventually you will be aware of feeling life goes on. The time scale varies depending on your ability to put it in perspective, to cope and deal with the response of others, and on your ability to support each other.

Q WILL I BE FORCED TO LOOK AT MY BABY AND HOLD HIM IF I DON'T WANT TO?

A No, you won't be forced to do anything you don't want to do. Please, however, give it serious consideration. You need to say goodbye to your baby. Also, the majority of people assume that because the baby has died, he or she is going to look deformed. This is simply not true. Dead babies just look as though they are sleeping. It is important to see your baby and remember how he or she looked, not spend the rest of your lives imagining your child. The staff caring for you will be supportive and will probably be keen for you to look and hold your baby, take photographs, hair locks, and footprints/handprints. Most parents are, with hindsight, very grateful that they did all these things.

Q HOW AM I SUPPOSED TO FEEL IF MY BABY HAS DIED?

A There is no "supposed to". As for how you can expect to feel – devastated, guilty, angry, lonely, isolated, grief-stricken, resentful, bitter – these are all natural feelings. Talk – the worst thing you can do is bottle up your feelings. Your main problem may be the reaction of others – few people may be able to bring up words such as baby, dying, and death, because they don't want to upset you, and worry how you will cope if they do. It will be up to you, probably, to bring up the subject, and don't feel you have to be nice about it all the time – the anger at your loss must be included with all your other feelings.

Q WHAT CAN I DO TO HELP MY PARTNER?

A You will probably find that in the first few days or weeks you distance yourselves from each other on one level, as you try to work out why it happened. Grieving is a process that has stages. It is unlikely that you will both be in the same place at the same time initially. Be prepared for this and, hard as it will be, try to allow each other the space to feel the way you need to at that particular time.

FUNERAL ARRANGEMENTS

The following information may vary in specific details depending on where you live. If your baby was born, lived for a short while and then died, you will have to register a birth and a death. If your baby was born dead after 24 weeks, then your baby was stillborn and will need to be registered as such. The staff caring for you will discuss this and advise you as to what happens at your hospital. This traumatic process is normally helped by a midwife or bereavement counsellor.

At the hospital
You may wish to arrange a naming ceremony and funeral for your baby. Representatives of most religions are available in many hospitals and will be able to offer you advice. You have the right to bury or cremate your baby, but if you choose not to, the hospital will make arrangements to dispose of your baby's body in a respectful way. They will normally offer a non-denominational service every few months for babies that have lost their lives at, or before, birth, and you would be invited to attend this.

Dealing with undertakers
If you decide to arrange a funeral yourselves, undertakers are usually very accommodating in these circumstances and will not find your particular requests unusual. Some, usually known to the hospital, may have special expertise in babies and children that have died. The first thing to do is decide between you and your partner what you would like to happen, and then discuss it with the funeral directors and whoever is your contact at the hospital. Once you know what direction you want to go, things will become much more clear.

AN ASSISTED DELIVERY

Q WHAT IS AN ASSISTED DELIVERY AND WHY IS IT DONE?

A Instruments such as forceps or a ventouse cup (see below) may have to be used in the second stage of labour if the cervix is fully dilated but your baby fails to make good progress down the birth canal. An assisted delivery may also be needed if your baby's head is facing the wrong way and is wedged in your pelvis, or if your baby is large, or shows signs of distress and has to be delivered fast.

Q WILL THE MIDWIFE OR AN OBSTETRICIAN ATTEND IF I HAVE AN ASSISTED DELIVERY?

A If forceps or a ventouse vacuum cup need to be used, an obstetrician will usually deliver your baby. Your midwife will remain with you and will help the doctors with the procedure. Your obstetrician's experience and personal preferences will probably dictate whether he or she assists the delivery by using forceps or a ventouse vacuum cup.

WHAT DOES AN ASSISTED DELIVERY INVOLVE?

An assisted delivery is carried out if your labour is prolonged or if there is a delay in the second stage and you or your baby have become distressed. You may also need an assisted delivery if you have an epidural and cannot push properly, or to deliver a breech baby. Occasionally, forceps are used to deliver a second twin. Forceps or ventouse gently pull your baby out while you continue to push.

How are forceps used?
Forceps can only be used when the cervix is fully dilated and the baby's head is low in the pelvic outlet. There are various designs of forceps but all are based on the principle of two separate metal tongs that can be placed around the baby's head and linked together so that there is little pressure on baby's head. A type of forceps called Kielland's forceps is used to turn the baby when the head is in the wrong position for delivery. Forceps called Neville Barnes' (or Wrigley's) are used when the baby is facing the right way and needs lifting out.

How does a ventouse vacuum cup work?
Ventouse can only be used when the cervix is fully dilated and the baby's head low in the pelvic outlet. The principle for the ventouse cup is very simple: a plastic or a metal cup is placed over the baby's head; a tube runs from the cup to a machine that uses either an electrical mechanism or a pump to build up a vacuum in the cup. Once a good seal has been established on the baby's head, the obstetrician will gently pull on the cup while you continue to push, until the baby's head and body begin to emerge from the birth canal.

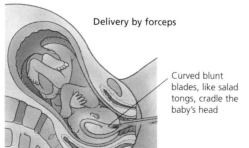

Delivery by forceps

Curved blunt blades, like salad tongs, cradle the baby's head

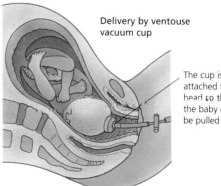

Delivery by ventouse vacuum cup

The cup is attached to the head so that the baby can be pulled out

Q HOW LONG HAVE THESE METHODS BEEN USED FOR DELIVERING BABIES?

A Forceps were invented in the sixteenth century by a British surgeon, a member of the Chamberlain family, who kept the method a closely guarded secret for over a century. The ventouse or vacuum cup is a more recent invention that became popular in the 1950s and 1960s.

Q HOW LONG DOES A FORCEPS OR VENTOUSE DELIVERY TAKE?

A The delivery itself rarely takes longer than ten minutes but it can take about 45 minutes to get you ready for the procedure. You may need an epidural or spinal anaesthetic, and you may be moved to a larger delivery room or operating theatre if a Caesarean delivery is necessary. You will also have to have a catheter tube inserted into your bladder to drain away any urine beforehand.

Q I'VE HEARD SO MANY STORIES ABOUT FORCEPS, ARE THEY TRUE?

A Such stories were associated with an early procedure called "high-forceps", which involved a doctor reaching up into the maternal pelvis to extract the baby, causing much pain and internal bruising. This method is no longer used. Now, forceps deliveries are undertaken only when the baby's head has descended well into the pelvis or is in the pelvic outlet. If the baby's head is not well positioned, a Caesarean section is carried out.

Q HOW MUCH PAIN WILL I FEEL WITH AN ASSISTED DELIVERY?

A You are usually given a spinal or epidural anaesthetic so that you feel little of what is going on. If you already have an epidural anaesthetic in position (see p. 162), it will be topped up, but if it is too late in the labour for you to be given an epidural, a local anaesthetic will be given to numb the perineum area. Rarely, a general anaesthetic is used.

Q WILL THE FORCEPS OR VENTOUSE LEAVE ANY MARKS ON MY BABY'S HEAD?

A Forceps may leave two bruises or red marks on either side of your baby's head, and ventouse commonly leaves a bump on top of the baby's head. The marks or bump should disappear within a few days, and the bruising within a week or so. Sometimes the swelling makes the head look elongated, but this isn't permanent.

Q WHAT IF MY BABY CAN'T BE DELIVERED BY FORCEPS OR VENTOUSE?

A If there is any question about whether the baby can be delivered vaginally, you will be taken to the operating theatre for what is known as a "trial of ventouse/forceps", to see whether a vaginal delivery is possible. If it is not, because your baby is in the wrong position, or is too large, a Caesarean will be necessary (see p. 196); if you are already in theatre, this can take place quite speedily.

HOW SAFE ARE ASSISTED DELIVERIES?

The use of instruments to deliver babies has been common practice for centuries and has undoubtedly saved babies who would otherwise have died in the birth canal. It is a very safe method of delivery as long as it is undertaken by competent doctors with the facilities to perform a Caesarean delivery, should the procedure fail.

Which method is safer for me?
Despite many clinical studies, no-one is absolutely certain which is the safer method for the mother – forceps or ventouse. The use of a vacuum cup can result in fewer tears and less need for an episiotomy than forceps, although it is perhaps more traumatic for your baby than a forceps delivery.

Your baby and forceps
With the blades acting as a protective "cradle", forceps are a little gentler on the baby's head as it descends through the birth canal. But if a delivery is particularly difficult, the nerves to the baby's arms may be temporarily damaged. Permanent damage is very rare, however, and the majority of babies are absolutely fine after a forceps delivery.

Your baby and ventouse
A ventouse vacuum extraction commonly leaves a swelling on the the top of the baby's head; this should, however, soon go down. A very large bump can sometimes turn into an extensive bruise and may even cause the baby to become jaundiced, but such complications are the exception rather than the rule.

A CAESAREAN BIRTH

Q WHAT IS A CAESAREAN BIRTH AND WHEN MIGHT I NEED ONE?

A A Caesarean birth is the delivery of your baby by an operation on your abdomen; instead of passing down your vagina, your baby is lifted out of your womb through your abdomen. You will have a Caesarean if your doctors decide that a normal vaginal delivery could threaten the health of you or your baby, or that it is impossible to achieve.

Q WHAT IS AN ELECTIVE CAESAREAN?

A An elective Caesarean is a planned procedure decided upon before you go into labour. There are a number of reasons why your doctor may suggest before labour that you should have a Caesarean, for example, if you have a medical condition, such as diabetes, or you are HIV positive. There are other conditions that indicate

that you will definitely need to have a Caesarean; these include severe cephalopelvic disproportion (CPD), where your baby is very large and your pelvis very small, or when the placenta is completely covering the cervix, known as placenta praevia (see p. 140).

Q WHEN IS AN EMERGENCY CAESAREAN NECESSARY?

A An emergency Caesarean takes place when a problem is discovered that threatens the life of the mother and/or her baby. This situation can arise before labour begins, for example, if you have an antepartum haemorrhage (see p. 188) or a cord prolapse, or otherwise an emergency Caesarean may be decided upon during labour if the mother's blood pressure becomes dangerously high, or if the doctors decide that the baby is in distress (see p. 188).

SOME COMMON WORRIES ABOUT CAESAREAN DELIVERIES

Do my doctors want me to have a Caesarean just because it's easier for them?
Obstetricians prefer normal deliveries because although Caesareans are safe, a vaginal birth is the safest, and you can recover more quickly. Caesareans are advised only if there is a valid medical reason.

If I have one Caesarean, will I ever be able to deliver vaginally?
About 75 per cent of women who have had a Caesarean can have a normal delivery with their next baby. Doctors used to worry that a Caesarean scar could rupture in subsequent labours, but this risk is now known to be low. However, you may have a very small pelvis or other condition that makes a Caesarean the safest option.

Will I be able to breastfeed?
Yes. However, if you have an elective Caesarean and are not in labour, it can take a little more time for your breasts to produce milk. Also, if you have a general anaesthetic, it will take a few hours for the drugs to be washed out of your body, so it is better for you to wait a while before feeding your baby.

My mother and sisters have had Caesareans, will I need one?
This is not usually the case unless all of your family are small, with small pelvic bones. Many quite short and slim women manage to have normal labours.

What if I need a general anaesthetic (GA)?'
A general anaesthetic is where you are put to sleep for the operation. You may feel "groggy" and sick for some hours as the general anaesthetic wears off, but many thousands of Caesareans are done every year under GA without a serious problem.

Will my baby have psychological problems if I cannot deliver him or her vaginally?
There is no evidence to suggest that this can affect your baby's psychological development. The best way for your baby to be born is the safest way, whether by a Caesarean or by a vaginal delivery.

Can I see my baby immediately after the birth?
Unless your baby needs to be taken to the special care baby unit (see p. 228) or you had a general anaesthetic, you can hold your baby straight away.

Q WILL I HAVE TO HAVE A GENERAL ANAESTHETIC IF I HAVE A CAESAREAN?

A It used to be common to have a general anaesthetic; but now you are likely to have an epidural or spinal anaesthetic (see p. 162). With an epidural, you are awake and can see and hold your baby when he or she is lifted out of your womb. You may feel sensations, but it is unusual to feel pain. With an emergency Caesarean, you will be given a general anaesthetic unless you had an epidural earlier.

Q HOW COMMON ARE CAESAREAN DELIVERIES?

A Caesareans are far more common today than they were 50 years ago. This is because techniques for this operation have greatly improved, and a Caesarean is now a very safe way for you to have your baby. In certain parts of Europe about 15 per cent of babies are currently born this way and the rate is even higher in certain parts of the US and South America.

WHAT HAPPENS DURING A CAESAREAN OPERATION?

You are prepared for a Caesarean by being shaved below the pubic hairline and given an epidural anaesthetic. An intravenous drip will provide you with fluids. Although this is a major abdominal operation, it is usually fairly quick, taking only about half an hour.

WHO CAN BE PRESENT
If you are awake, a screen will be set up so that you can't see the operation and, if your birth partner is squeamish, he or she can also sit behind the screen and remain with you without seeing the operation.

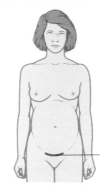

THE INCISION
A side-to-side cut is usually made below your shaved pubic hairline. This is better than an "up and down" incision from the navel downwards because it heals more quickly.

Horizontal incision

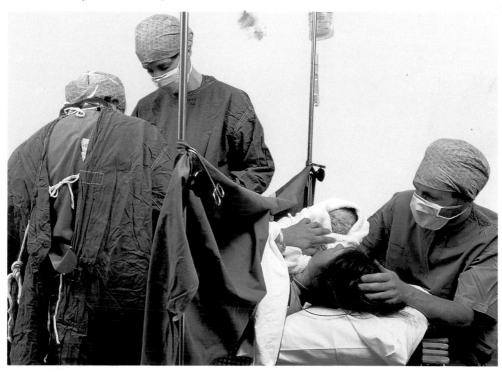

A BREECH BIRTH

Q WHAT IS A BREECH BABY?

A At around 32 to 34 weeks, most babies settle into position in the womb with their head down; this is called the cephalic position (see p. 67). If your baby is "breech" this means that your baby is bottom down inside your womb. If the baby stays in this position, this could cause complications during the birth, for example, if the baby's head becomes stuck during the second stage of labour (see box). You are therefore more likely to have a Caesarean delivery. As the pregnancy progresses, most babies turn and become head down; at term, only about three per cent of babies are still in the breech position.

Q WILL I NEED AN EPIDURAL?

A It is not essential but, because you may need an assisted birth or a Caesarean, your doctors may suggest an epidural so that you are already anaesthetized for these procedures.

Q WHICH IS SAFER FOR A BREECH BIRTH, CAESAREAN OR VAGINAL DELIVERY?

A A recent large study suggested that breech babies are delivered more safely by Caesarean section than by vaginal delivery. Almost certainly, this will result in far fewer vaginal breech births, and less experience in dealing with them amongst midwives and doctors.

HOW DOES A BREECH BIRTH DIFFER FROM A NORMAL ONE?

Breech deliveries are more complicated than cephalic ones, and therefore need experienced doctors and midwives. Recently, there has been a trend for breech babies to be delivered by a Caesarean and, therefore, there are now fewer staff who are experienced enough to deal with vaginal breech deliveries.

What are the problems?
The main potential problem with a vaginal breech delivery is that your baby's head may become stuck in the pelvis in the second stage of labour, depriving your baby of oxygen, which increases the risk of fetal distress. Your labour may also be slower because your baby's head isn't pushing down on the cervix, and there is a higher risk of tears or bleeding occurring.

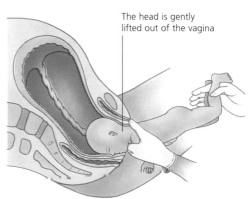

The baby's body is carefully supported

The head is gently lifted out of the vagina

DELIVERING YOUR BABY'S BODY
With a breech delivery, your baby's buttocks will be delivered first and then the legs will emerge. You may need an episiotomy before the head is delivered.

DELIVERING YOUR BABY'S HEAD
Once the rest of the body is delivered, the head will be drawn down the vagina and, at this stage, forceps can be used to complete the delivery.

TWINS AND MULTIPLE BIRTHS

Q HOW DOES A TWIN DELIVERY DIFFER FROM THE DELIVERY OF ONE BABY?

A A twin delivery, like a twin pregnancy, is "high risk" so you will be delivered in hospital by one or more obstetrician, two paediatricians, and probably two midwives. Athough many twin deliveries do proceed without any complications, there is a higher chance that the birth will need assistance with forceps, or ventouse (see p. 194), or that you will have a Caesarean delivery (see p. 196).

Q WHO WILL DELIVER MY BABIES?

A With a normal vaginal delivery, the midwife can deliver your babies with an obstetrician in attendance. If there are complications, the obstetrician will probably deliver your babies or carry out a Caesarean section.

Q WILL I NEED TO HAVE AN EPIDURAL WITH TWINS OR TRIPLETS?

A This is not obligatory but sometimes it is advisable because, should you need help in the second stage of labour (such as forceps or ventouse or a Caesarean), your pain relief will be in place and the delivery will not be further delayed.

Q ARE THERE LIKELY TO BE PROBLEMS WITH THE SECOND TWIN'S DELIVERY?

A After your first baby is born, your contractions may die away and there may be a pause before they pick up again, delaying the birth of your second baby. If this wait seems to be over-long, you may be given a drug called syntocinon (see p. 170) to increase the regularity and strength of your contractions. Once this baby is coming down the birth canal, the waters are broken to speed up the delivery.

Q I'M EXPECTING TRIPLETS, WILL I NEED TO HAVE A CAESAREAN?

A Yes, a Caesarean is the least traumatic way for triplets to be delivered. This is because the babies may be in an awkward position, or are premature and very small and therefore unable to cope with the extra strains involved in a normal vaginal birth. They will also probably need special paediatric care after the delivery.

PRESENTATION OF TWINS

The position of your twins can influence the kind of delivery you will have. If both twins are in the same position, the outcome is much easier to predict. In some rare circumstances, the first twin may have a vaginal delivery, but your second twin may be breech or get distressed and have to be delivered by emergency Caesarean section.

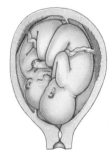

CEPHALIC TWINS (left)
With this presentation a vaginal delivery may be possible for both babies.

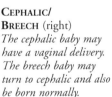

CEPHALIC/ BREECH (right)
The cephalic baby may have a vaginal delivery. The breech baby may turn to cephalic and also be born normally.

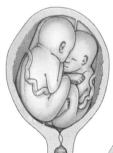

BREECH TWINS (left)
With both babies feet down there is a strong chance of a Caesarean.

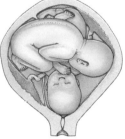

CEPHALIC/ TRANSVERSE (right)
Both babies are delivered by a Caesarean.

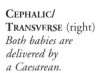

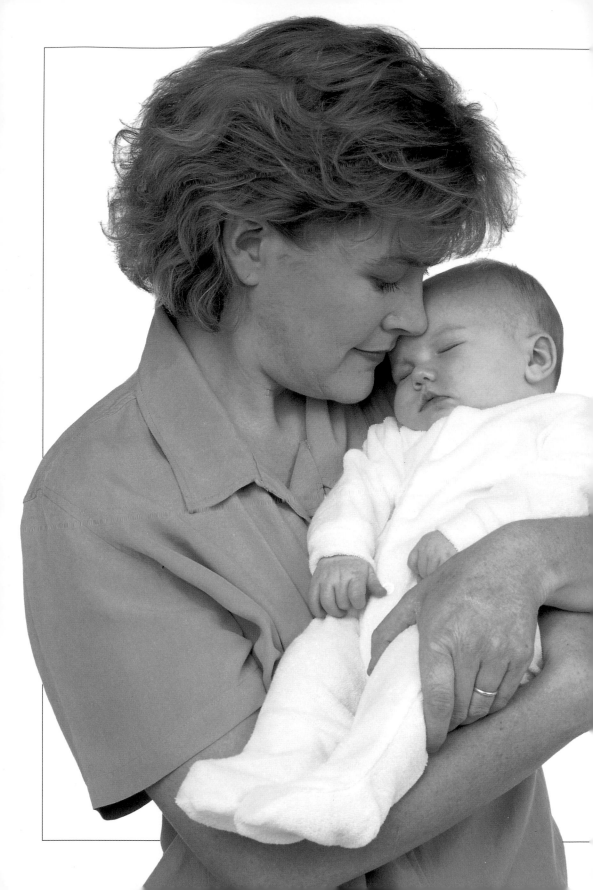

THE
FIRST SIX
WEEKS

A baby to hold, love, and care for is all a parent-to-be longs for – but you are now responsible for this tiny new life and this can seem daunting at first. The baby's arrival will change your lives forever – but few would ever consider that the hard work, lack of sleep, and the ever-present demands of their baby were not worth it. As well as answering your questions about your own recovery and the well-being of your newborn, including problems with post-natal depression, premature babies, or babies needing surgery, this chapter offers practical advice and reassurance to help you and your partner find your feet during the first few weeks following the birth.

YOUR FIRST 48 HOURS

Q WHAT CAN I EXPECT TO HAPPEN IN THE FIRST FEW DAYS?

A In the first 48 hours, your biggest concern will probably be about how tired and sore you feel. You may also feel relief and euphoria that it is all over (see below). Your baby will probably sleep a great deal at first, so make the most of this and catch up on your rest. If you had a home birth, you will be able to relax in your own familiar surroundings and your midwife will come back to see you twice a day for the first few days.

Q CAN I DRESS MY BABY, AND WHAT KIND OF NAPPY SHOULD I USE IN HOSPITAL?

A Most hospitals are agreeable to your bringing your own baby clothes. You can dress your baby in these as soon as you feel up to it. If you do not feel up to par, the midwife will offer to dress your baby. In these first few days, and particularly in hospital (where there are no clothes washing facilities), most women opt for disposable nappies.

Q HOW OFTEN DOES MY BABY NEED TO BE FED?

A It is common for babies to feed little in the first 48 hours because they are quite sleepy; some forms of pain relief (pethidine and other opiates) given to you before delivery can cross the placenta and make a baby even more sleepy. If your baby sleeps for much of the time, wake him or her up every four hours or so to feed, particularly first thing in the morning. Your baby may want to suckle frequently, probably more for comfort than from hunger. If you are bottle-feeding, feed about every three to four hours.

Q HOW MUCH WILL MY BABY TAKE IN AT EACH FEED?

A If you are breastfeeding, your baby will need relatively little of the pre-milk (colostrum) that comes in the first two days, because it is so rich and high in protein. If bottle-fed he or she will need more feeds as the food will be less rich.

HOW YOU FEEL EMOTIONALLY

Nothing quite prepares you and your partner for the mixed emotions and sudden mood swings that you will experience during the first few days after the birth of your child. One minute you feel on top of the world, and the next exhausted and tearful. The arrival of a new baby creates conflicting feelings of joy, responsibility, and pride, possibly even fear. Or you may feel so overwhelmed by the whole event that you experience a sense of anticlimax. After a painful labour, you may feel resentful and detached – this too is quite common. Just remember that you have done an amazing thing – brought a new life into being.

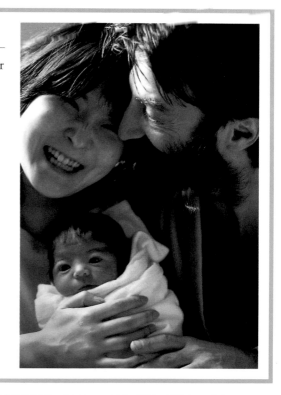

NOW COMES THE JOY
Who would have thought that such a small bundle could bring such joy and wonder to you both.

What can I expect to happen in hospital?

When you stay in hospital after the birth, your midwife accompanies you to the post-natal ward where you will be welcomed by the ward staff and made comfortable in a bed with your baby beside you.

Can my partner come in to see me at any time?
Every hospital has its own visiting hours but these do not usually restrict partners from visiting from morning until late at night. Most hospitals will not allow partners to stay overnight because they do not have the accommodation facilities.

How is my baby identified?
Your baby will have one name band around one wrist, and another one around an ankle. The details on the bands will include the baby's name and hospital number, and the date and time of birth. When the time comes to remove the bands, keep one as a memento, because later, when your baby has grown, you will be able to see just how tiny he or she was.

Will I have to adapt to the routine of a post-natal ward?
Most hospitals have a set ward routine that may not allow for as much rest as you would like, unless you have a private room where you may not be quite so aware of it. Your day can begin as early as 6.30am, and each day might seem like an endless round of feeding, changing, checks, and visits from doctors and other staff, as well as from family and friends. Try not to let the first few days with your baby be marred by these irritations. Some ward sisters will try to be flexible if certain routines really don't suit you – ask.

I need a good night's sleep but can't stay asleep for long. Why?
Apart from a crying baby, there are several possible reasons for this: first, you may still be on an adrenalin "high" from the delivery and need to calm down; you are finding that the hospital ward is too strange or noisy at night for you to get unbroken sleep; or you may unconsciously fear sleeping too deeply in case your baby needs you. Talk to your midwife or doctor if you feel that this lack of sleep is becoming a problem. You should also try to take naps during the day while your baby is asleep.

This is my first baby – how do I begin?
First, don't compare yourself with the more experienced mothers, or feel inadequate when you see the confidence with which other women handle their babies. The nurses and midwives will help you to feed and change your baby and you will be able to ask them questions; you should find them supportive rather than critical. There's much to be said for the companionship that exists between mothers in maternity wards; you can share your worries, experiences, and observations, as well as form lasting friendships. All hospitals show new mothers how to "top and tail" their babies (see p. 212), bath them, and make up feeds.

How long do I have to stay in hospital?
Doctors used to think that long stays in hospital were essential, but it is now recognized that a woman with an uncomplicated delivery does not need to stay in for long: two to five days is standard for a first baby; some systems allow you to go after six hours. If you're anxious to get home, and feel that you and your baby are well, then discuss the possibility of an early discharge with your midwife. When it is agreed that you can go, your baby will be examined by a paediatrician. This is a routine part of the discharge procedure and does not mean that anything is wrong.

Why am I so anxious about going home with my new baby?
Taking a newborn baby home for the first time can be a stressful experience. Before leaving the hospital, make sure that you are happy about dealing with basic babycare; if there's anything you're not sure about, ask your midwife. You'll need suitable outdoor clothing for you and your baby to travel home in. At home, there should be a supply of nappies and other basic needs (see p. 210). It is a good idea to have someone – either your partner, your mother, an aunt, or a friend – available to help you for at least the first few days, and preferably for longer.

Should I inform my doctor that I'm leaving hospital?
This isn't necessary; the hospital sends your doctor a summary of your labour, delivery, and subsequent recovery and discharge. He or she will probably visit you at home.

YOUR NEWBORN BABY

The labour is over and you are holding the baby you have dreamed about for so long. But your baby's appearance may be a shock. Instead of the beautiful baby you imagined, your baby emerges with visible signs of the birth, from bloody hair and minor bruising to blotchy, wrinkled skin; it takes a little time for your baby to "smooth out" and become a perfect baby. Your baby will be checked for any problems (see opposite).

WHAT MIGHT MY BABY LOOK LIKE?

As well as being covered with blood and vernix, your baby may be bruised and marked from the birth, especially if a fetal scalp electrode was attached or forceps were used. The skin can be an alarming, dull bluish-grey in the first minutes after the birth, but soon becomes pinker. Add to this a red, wrinkled face, and a strangely shaped head from the pressure of birth, and you have a realistic picture of a newborn. The body's systems are not effective yet, so you will notice blotches, and colour changes that may worry you, but are perfectly normal. Most blemishes will disappear by the time your baby is two weeks old.

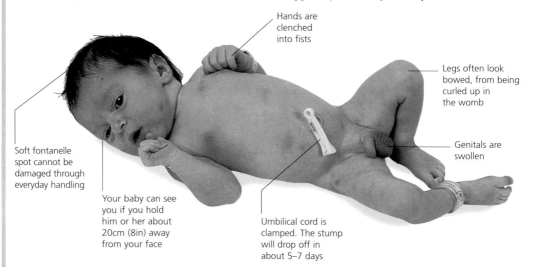

Hands are clenched into fists

Legs often look bowed, from being curled up in the womb

Soft fontanelle spot cannot be damaged through everyday handling

Your baby can see you if you hold him or her about 20cm (8in) away from your face

Umbilical cord is clamped. The stump will drop off in about 5–7 days

Genitals are swollen

The head
Pressure exerted during the birth can distort the shape of the head for the first two weeks. The bones of the soft spot (fontanelle) on the top of the head have not yet knitted together; this will not happen until about 18 months.

The hands and feet
If your baby's circulation is slow to start, the hands and feet may appear bluish, but should turn pink if you move your baby into another position. Fingernails can be long at birth.

The eyes
Blue at birth; true eye colour may not develop until your baby is six months old. Puffy eyelids are caused by the pressure of birth, and squinting is common. Your baby may even look cross-eyed at times in the first months.

The skin
The thick white grease (vernix) that protected the skin in the womb is absorbed or rubbed off. Spots, rashes, and dry skin should clear naturally. Body hair (lanugo) rubs off within two weeks.

The breasts
Your baby's breasts may be swollen and even leak a little milk. This is perfectly normal in both sexes. The swelling should go down within two days. Do not try to squeeze the milk out.

The genitals
Swollen genitals are common in both sexes. A baby girl may have vaginal discharge but this should soon disappear. The testicles of a baby boy are often pulled up into his groin and will descend later.

WHAT IS THE DOCTOR LOOKING FOR?

A doctor will examine your baby from head to toe at least once during the first six days. As well as checking for any physical abnormalities, the doctor looks for signs of infections or other problems.

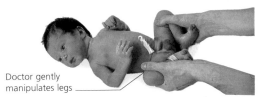

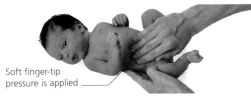

Doctor gently manipulates legs —————

HIPS
The hips are checked for signs of dislocation by bending the legs up and gently swivelling them.

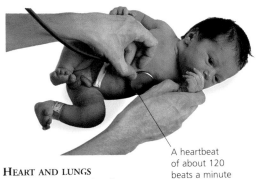

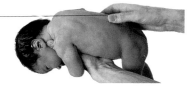

Soft finger-tip pressure is applied —————

ABDOMINAL ORGANS
The abdomen will be gently palpated so that the size of the abdominal organs can be checked.

HEART AND LUNGS
A stethoscope is used to listen to the heart and lungs.

A heartbeat of about 120 beats a minute is normal

Any spinal problems can be detected at this stage —————

The Guthrie test
Seven to ten days after the birth, a blood sample is taken by pricking your baby's heel. The sample is tested for phenylketonuria (a rare cause of mental handicap) and for thyroid deficiency.

SPINE
The doctor will run his thumb along the length of the back to check that the vertebrae are in the correct place.

WHAT CAN MY BABY DO?

Although newborn babies are entirely dependent on an adult for food and warmth, they are not completely helpless: they can breathe for themselves, cry to get your attention, grasp with their fingers and toes, see your face at close range, and hear and possibly distinguish your and your partner's voice from other voices. Newborn babies are not, however, able to control their bodily functions.

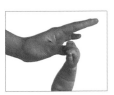

GRASP REFLEX
A newborn's grasp can be tight enough to support his or her whole weight – although you should never try this.

Hands reach out as if to catch hold of something —————

STEPPING REFLEX
Your baby will perform a walking action when supported under the shoulders in an upright position, feet touching a firm surface.

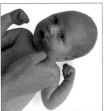

ROOTING REFLEX
Stroke your baby's cheek and he or she will turn towards your finger, mouth open and ready to suck.

STARTLE REFLEX
If you let your baby's head flop back, he or she will think they're falling and stretch out their arms and legs.

Reflex stepping movements

THE FIRST SIX WEEKS

YOUR RECOVERY

Q WHY DOES BREASTFEEDING GIVE ME STOMACH PAINS?

A You are probably experiencing afterpains, firm contractions of your womb that feel like period pains. Afterpains are more pronounced during breastfeeding because nipple stimulation provokes the release of oxytocin – the hormone that causes contractions. These contractions mean that your womb is shrinking and returning to its normal position in your pelvis. For severe spasmodic cramps, you may need to take pain relievers before starting to breastfeed.

Q I HAVEN'T HAD A BOWEL MOVEMENT SINCE THE BIRTH – IS THIS A PROBLEM?

A Many women find that they cannot open their bowels for three to four days after delivery. This is normal: you probably passed some motions while in labour, and haven't had much to eat since the birth. If you're concerned about being constipated, increase the fibre content in your diet.

Q WILL A BOWEL MOVEMENT TEAR MY STITCHES?

A If you are scared to go to the lavatory because you're worried about tearing your stitches, try to relax – your stitches are tough enough to cope with bowel motions. Ask your doctor or midwife to prescribe a soothing cream or some pain relievers to help with any discomfort. You could also try making a pad of toilet tissue and supporting your vaginal area with this during your bowel movement – it will give you reassurance that your stitches are not about to burst.

Q I'M PASSING A LOT OF BLOOD SINCE THE BIRTH, IS THIS NORMAL?

A The bleeding that you see after the delivery is lochia that is discharged via your vagina as your womb contracts. For the first few days or weeks, the lochia is heavily bloodstained, and thereafter, over the following few weeks, it becomes pinkish and finally colourless. Occasionally, you may pass blood clots in the first day or so; bring this to the attention of your midwife as it sometimes means that a small piece of placenta or membrane is left behind in your womb. Usually, however, this settles on its own.

POST-NATAL CHECKS

Whether at home or at hospital, your post-natal check will be carried out by a midwife. She will ask you questions and examine you to confirm that you are recovering from the birth, that you show no signs of infection (for example in your womb or breasts), and that you are well emotionally. Initially, the checks will be daily, whether at hospital, or at home, and your progress written on a record sheet. If you had forceps, ventouse, or Caesarean delivery, or a medical problem, such as high blood pressure, a doctor will check your recovery during routine rounds.

What do the checks entail?
■ You will be asked questions about your breasts, your bleeding (lochia, see below, left), how you feel, if you are passing water and have good bowel movements, how your stitches feel, your contraceptive plans, and any worries you have.
■ Your breasts, nipples, and womb will be examined, your stitches looked at, your legs checked for swelling, and your temperature as well as your pulse and blood pressure taken.
■ Your haemoglobin level and, if necessary, your immunity to rubella will be checked.

Problems to look out for
■ You have a temperature soon after delivery.
■ You experience pain on passing water, or if your bleeding smells odd.
■ You have a persistent gush of heavy bleeding.
■ You feel faint and fall over, or lose consciousness for a few seconds.
■ You can't pass urine despite feeling really uncomfortable, as if your bladder is too full.
■ You feel breathless or develop chest pain.
■ Your calf or leg becomes tender and/or swollen.
■ You are concerned about your baby.
■ Your breasts are particularly painful and engorged (mastitis).

Q WHY IS MY ABDOMEN STILL LARGE AND MY HANDS AND FEET STILL SWOLLEN?

A Your baby was only part of your overall weight gain in pregnancy; you also gained extra fat and probably have significant fluid retention – which is why your fingers, toes, and possibly legs are still swollen. This swelling (called "oedema") can last for several days but it will go down gradually as you pass more urine. To speed up this process, try to rest with your feet up whenever possible, and avoid standing for long periods.

Q IS IT NORMAL TO HAVE A HEADACHE AFTER AN EPIDURAL?

A You may get a mild headache after you've had your baby, but there is no concrete evidence as to whether this is due to the epidural or the delivery itself. Very rarely, you may get a severe headache because the epidural needle has made a hole in the thin membrane of the spinal cord, and caused a leakage of cerebrospinal fluid (CSF). This is not dangerous, but it is uncomfortable. It is known as a "spinal" or "epidural" headache.

Q WILL I NEED TREATMENT FOR A SEVERE EPIDURAL HEADACHE?

A You will be advised to lie flat, drink plenty, and take a recommended dose of pain relievers, such as paracetamol, for at least two days, while the hole heals itself. If the symptoms are severe, an anaesthetist may perform a simple procedure called a "blood patch". Using a needle, he or she will squirt a few drops of your blood into your spine where the hole is; this forms a clot and plugs the hole. Recovery is normally rapid and complete after this.

Q DO I HAVE TO HAVE A CATHETER IN AFTER AN EPIDURAL?

A If you have had a catheter inserted into your bladder during the epidural (see p. 162), it stays in for a few hours after the epidural is removed. This allows time for the nerve supply to your bladder to return to full working order; while these nerves are still numb, you can't tell whether or not your bladder is full, so the bladder may get distended and damaged. Once the epidural stops working, you should urinate within a few hours.

AFTER A CAESAREAN BIRTH

When can I go home after a Caesarean?
The normal length of stay in hospital after a Caesarean is five to seven days, but you may be able to go home earlier. Ask your midwife or doctor about this. After six to seven days, your stitches will be removed by your community midwife at your home. While the removal of stitches is not painful, it may be uncomfortable.

What kind of discomfort might I experience?
Your first few attempts at getting out of bed and walking around will be painful, and you may feel dizzy, but don't give up – the more you try, the sooner you will be able to move around without any assistance. Although you will not be able to lift your baby straight away, you can cuddle and breastfeed by placing a pillow on your lap to support your baby (see p. 216). It may take a few days before you have a bowel movement, and you may suffer with trapped wind, which can cause considerable discomfort as it presses against your incision line. The best solution is to pass as much wind as possible to reduce this discomfort. Coughing can also hurt a lot.

Why are there lumps on my scar?
The skin around your incision line can feel quite lumpy for days, or maybe even weeks, after a Caesarean operation. These lumps will eventually become bruises and the skin will return to normal. The lumps are caused by slight bleeding under the skin after the operation.

Why is the skin around my wound numb?
Small nerves just beneath your skin were cut during the operation, and this causes numbness just around the scar. These nerves will grow back over the next couple of months, and normal sensation will return.

How can I look after my wound at home?
Just keep your wound dry and ventilated; it may leak a little in the first few days, but this is nothing to be concerned about. You can bathe once the dressing has been removed by your doctor, but dry the wound with a separate clean towel. If the scar becomes tender or red, show this to your midwife or doctor, because you may have developed a mild infection that needs antibiotics.

AT HOME WITH YOUR BABY

Q HOW AM I GOING TO COPE WITH MY FIRST FEW DAYS AT HOME?

A It's only natural to feel anxious about your new responsibilities when you arrive home with your new baby. Your midwife will visit you for ten days, to help with any babycare problems. You're obviously not going to be able to run the home in your normal way for a few weeks or months – your main priority is to look after yourself and your baby. Don't struggle on with the day-to-day domestic chores at the expense of your own well-being. Get help. If your partner is entitled to some paternity leave he may be able to help you for a week or two, or perhaps your mother or a friend can stay for a while.

Q MY BABY WAS WEIGHED TODAY AND HAS LOST WEIGHT – IS THIS NORMAL?

A This is entirely normal. If you think of the tiny amounts your baby has eaten, and of the contents of all those nappies, it is not surprising that your baby has lost weight. Newborn babies are expected to lose up to ten per cent of their birth weight in the first few days after delivery. Your baby should regain this lost weight and will probably be back to his or her birth weight by about ten days after the birth.

Q MY BABY VOMITED BITS OF DRIED BLOOD AFTER FEEDING – IS THIS SERIOUS?

A What you are seeing is mucus mixed with blood from the delivery which your baby has swallowed and cannot digest. The best thing for your baby to do is to bring it up. Try to feed your baby again and tell your midwife about the incident. Sometimes the midwife will suggest a "stomach wash-out", which involves her running warmed sterile water through a tube into the baby's stomach to bring out any residue of mucus or blood that may be lying there.

Q WHEN I CHANGED MY BABY'S NAPPY, IT WAS STAINED PINK – IS THIS BLOOD?

A Pink stains are simply the urates (acids in the urine), which a newborn baby passes at first and this is quite normal. However, blood in the urine is very uncommon and should always be reported to your doctor.

POST-NATAL VISITS AND CHECKS

What the midwife does
A community midwife will be given details of your discharge from hospital and she then has a legal obligation (in the UK) to visit you and your baby at home for at least ten days after your delivery. The midwife's role after the birth is to establish that you are recovering from the birth and that your baby is thriving.

Your baby's health checks
The post-natal checks establish that your baby is well or pick up any problems. The midwife asks about your baby's feeding, sleeping, and toilet habits and will weigh your baby at regular intervals (see below); she will also check on the umbilical cord and any delivery marks.

Looking after your baby
Ask the midwife questions about your baby, or about any aspects of babycare, from sterilizing your feeding equipment to what type of nappies to use and how often to feed your baby. Your midwife will also show you how to bath and top and tail your baby if needed.

How often should my baby be weighed?
The usual practice is for your midwife to weigh your baby about three times a week for the first two weeks. Because babies lose and regain ten per cent of their birth weight during the first ten days after the delivery, your midwife may not be concerned with the baby's weight gain as long as he or she is feeding well, until after ten days.

Should my baby be given vitamin K?
Yes, because newborn babies are low in vitamin K and this helps blood clot and protects against haemorrhage (especially into the brain). Vitamin K can be given by mouth or injection but if you had a forceps, ventouse or Caesarean delivery, or gave birth prematurely, your baby should be given the injection. Earlier concerns of a link between the vitamin K injection and childhood cancer are almost certainly unfounded.

Q MY BABY'S BOWEL MOTIONS ARE GREENISH-BLACK – IS ANYTHING WRONG?

A Your baby is completely normal! The first few bowel movements are made up of "meconium", the sticky, dark substance that lined your baby's bowel during the pregnancy and is now being excreted. This may take up to 48 hours to pass through, after which your baby's motions will be more solid, and yellow in colour.

Q HOW OFTEN SHOULD MY BABY PASS URINE AND EMPTY HIS OR HER BOWELS?

A How much a newborn baby urinates can vary considerably but as long as it happens at least once every 24 hours all is well. Usually, however, because their bladders are so tiny, newborns tend to urinate every hour. Bowel movements also vary greatly but again should occur at least once a day. It may be that your baby had a big bowel movement just before, during, or just after birth and so may not need to have another bowel movement for some time. The first bowel movement is significant because it confirms that the anus is open. The same goes for urinating; it shows that the baby's kidneys, bladder, and all the other plumbing are working properly.

Q WHEN WILL MY BABY SETTLE INTO A ROUTINE?

A You will end up feeling very frustrated if you try to make your baby conform to a set pattern at this stage. Just go with the flow in these early days, taking each very different day as it comes. Old-fashioned ideas of imposing discipline and a routine on very young babies serve no real purpose and usually fail. Babies have different sleep patterns (see p. 214); some sleep for long periods of time, others sleep fitfully, but after a few weeks or months a sleeping and waking pattern will gradually emerge.

HANDLING YOUR NEWBORN

You may be afraid to handle your newborn baby at first because he or she seems so small. The important thing is to support the baby's head, because the neck muscles are still quite weak. Because it is reassuring and helps you to develop a relationship with your baby, talk to your baby when changing a nappy or giving a bath. You will soon gain enough confidence to be able to relax when handling your baby.

PICKING UP YOUR BABY

Carefully slide your hands under your baby's head and bottom

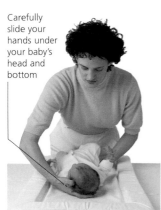

Gently support your baby's head in your hand

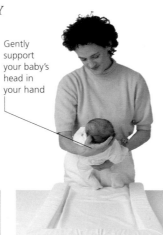

Cuddling your baby will stop him or her crying

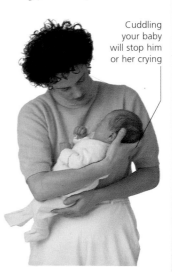

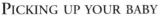

1 Lift your baby by placing one hand under the head and one under the bottom.

2 Lift slowly and gently while supporting your baby's body and head with each hand.

3 Turn your baby so that the head and the back are supported by your arms.

CARING FOR YOUR BABY

Q HOW CAN I MAKE SURE THAT MY BABY IS COMFORTABLE AND CONTENT?

A Your baby has simple, but time-consuming needs during the first few weeks of life. Making sure that your baby is warm, comfortable, and satisfied will keep him or her content. You'll be feeding and holding your baby constantly, and spending a lot of time changing nappies after feeds, when your baby wakes, and before your baby sleeps. These basic tasks can be enjoyable for both of you if you play games, chat to, and cuddle your baby as you do them.

Q I DON'T LIKE TOUCHING MY BABY'S CORD, DO I HAVE TO CLEAN IT?

A Your baby's cord will dry up, wither, and drop off naturally about five to seven days after the birth. However, keep the cord as dry as possible, even if you do not actively clean it: make sure that the nappy isn't covering the cord and dry the cord thoroughly after bathing your baby. Some midwives recommend applying surgical spirit or antiseptic powder, or give you sterile swabs to clean it. If the cord or navel area gets swollen, red, smelly, or weepy, tell your midwife or doctor.

ESSENTIALS FOR YOUR NEWBORN BABY

Preparing for the arrival of your baby can be one of the most enjoyable parts of your pregnancy, as you shop for clothes and equipment. Remember, when buying baby clothes, that your baby will grow quickly, so buy only a few of the smaller sized items to begin with. Below are some suggestions for the basic items you will need.

PRACTICAL ITEMS

■ Several packs of disposable nappies (or 2 dozen towelling nappies with plastic pants and liners, 2 nappy buckets and sterilizing powder, and some safety pins)
■ Barrier cream (e.g., zinc and castor oil or petroleum jelly)
■ Plastic changing mat
■ Cotton wool
■ Baby soap/shampoo/liquid soap/baby lotion/oil (for dry skin)
■ Waterproof apron
■ Baby bath
■ Sponge/flannel
■ Large, soft towel
■ Baby brush

Shaped fabric nappy

Cotton wool

Cream

Disposable nappy

SLEEPING

■ Cot or Moses basket
■ Cot and mattress (when your baby is older)
■ 4 cotton sheets for cot/pram
■ 2 soft, lightweight blankets
■ Baby alarm (optional)

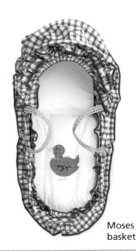
Moses basket

CLOTHES

Choose machine-washable clothes in natural fabrics
■ 4 stretchsuits/rompers
■ 3 vests/bodysuits
■ Light cotton nighties (if too hot to sleep in bodysuit; makes it easier to change nappies)
■ 2 pairs of socks and bootees
■ Shawl (optional)
■ Scratch mittens, bibs
■ In winter: cardigan, woolly hat
In summer: light summer hat

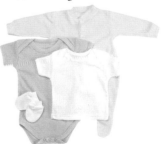
Stretchsuits, vests, and mittens

Q WHAT TYPES OF NAPPIES ARE AVAILABLE AND WHICH SHOULD I CHOOSE?

A There are two types of nappy: fabric, which you can wash and are reusable; or disposable. Disposable nappies are more costly over a period of time, but are convenient to use. There is a wide range available for boys or girls and from newborn to toddler sizes. Occasionally, babies are sensitive to disposables and develop a mild rash, so you may need to change your brand of nappy. Although fabric nappies involve more work, they do work out cheaper in the long run. And you can choose between buying terry towelling squares or shaped fabric nappies. You will need to buy 20 or more and will have to wash and sterilize them after each use, using special nappy-cleaning powder and nappy buckets to soak the fabric nappies in.

Q DO I NEED TO USE BARRIER CREAM EACH TIME I CHANGE A NAPPY?

A After the birth, using a gentle barrier cream, like petroleum jelly, can make it easier to clean off meconium (see p. 66) from your baby's bottom. After a few days, when your baby stops passing meconium, you may need to use a small amount of cream if your baby develops a rash or soreness.

Q HOW DO I KNOW IF MY BABY IS WARM ENOUGH?

A The hands and feet are cooler than the rest of the body so, to find out if your baby is cold, feel the chest, head, or back of neck. If the skin is cool, it is better to put an extra layer of clothes on your baby rather than turn up the heating, because these can be easily removed if your baby overheats.

CHANGING YOUR BABY'S NAPPY

Keeping everything you need in one place will make the task much easier. When putting on a fresh disposable nappy, avoid touching the front of the nappy if you have cream or oil on your fingers as this may stop the tabs from sticking.

Cleaning a boy
Wipe gently, don't drag on the skin of the penis or pull the foreskin back.

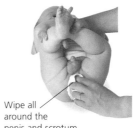

Wipe all around the penis and scrotum

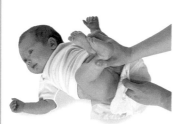

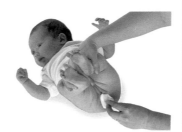

1 Open the soiled nappy and remove any faeces with a clean part of the nappy, then discard.

2 Clean the bottom: wipe in the skin creases using several pieces of wet cotton wool. Dry carefully.

Cleaning a girl
To prevent the spread of bacteria from the anus to the vagina, always wipe from the front to the back.

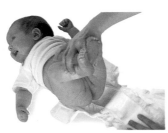

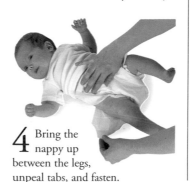

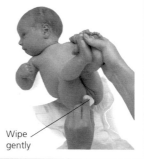

3 Lay the new nappy flat beneath your baby, and line the top up with your baby's waist.

4 Bring the nappy up between the legs, unpeal tabs, and fasten.

Wipe gently

THE FIRST SIX WEEKS

BATHING AND DRESSING YOUR BABY

With a little care and organization, washing your baby can be a playful experience, and dressing your baby in snug-fitting clothes can be a simple procedure. Gather everything you need before you start because you should never leave your baby unattended. If you still have to move away to get something or, for example, to answer the telephone, take your baby with you. As you clean and change your baby, always remember to keep talking to and cuddling him or her.

TOPPING AND TAILING YOUR BABY

Your baby's face, hands, and bottom are prone to irritation from sweat, urine, and soiling, and must be cleaned daily. Topping and tailing enables you to clean these areas without giving your baby a full bath. To reduce the risk of infection, start with the face and finish with the bottom.

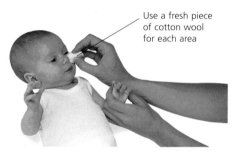

Use a fresh piece of cotton wool for each area

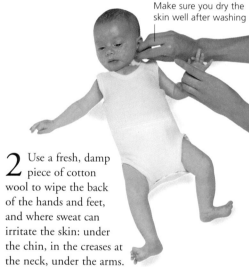

Make sure you dry the skin well after washing

1 Cool some boiled water. Wipe each eye from the corner out, using a new piece of cotton wool for each eye. Wipe over and behind, but not inside, the ears, and then clean the face and around the nose.

2 Use a fresh, damp piece of cotton wool to wipe the back of the hands and feet, and where sweat can irritate the skin: under the chin, in the creases at the neck, under the arms.

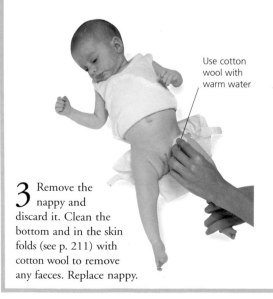

Use cotton wool with warm water

3 Remove the nappy and discard it. Clean the bottom and in the skin folds (see p. 211) with cotton wool to remove any faeces. Replace nappy.

Cleaning the cord

Using cotton wool and surgical spirit, clean in the creases around the stump. Dry with a fresh piece of cotton wool.

Don't pull on the stump or try to remove it

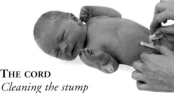

THE CORD
Cleaning the stump will help to prevent any infection.

BATHING YOUR BABY

Put cold, then hot water in the bath; test the water temperature with your elbow: it should be warm, not hot. With the vest on, clean the face and neck (see opposite). Remove the vest to wash the hair, and remove the nappy to bathe your baby.

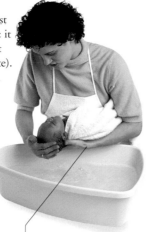

1 With your baby wrapped in a towel, lower the head over the tub and gently pour water over your baby's hair. Gently rub shampoo into the hair and rinse away with water, avoiding the face.

Support your baby's body with your arm, and the head and neck with your hand

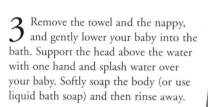

2 A baby can lose a lot of heat through his or her head, so dry your baby's head immediately by gently patting it with a towel.

Comfort your baby by talking constantly to him or her

3 Remove the towel and the nappy, and gently lower your baby into the bath. Support the head above the water with one hand and splash water over your baby. Softly soap the body (or use liquid bath soap) and then rinse away.

Keep the head above the water

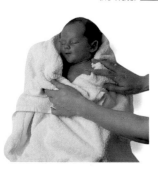

4 Place your baby in a soft, dry towel. Pat your baby dry, making sure there is no dampness between the skin creases. If you wish, apply cream or talcum powder but not both.

DRESSING YOUR BABY

You can ease your baby gently into close-fitting clothes, such as vests or bodysuits, by stretching and rolling the neck and arm openings. Babies often cry while being dressed, but this is usually because they don't like to feel the air on their skin. Never lay your baby near the edge of a surface because he or she could roll off.

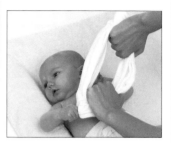

1 Roll the vest up and pull the neck wide so that it is ready to slip over your baby's head.

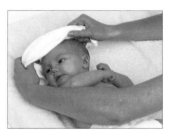

2 Bring the vest over the head, making sure that it doesn't drag over your baby's face.

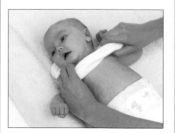

3 Stretch the armholes and guide the arms through; roll the vest down over the body.

SETTLING YOUR BABY

Q HOW CAN I HELP MY BABY TO ESTABLISH A ROUTINE?

A As your confidence in your ability to look after your new baby grows, the way you approach some tasks can help your baby to recognize a pattern. For example, if your baby needs feeding in the night try to do this swiftly and don't "play" with your baby. He or she will then begin to associate play and stimulation only with the day and will sleep more easily if he or she does not expect this kind of attention at night.

Q SHOULD I ATTEND TO MY BABY EVERY TIME HE OR SHE CRIES?

A Yes, you should always attend to your crying baby. At this very early stage your baby will cry for specific reasons; crying is your baby's only means of communicating his or her discomfort or distress to you. Your baby has not yet learned that by crying he or she can always get your attention.

Q WHAT IS THE MOST LIKELY REASON FOR MY BABY'S CRYING?

A Apart from hunger or a nappy change, your baby may be uncomfortable because he or she is suffering from colic (see p. 227). Once older, your baby may cry for less specific reasons, perhaps just to get your attention or for a cuddle.

Q MY BABY ISN'T HUNGRY OR WET, SO WHY IS HE OR SHE STILL CRYING?

A Your baby could be too hot or too cold. Feel the chest or the base of the neck; if the skin feels either flushed and hot, or chilled, add or take away layers of clothing as needed. If your baby has been fed recently, he or she may have wind; place your baby against your shoulder and gently pat on the back (see p. 222). If none of these measures help, your baby is possibly unwell, in which case you should contact your doctor, or take your baby to the baby clinic (see p. 227).

ENSURING YOUR BABY SLEEPS SAFE AND WELL

When you put your baby to bed, you will obviously want him or her to be safe and comfortable. To allay your own fears, there are some general precautions that you can take to help your baby to sleep safe and well; these precautions are also recommended in order to reduce the likelihood of cot death.

■ Put your baby on his or her back or side to sleep, not on the front. When your baby is big enough to need a cot (around three months) make sure you lay him or her in it correctly (see below).
■ Make sure your baby's room is warm, ideally 17–20°C (62–68°F) and well ventilated.
■ Ensure that your baby does not overheat, keep the bedclothes light, and remove layers as needed.
■ Never allow anyone to smoke near your baby.
■ If you feel happier, let your baby sleep in your room for the first six months.
■ Make sure that your baby's mattress is firm and also that it is clean and well aired, so that your baby is not breathing in dust.
■ Breastfeed if you can; it has been suggested that this may reduce the risk of cot death.

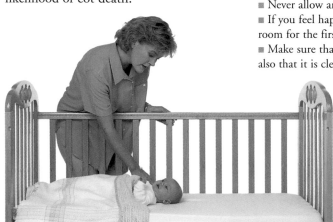

LAYING YOUR BABY DOWN
Ensure that your baby's feet touch the end of the cot so that he or she can't wriggle under the bedclothes. Use blankets and sheets so that you can add or remove layers.

Putting your baby down to sleep

Your new baby is unlikely to get into a sleep routine straight away, but instead will sleep whenever he or she feels the need to, especially after a satisfying feed. Most young babies tend to sleep for three or four hours, then wake for a change or a feed. Try to establish a bedtime routine early on, so that your baby associates certain events with the day's end.

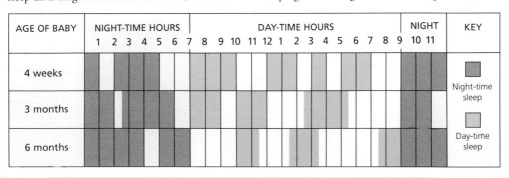

Cradling your baby can help to settle

Your baby should sleep on his or her back or side

Relaxing your baby
To help your baby drop off to sleep, try gently rocking in your arms, which will have a soothing effect. You can also try singing or gently rubbing your baby's back.

What your baby sleeps in
In the first few weeks of life, your baby is so small that a Moses basket is perfectly adequate; it is also cosy and portable. Later on you will need a cot; make sure that the cot you buy conforms to legal safety standards.

Your baby's sleep pattern

The chart below shows how, in the first weeks, your baby's sleep pattern may be erratic. Babies sleep an average of 18 hours out of 24, and not necessarily at night. In the next few months, your baby should establish a more regular sleep pattern, sleeping more at night and less during the day.

AGE OF BABY	NIGHT-TIME HOURS 1 2 3 4 5 6	DAY-TIME HOURS 7 8 9 10 11 12 1 2 3 4 5 6 7 8 9	NIGHT 10 11	KEY
4 weeks				
3 months				Night-time sleep
6 months				Day-time sleep

THE FIRST SIX WEEKS

BREASTFEEDING YOUR BABY

Q **I DON'T KNOW IF I CAN DO IT – WILL I BE SHOWN HOW TO BREASTFEED?**

A Yes; for many mothers, breastfeeding is a natural activity, but for others it can prove difficult. It can take several weeks before you feel confident with the process but once you do, it can become second nature. As the subject is usually covered in antenatal classes, you'll have some idea of what to expect, and the midwives in the hospital and in the community will show you what to do. There are support groups with counsellors to help mothers who are finding it hard to breastfeed (see p. 256).

Q **CAN I FEED MY BABY STRAIGHT AFTER THE BIRTH?**

A As long as your baby is able to suck, yes, you can and should breastfeed immediately after delivery to trigger milk production. The sucking action on your nipple stimulates the hormone oxytocin, which causes the muscle fibres in the milk glands to contract and squeeze milk into the milk ducts. This is known as the "let-down reflex". Most babies do not need to feed much in the first 48 hours because the first milk, colostrum (see opposite), is very rich.

GETTING STARTED

When you start to feed your baby, make sure you are comfortable and can sit without having to get up for at least 30–45 minutes. Your baby will feed best when cradled in your arms, his or her body held close to yours; the head should be level with your nipple. Brush your nipple along your baby's lips to trigger the "rooting reflex", which makes your baby open his or her mouth wide to accept your nipple.

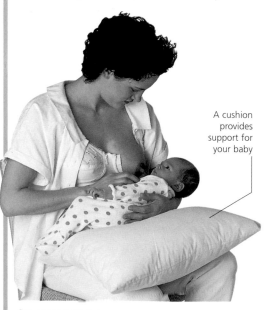

A cushion provides support for your baby

SIT COMFORTABLY
Get into the habit of settling yourself comfortably before feeding, perhaps with a drink by your side; try not to hunch over your baby.

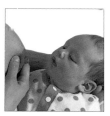

OFFERING YOUR NIPPLE
Cup your breast and offer – rather than push – your nipple to the side of your baby's mouth or brush it across his or her lips. Your baby should open his or her mouth wide to take it.

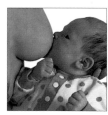

LATCHING ON
To prevent your baby chewing on the sensitive tip of the nipple, encourage him or her to take the whole nipple and areola into the mouth. Your baby should suck hard and rhythmically.

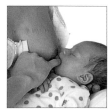

REMOVING YOUR NIPPLE
When finished with one breast, place your little finger in your baby's mouth and push gently down on the lower jaw. This will break the suction and avoid painful pulling on your nipple.

Q WHAT IS COLOSTRUM AND WHY IS IT SO IMPORTANT?

A Colostrum is the thick yellow "premilk" that your breasts produce for the first few days after delivery. This premilk contains water, protein, and minerals in the correct proportion to take care of your newborn's nutritional needs at this early stage. It is also high in antibodies and rich in lactoferrin, a substance which is, in effect, a natural antibiotic.

Q WHEN WILL I START PRODUCING PROPER BREAST MILK?

A By the third day after delivery, your breasts will produce real white breast milk, which is high in fat, carbohydrate, and protein – all vital for your baby's growth – as well as substances that protect against disease and infection. When the milk first comes in, your breasts may expand suddenly as they produce a lot of milk, which causes discomfort. This is normal, and usually only lasts for about 24 hours. Your body then adapts to your baby's needs, producing just enough milk to nourish your baby.

Q SHOULD I GIVE MY BABY BOTH BREASTS AT ALL FEEDS?

A This is not necessary because your breast milk is different at the beginning and end of feeds. The watery "foremilk" is thirst-quenching and the "hindmilk" has far more fat and is nourishing. It's important that your baby gets both kinds of milk from one breast rather than the foremilk from both.

Q FOR HOW LONG AND HOW OFTEN SHOULD MY BABY FEED?

A There's no official time limit – it can be as little as five minutes or as much as 15–20 minutes. It depends how hard your baby sucks and how quickly he or she swallows the milk. This, in turn, depends on how alert your baby is (which varies at different times of the day), and how comfortable. Time is not a good yardstick. You will learn to tell when your baby is content because he or she releases the nipple; also, your breasts will feel less full. The number of times you feed your baby will depend on your milk and your baby's appetite.

Q WHY IS IT IMPORTANT TO BE COMFORTABLE AND RELAXED?

A Feeling tense can stop milk reaching the milk ducts. You are also likely to be in one position for a while, so find a comfortable one: lie on your side facing your baby; sit up with your baby resting in the crook of your arm; or rest back on cushions.

CAN I BREASTFEED AFTER HAVING A CAESAREAN?

Yes, you can breastfeed your newborn after having a Caesarean section delivery. Indeed, if you are both fine, you will be encouraged to breastfeed as soon as you can. But you will have to wait for a while if you are feeling groggy after a general anaesthetic, or if your baby needs special care.

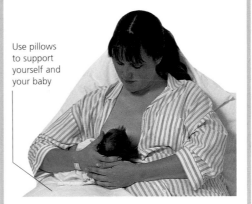

Use pillows to support yourself and your baby

FEEDING WITHOUT PAIN
It is often uncomfortable to breastfeed after a Caesarean section delivery, because of the pressure on the incision, and sore stomach muscles. To alleviate this, place a pillow on your lap under your baby for support.

Q DO I HAVE TO EAT MORE THAN USUAL IF I'M BREASTFEEDING?

A Yes, you do, because the quality of your breast milk depends on your diet; you will also probably be feeling hungrier. You need to make sure that there are enough nutrients both for the manufacture of milk and for your own needs. Eat a varied and well balanced diet of about 2,500 calories a day and make sure that you include plenty of protein (see p. 104).

Q WILL BREASTFEEDING CAUSE MY BREASTS TO SAG, AND RUIN MY FIGURE?

A If you always wear a good supporting bra while pregnant and breastfeeding, your breasts should return to their normal shape when you stop breastfeeding. Your figure will return to its pre-pregnant size quicker if you breastfeed because it uses your body's fat stores laid down in pregnancy.

BREASTFEEDING AND YOU

Q CAN I MAKE BREASTFEEDING EASIER OR LESS DEMANDING?

A Breastfeeding can present physical and practical problems. Expressing your milk and knowing how to deal with sore breasts can help.

Q WHY MIGHT I WANT TO EXPRESS MY MILK?

A Expressing breast milk into a bottle gives you flexibility, allowing you to store your milk and enabling your partner or other carer to help with feeds. For a baby in special care, expressed milk ensures that the mother's natural immunity is passed on via her breast milk. Expressed milk is useful when you and your baby cannot be together: if you go out for an evening, or later on when you return to work.

Q WHEN IS THE BEST TIME TO EXPRESS – BEFORE OR AFTER FEEDING MY BABY?

A It is best to express milk between feeds. If you express before feeding, there may not be enough to satisfy your baby, and if you express afterwards there may not be much milk left. Or you could feed with one breast entirely and express the milk from the other one.

Q HOW DO I STORE EXPRESSED MILK?

A You can store it the same way as formula: in the fridge or the freezer. The milk keeps for up to 72 hours in the fridge; you should not "top up" an existing supply. It will keep in the freezer for up to six months, stored in ice cube trays or bags.

HOW TO EXPRESS YOUR MILK

There are two ways to express your breast milk: either with your hands or by using a pump (see below). Expressing by hand is fairly easy and painless but very slow, whereas a pump is often quicker and less tiring. Hand expressing may help to relieve sore, engorged breasts, and may be less painful than expressing by pump.

By hand

Wash your hands, have a sterile bowl ready, support your breast in one hand and massage around the entire breast, including the underside, at least ten times. Stroking and gentle pressure towards the areola squeezes the milk out through the nipple.

By pump

Pumps can be manual or battery-operated. All pumps vary slightly but work on the same principle: a funnel forms a seal over your nipple, you then pump the milk out by suction. The milk collects in the bottle attached to the pump.

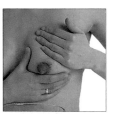

MASSAGE FIRST
In order to encourage the flow of milk though the milk ducts, massage around the entire breast at least ten times.

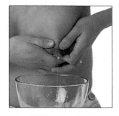

SQUEEZE LAST
Squeeze areola with the thumbs and forefingers together, while pressing backwards; the milk should begin to spurt out. Continue this action for several minutes.

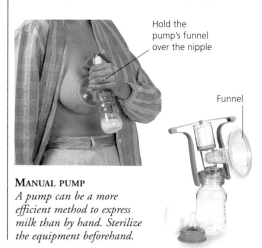

Hold the pump's funnel over the nipple

Funnel

MANUAL PUMP
A pump can be a more efficient method to express milk than by hand. Sterilize the equipment beforehand.

IF YOU HAVE PROBLEMS

If you have any difficulties with your breasts or breastfeeding, you should seek professional help as soon as possible. Never struggle on alone or give up – persevere, because it will be worth it. You could ask your midwife or health visitor for advice or talk to a support group (see p. 256).

CARING FOR YOUR BREASTS

Let the air get to your nipples often, and wash your breasts every day – but don't use soap, which can be drying. Gently pat yourself dry. Support your breasts with a good maternity bra, and wear it day and night in the early weeks. If milk leaks between feeds (and this is common), buy some breast pads and wear them inside your bra for protection. Change the pads frequently.

LEAKING BREASTS
A disposable breast pad will absorb any drips and small leaks.

Front-opening maternity bra

Engorgement
The production of milk is a finely tuned "supply and demand" process, but when your milk first comes in, it takes a while to achieve a balance. Your breasts may become hard, swollen, and sore (known as engorgement) because they are producing too much milk; this can raise your temperature and make you feel feverish and weepy.

Can expressing milk relieve engorgement?
If your breasts are engorged, nursing is difficult for your baby and painful for you. Expressing large amounts of milk is not the answer because your body will keep producing milk to this capacity. However, expressing a small amount of milk can bring relief. You could also try applying alternate warm and cold cloths, or use the showerhead to spray warm and then cold water on your breasts. A pain reliever such as paracetamol may help.

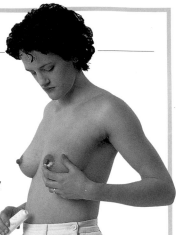

NIPPLE CREAM
A calendula-based cream may help to relieve the soreness.

Sore and cracked nipples
It is normal to have tender nipples for the first few days, as they take time to toughen up. If your baby isn't latching on properly (see p. 216), he or she may be chewing your nipples and damaging soft tissue, even making them bleed. If you are not in too much pain, it is safe to continue feeding. Your milk contains natural antiseptics, so after every feed, rub some of your milk around the nipple and allow it to dry naturally. You may need to use a special nipple cream, such as a calendula cream; consult your midwife or doctor.

Breast inflammation
If one or both breasts become red, patchy, and very sore, you may have a condition called mastitis, when the flow of milk is blocked, causing stagnation. The milk and surrounding tissue may become infected by bacteria that have entered the milk ducts through your nipple.

Can breast inflammation be relieved?
In its early stages, this condition may respond to antibiotics and pain-relieving drugs. It is important to continue breastfeeding in order to empty the breasts and relieve pressure. If you have a high temperature and feel nauseous and dizzy, and have a hot, firm lump in your breast, this is an abscess; you will need to go to hospital to have the lump drained.

Pain-relieving drugs and breastfeeding
It is safe to take most drugs that are based on paracetamol, because only a very small amount passes across in the milk and reaches the baby. However, aspirin is best avoided because it has been linked to a rare condition (Reye's syndrome) that can affect babies.

THE FIRST SIX

BEGINNING BOTTLE-FEEDING

Q I HAVE DECIDED NOT TO BREASTFEED, DO I NEED TO TELL MY MIDWIFE?

A If you are having a hospital birth, tell your midwife who will advise hospital staff. They will provide bottle-feeding equipment and formula and show you how to use it. However, your midwife will not supply bottle-feeding equipment for a home birth; she will discuss this with you before the birth and advise you to buy the equipment and formula.

Q WHICH FORMULA SHOULD I BUY?

A Most of the wide variety of baby formulas now available are based on cows' milk and contain vitamins and minerals. If you don't want your baby to have animal products or your baby develops an allergy to cows' milk, there are soya milk formulas. Dry powder formulas are cheaper, but ready-made formulas are more convenient.

Q WHY IS IT SO IMPORTANT TO CLEAN AND STERILIZE ALL THE EQUIPMENT?

A Clean equipment is crucial because milk is an ideal breeding ground for the bacteria that cause gastroenteritis, a disease that can be life-threatening in a young baby. You must sterilize everything that comes into contact with the feed.

Q HOW DO I MAKE SURE THAT THE EQUIPMENT IS STERILE?

A Wash everything in warm, soapy water. Scrub bottle rims, clean right to the bottom of the bottles, and turn the teats inside out to wash them. Use a plastic brush to scrub away any build-up of milk inside a teat. Then sterilize the equipment, either by placing the bottles and teats in a steamer, immersing them in sterilizing fluid, or microwaving them. Keep the equipment below water level, and remove any air bubbles. Replace the fluid daily.

WHAT EQUIPMENT DO I NEED?

Essential equipment for bottle-feeding includes four to six bottles and teats. To make a feed you need a measuring jug, a funnel, a plastic spoon, and a plastic knife for levelling off the formula. To sterilize equipment you need a bottle brush, and either sterilizing fluid/tablets, or a steam sterilizer.

Other equipment

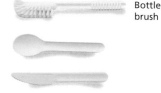

Bottle brush

Plastic spoon and knife

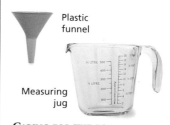

Plastic funnel

Measuring jug

Feeding equipment

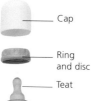

— Cap

— Ring and disc

— Teat

TYPES OF BOTTLE AND TEATS
Bottles are usually made of plastic. One system consists of disposable bags that fit inside a plastic tube. Teats can be made of latex or silicone and come in several shapes: experiment to find the one that suits your baby best.

Wide-necked bottle with silicone teat

With this system, only the teat needs to be sterilized

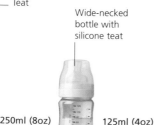

250ml (8oz) bottle

125ml (4oz) bottle

Disposable plastic bottle liner

CARING FOR THE EQUIPMENT
Keep all equipment scrupulously clean. Rub the inside of teats with a plastic brush, clean bottles with a bottle brush. Sterilize all equipment. Plastic or glass is best.

How do I make up a feed?

When making up your baby's feed, it is important to follow the directions on the can (or packet) exactly. Do not add extra scoops, or dilute the formula further, or add cereals to your baby's feed. To do so changes the specific concentration and could lead to obesity or even serious illness in your baby. Always use previously boiled tap water.

──────── **REMEMBER** ────────

■ *Read the instructions on the formula can (or packet) carefully and follow them closely.*
■ *Wash your hands before beginning.*
■ *If you become distracted when measuring the formula, throw the milk away and start again.*
■ *Don't keep unfinished feed.*
■ *Don't reheat unused milk: this is a dangerous source of bacteria.*
■ *Don't warm up milk in a microwave oven.*

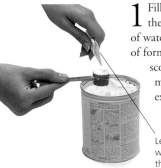

1 Fill the jug with the correct amount of water. Open the can of formula and use the scoop provided to measure out the exact amount.

Level each scoop with the back of the knife

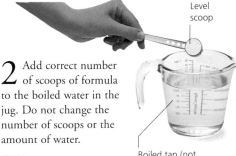

Level scoop

2 Add correct number of scoops of formula to the boiled water in the jug. Do not change the number of scoops or the amount of water.

Boiled tap (not mineral) water

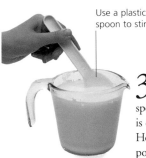

Use a plastic spoon to stir

3 Stir the formula well with a plastic spoon until the powder is completely dissolved. Hot water will help the powder dissolve faster.

Pour the formula through a funnel to avoid spillage

4 Pour the formula milk into the clean bottles through the plastic funnel.

Storing feeds

You can make up a batch of feeds that can be stored for 24 hours; this is particularly useful for night feeds. Make up several jugs of formula and pour into bottles. Put the teats on upside down, but don't let them dip into the milk. If they do touch the milk, put the teats the right way up. Cover with the discs and screw on the rings. Cool the bottles and place them in a fridge immediately. Breast milk expressed into bottles can also be stored in this way.

Do not let the teat touch the milk

TIME LIMIT
Store prepared formula in the fridge for no longer than 24 hours.

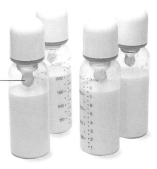

THE FIRST SIX WEEKS

BOTTLE-FEEDING YOUR BABY

Q HOW OFTEN SHOULD I FEED MY BABY?

A Bottle-fed babies should be fed, like breastfed babies, on demand, not at set times; this can vary from day to day, depending on how big your baby is, and how hungry. You will not spoil your baby by answering his or her hunger cries. A baby's feeding clock works on a 24-hour basis, and most have an average of six to ten feeds during that time. As your baby will expect to be fed as often during the night as during the day, you will probably get no more than two to three hours sleep at a time.

Q HOW LONG SHOULD A FEED TAKE?

A Just as there are no set times for feeding your baby, there is no set time for how long a feed should take. Always let your baby set the pace. Sometimes he or she will be feeling playful and will want to pause to look around or touch the bottle; when this happens, a feed can take anything up to half an hour. When your baby lets go of the teat, or finishes all the milk, take the bottle away. If he or she still wants to suck, offer your clean little finger.

GIVING YOUR BABY A BOTTLE FEED

Before you give your baby a feed, check that the milk is at the correct temperature by shaking a little on to your wrist; it should feel just warm.

FEEDING YOUR BABY

It is always best to feed your baby while cradling him or her in your arms, with the head tilted back slightly. Make sure the teat is always full of milk and that there are no air pockets. To give your baby the comforting feeling of skin-to-skin closeness, you could remove your blouse during the feed.

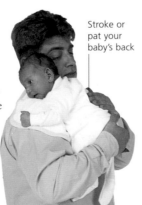

HOLDING THE BOTTLE
Hold the feeding bottle firmly so that your baby can pull against it slightly to get a good sucking action.

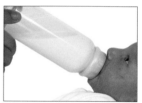

AVOIDING WIND
To stop your baby sucking in air, keep the milk level up.

WINDING

Bottle-fed babies need winding more often than breastfed babies because there is a tendency to gulp down air or milk if the rate of flow is not quite right.

OVER THE SHOULDER
Wind your baby over your shoulder. Some milk may come up ("possetting"), so protect your clothes.

Stroke or pat your baby's back

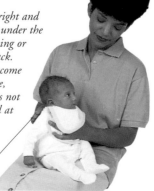

SITTING UP
Sit your baby upright and support the head under the chin, gently rubbing or patting on the back. If wind does not come up after a minute, then give up. It is not necessary to wind at every feed.

Always be gently, or the entire feed can come back up

Q CAN MY BABY AND I STILL ENJOY A SENSE OF CLOSENESS IF I BOTTLE-FEED?

A Yes, you can enjoy the same intimacy as a breastfeeding mother enjoys with her baby. Hold your baby close (if you like, against your naked skin) and smile and talk to your baby. Never leave your baby to drink from a bottle propped up in the cot or pram because this can cause choking.

Q WHAT IF MY BABY FALLS ASLEEP WHILE BOTTLE-FEEDING?

A If your baby dozes off, it may be because he or she has had enough milk, or wind has made your baby feel full. Take the bottle away, wind your baby (see opposite), then start to feed again. Winding is not always needed; your baby will usually seem uncomfortable when he or she needs winding.

Q MY BABY RARELY FINISHES THE BOTTLE, IS HE OR SHE GETTING ENOUGH MILK?

A This may be the result of making too much milk per feed. Ask your midwife or health visitor how much milk your baby should receive according to his or her weight, and have your baby weighed. It is possible to overfeed a bottle-fed baby but not a breastfed one because the strength of breast milk varies and it is thirst-quenching. If you bottle-feed, give your baby some water between feeds if he or she seems thirsty. Poor feeding could indicate an illness that needs attention. If your baby gains weight, he or she is probably feeding well.

Q HOW DO I CHANGE FROM BREAST-TO BOTTLE-FEEDING?

A Make a gradual transition by replacing one breastfeed every third day; replace a lunchtime breastfeed with a bottle. If your baby won't take the bottle, try again at the same feed the next day. You may need to try different types of teat, or moisten the teat with breast milk to encourage your baby. After three days with one bottle-feed each day, replace a second daytime feed with a bottle; do this for another three days before tackling a third feed. Do this until eventually your baby is being bottle-fed for all his or her feeds. If your baby persists in not taking the bottle, get someone else to give the bottle so that your baby cannot smell you.

Q HOW LONG WILL MY MILK TAKE TO DRY UP ONCE I STOP BREASTFEEDING?

A You may be uncomfortable for a few days while the milk dries up. Take paracetamol if your breasts are full and sore, but they should return to normal after about five to ten days.

DISCUSSION POINT

IS BREAST OR BOTTLE BEST?

Protecting your baby from illness

An important argument in favour of breastfeeding – at least for the first few days – is that the thick yellow "premilk" (colostrum) produced immediately after delivery contains antibodies to protect your baby against certain types of illness (especially stomach, respiratory, and viral infections), and may protect against allergies such as asthma. Today's baby formulas try to replicate the nutrients found in normal breast milk but are unable to reproduce these antibodies.

Preparing for a feed

Breast milk is convenient because it's always available, already sterile, and is the correct temperature and strength, whereas if you bottle feed, you need to spend time ensuring that the equipment is scrupulously clean and is sterilized so that your baby is not exposed to infections.

Bonding with your baby

Breastfeeding with regular skin-to-skin contact does allow you to share a special closeness with your baby. If your partner feels excluded from this process, expressing your milk into a bottle will enable him to help with feeds.

Making a choice

Breastmilk is preferable because it contains all the nourishment your baby needs. It has also been suggested that breastfeeding may reduce the risk of cot death. However, you may have reasons why you do not wish to breastfeed; for example, breastfeeding may simply not be comfortable, or bottle-feeding may be more convenient for you if you are planning to return to work. If you are HIV positive, it is best not to breastfeed because of the increased risk of passing the infection to your baby (see p. 130).

FAMILY CONCERNS

Q HOW DO WE KNOW IF WE WILL MAKE GOOD PARENTS?

A How can any of us know whether we will make good parents? This is something you have to learn "on-the-job", so all you can do is take each day at a time until your confidence grows through experience. Your insecurity may have something to do with the fact that you feel isolated at the moment. Once you have the opportunity to get out more, join a local mother-and-toddler group so that you can share your experiences with others.

Q HOW DO WE COPE WITH EVERYONE GIVING US ADVICE?

A Friends and relatives who have already survived the trials of parenthood, naturally assume that you will want the benefit of their experience. This advice is well-intentioned and often useful but may also be old-fashioned, or conflict with your own ideas of parenthood. It is hard to tell those who mean well that you want to do things your own way, but you must make yourself clear from the outset.

ADJUSTING TO FATHERHOOD

The enormous responsibility of fatherhood, and the fears this evokes, can prevent you from getting the most out of family life initially, but if you learn to play an active role, helping with nappy-changing, bath time, or putting to bed, you will soon feel relaxed and confident with your baby.

Feeling neglected

It's a simple fact that newborn babies can take up every second of a mother's time in the early weeks, and that fathers often feel neglected, or even jealous of the baby. This is only natural because your partner now has a new focus to her life and it is not you. Tell your partner how you feel before this builds up into resentment and causes harm to your relationship. You could also take a more active role in caring for your baby.

Feeling left out

Many new fathers wrongly assume that their partner is coping perfectly well without any help from them but you may be surprised to learn just how much she needs you. Just knowing that you are there helps your partner. If you feel excluded because you cannot share in breastfeeding, perhaps your partner could express some milk into a bottle so that you can help with the feeding too, including in the middle of the night.

Being scared of your baby

Babies seem to be fragile little creatures, and many men are scared to do anything other than hold them unless they have had younger brothers and sisters. Babies are, in fact, quite resilient to inept handling – as long as you don't drop them on their heads. Try to overcome your fears by watching your partner or midwife and then offer to help bathe and change your baby to give your partner a rest.

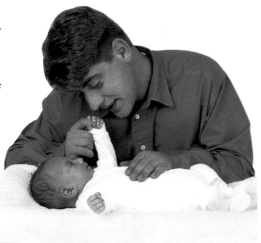

GETTING TO KNOW YOUR BABY
You will come to feel close to your baby through the daily loving contact and care: by changing nappies, giving baths, cuddling, stroking, and talking.

Q HOW WILL OUR OTHER CHILD/ CHILDREN REACT TO THE NEW BABY?

A Other children often see a new arrival as an exciting event. Alternatively, the new arrival may inspire feelings of jealousy in your other offspring; these jealous feelings may not be evident, as you may have expected, straight after the birth, so be prepared to deal with them if they emerge later. There should not be too many problems, as long as your children still get their share of attention and do not feel excluded (see below).

Q HOW CAN WE ENSURE THAT OUR OTHER CHILDREN DO NOT FEEL LEFT OUT?

A As soon as you bring your baby home, try to include your other child or children in everything that's going on by explaining what you are doing, and why, and getting them to help with simple chores. However demanding your new baby is, you should try to make some special time for your other offspring – without the baby – and to honour some of their established routines. For example, if you always read bedtime stories, you or your partner should continue to do so.

Q I FEEL MOODY AND LOW, IS THIS NORMAL?

A In the first few days after the birth you may not feel your usual self; your partner may also be worried that you seem depressed. However, this is quite normal and is probably just a case of the "baby blues" (see p. 249). Physically, you may be tired and sore, and you are possibly mentally overwhelmed by your new responsibility. Your body has undergone an hormonal upheaval, and you may also be anxious about your ability to care for your new baby. Talk to your partner about your feelings, so that he understands how you feel. He too, may be feeling a little exhausted or low as he adjusts to the ups and downs of a newborn baby in his life.

Q I'VE BEEN FEELING DEPRESSED FOR WEEKS, IS THIS NORMAL?

A Although it is normal to feel a bit weepy and low straight after the birth, if these feelings persist beyond the first week, you may be suffering from post-natal depression (see p. 249), which can be a serious problem. You and your partner should talk to your health visitor or doctor about your symptoms, so that you can both understand what you are going through and discuss ways in which you can work together to overcome the depression.

Q HOW CAN MY PARTNER AND I REKINDLE OUR ROMANCE?

A In all the excitement and stress caused by the arrival of your baby, it is easy to neglect each other's needs. It can be difficult to feel romantic in the hectic early round of breastfeeding, changing nappies, and interrupted sleep, but once you have established a routine of caring for your baby, you can begin to think of simple ways to recapture the closeness you and your partner enjoyed before the birth. Ask someone you trust to babysit occasionally so that you and your partner can go out for a meal. Set aside time to express all the mixed feelings you've both had since the arrival of your baby; just cuddle if you are too tired to make love; have a nap or a bath together at the end of the working day; try to make time to give each other a relaxing massage. Be prepared, though, for interruptions!

Q HOW WILL OUR NEW BABY AFFECT OUR SOCIAL LIFE?

A Your baby's demands will naturally take precedence over your social life in these early weeks, although you will probably find that you have plenty of visitors, and that it is also relatively easy to see friends with your new baby. You may also find that you make new friends through your baby as you meet other mothers with young children. Most mothers, however, do not have the energy for late nights at this early stage, but rest assured that your social life will eventually return to a semblance of normality once you all settle into a routine together.

Q WHEN WILL WE SETTLE DOWN AGAIN?

A The first six weeks after the birth are a continual round of bathing, changing, and feeding routines, and you will constantly feel tired. This is the downside of having a newborn baby, but you'll soon begin to experience the joys of parenthood as new patterns become established, as your confidence in handling your baby increases, and as your body begins to make a full recovery from the rigours of pregnancy and labour. You'll also find that your baby will start to distinguish between night (time to sleep) and day (time to wake up and be sociable), which gives you both more time for rest. As your energy returns, your family life will begin to live up to your expectations, and you and your partner will be able to focus on all the positive aspects of parenthood.

CONCERNS ABOUT YOUNG BABIES

Q MY BABY'S FACE IS VERY SPOTTY, IS THIS NORMAL?

A Babies are often spotty but this is rarely serious. Your baby's face may also have small, white spots (milia) caused by hormonal changes. These do not need treatment, and should disappear within a few days or weeks. If the spots are infected and red, leave them alone unless they burst; if this happens, gently clean them with cool, boiled water and apply antiseptic cream. If the infection persists or spreads, consult your doctor.

Q MY BABY'S BOTTOM LOOKS RED AND SORE, WHAT SHOULD I DO?

A Nappy rash is usually caused by the ammonia in urine irritating the skin, so check your baby's nappy often. A young baby's skin is very sensitive, especially to perfumed, chemical products; if a rash (not caused by wet nappies) develops, it may be due to the overuse of, or your baby's sensitivity to products such as baby cream or wipes (especially if they are not hypo-allergenic), and you may have to change or stop using the product. Wash your baby's bottom gently with non-perfumed baby soap and water and pat it dry. Zinc and castor oil cream can ease soreness, and protect against further irritation.

Q MY BABY USUALLY BRINGS UP A LITTLE MILK AFTER A FEED, AM I OVERFEEDING?

A Young babies don't realize when they have had enough milk and often just carry on feeding until they are too full, and then bring up some of their feed. It is also common for babies to vomit when they are trying to get rid of some wind.

Q MY BABY VOMITED WITH GREAT FORCE, IS THIS NORMAL?

A This is called "projectile vomiting". If it happens only once or within 72 hours of the birth, when your baby may still have mucus in his or her stomach, then it is probably not serious. Just feed and wind your baby well (see p. 222). If it happens after every feed, your baby may have a blockage in the outlet of the stomach, known as pyloric stenosis, which needs medical attention. However, this is a very rare condition.

Q WHY IS THERE A BLISTER ON MY BABY'S TOP LIP?

A This is probably a "sucking" blister, caused when the lips tighten around your nipple or a teat. The blister is not serious and needs no treatment; just leave it alone and it should disappear.

HOW DO I PREVENT MY BABY'S FACE GETTING SCRATCHED?

Since babies tend to wave their fists about and touch their faces a lot, they can scratch themselves with the sharp edges of their nails. These scratches are very superficial, and unlikely to cause your baby any lasting harm; they probably cause you more concern because they look sore. To stop this happening, you can buy "scratch" mittens; some stretchsuits have sleeves that cover your baby's hands.

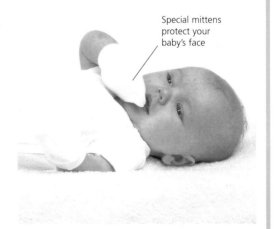

Special mittens protect your baby's face

CUTTING YOUR BABY'S NAILS
Your baby's fingernails are not yet growing independently of the fingers so are not ready to be cut.

Q MY BABY CRIES A LOT AND SEEMS VERY UNCOMFORTABLE, WHAT IS WRONG?

A This may be a condition called colic, which is caused by trapped wind. Colic makes babies cry hard, pull their knees up to their abdomen, and also makes them reluctant to feed or to settle. You can help to relieve the pain by massaging the abdomen, or putting your baby against your shoulder and rubbing the back. Ask your midwife, health visitor, doctor, or a pharmacist at the baby clinic, for medication to ease the colic.

Q MY BABY'S STOOLS ARE VERY LOOSE, IS THIS NORMAL?

A Loose stools are quite common, although babies who are breastfed are much more likely to have looser stools than those who are bottle-fed. However, if your baby's stools are green as well as watery, your baby probably has diarrhoea. This could be serious because it means that your baby is losing fluids, which can lead to dehydration, and this may need medical attention. If your baby has severe diarrhoea, a dry mouth, is lethargic, refuses to feed, and the fontanelle is sunken, contact your doctor at once.

Q WHAT CAN I DO IF MY BABY'S SCALP IS DRY AND SCALY?

A This is a condition called cradle cap, which often occurs in young babies. It looks unpleasant but is not at all serious and shouldn't cause your baby much discomfort. Cradle cap can spread to other parts of your baby's body but usually clears up within a few days. You can treat it by gently rubbing baby oil on to the scalp; leave the oil on for up to 24 hours before using a baby comb to comb the hair and loosen the scales. If, after washing your baby's hair, the scaliness persists, consult your doctor.

Q WHY ARE MY BABY'S EYES STICKY AND "GLUED UP"?

A It is possible that your baby has conjunctivitis, which is a mild eye infection. This can occur in newborn babies if fluid or blood gets into the eye during the delivery. Gently wipe your baby's eyes with cotton wool soaked in cool, boiled water, using a different piece for each eye. If the condition does not clear up, some midwives believe that placing a few drops of breastmilk into the affected eye may help to clear up the infection, but check with your doctor first. If the condition persists, your doctor can prescribe an antibiotic cream.

Q IS OUR SMOKING HARMFUL TO MY YOUNG BABY?

A Yes, a baby's lungs and nose are very sensitive to irritants. Smoke is an irritant, and although your lungs may be used to nicotine, carbon monoxide, and other noxious fumes, your baby's won't be. The fumes from cigarettes paralyse the lining of fine hairs in the nose, throat, and lungs that constantly sweep foreign particles out from the chest and help keep the lungs clear. There may be a link between a very smoky environment and cot death, but smoking around your baby will certainly increase his or her chances of developing respiratory problems such as asthma, chronic cough, and chest infections later on in childhood.

WHEN TO CONSULT A DOCTOR

On occasions your baby is likely to give you cause for concern, but you will soon learn to deal with most situations. However, in any of the situations listed below, your baby will need treatment, and should be taken to a doctor.

Contact your doctor if your baby:
- Is passing green, watery stools.
- Wheezes, and has a dry, rasping cough.
- Has an unusually low temperature.
- Has a skin rash.
- You suspect an infection is present.
- Has been vomiting more than usual.
- Is very lethargic.
- Is generally irritable and is not feeding well.

Contact your doctor or hospital immediately if your baby:
- Is breathing either very quickly, with a noisy grunting sound, or very slowly and irregularly.
- Seems to be having a fit: his or her back is arched and/or the limbs are moving jerkily.
- Has turned blue.
- Is acting strangely and doesn't recognize you, or becomes unrousable or extremely sleepy.
- Has sunken fontanelles.
- Develops a high temperature, especially in conjunction with any of the above.

If you can't contact your doctor, go straight to your local hospital's emergency department or, if you have no transport, ring for an ambulance.

THE SPECIAL-CARE BABY

Q MY BABY HAS TO GO INTO SPECIAL CARE – WHAT DOES THIS MEAN?

A It may be a confusing and frightening moment for you if your baby is taken into special care immediately after the birth, but there are many reasons why this care may be needed, and it does not necessarily mean that the problem is serious. Special care can range from the observation of a minor problem such as breathing difficulties, to (very rarely) intensive life-support in a neonatal intensive care unit (NICU). The time a baby needs to spend in special care varies from a few hours to a few weeks, depending on the seriousness of the condition, and the age and weight of your baby.

Q WHY MIGHT MY BABY NEED SPECIAL CARE?

A Special care is needed if your baby is born with any problem that requires immediate observation or treatment. Most premature babies (see p. 234) are placed in special care. If your baby has a problem related to the delivery itself, or arising after the birth, for example, jaundice, or if your baby has inhaled meconium, special care will also be needed.

Q DOES MY BABY HAVE TO GO TO A SPECIFIC PLACE FOR SPECIAL CARE?

A Yes, your baby may need to be in a special-care baby unit (SCBU), which is a separate ward staffed by specialist nurses and paediatricians. On this unit there is usually one nurse looking after every four babies, compared to the one midwife for every ten or more babies on a post-natal ward, so if your baby requires treatment or tests, this unit is the best place to be. Your baby may be placed in a cot or in an incubator. Within the unit there is also the neonatal intensive care unit (NICU), which deals with more serious problems in young babies.

Q WHO DECIDES WHETHER MY BABY NEEDS SPECIAL CARE?

A If the doctors caring for your baby believe that special care is needed, they will suggest this, although the ultimate decision rests with you. It may be a hard to let your baby be taken away from you at this point but the important consideration is to do what is best for your baby.

Q WHY DOES MY BABY HAVE TO BE IN AN INCUBATOR?

A Incubators may look very frightening but they are really just cots with lids that provide controlled conditions (see right). A small baby (particularly if premature) loses heat quickly and is vulnerable to bacteria; an incubator shields the baby from these and provides an environment in which a baby can develop and get stronger.

Q WHAT IS A VENTILATOR FOR AND WHY DOES MY BABY NEED IT?

A A ventilator is a machine that helps your baby to breathe. Your baby may need this help if he or she is born with respiratory problems due to underdeveloped lungs (see p. 234)), or suffers from a diaphragmatic hernia where the intestines put pressure on the lungs. Other breathing problems can occur during, or after the birth, such as a chest infection, or if there are drugs still in your baby's system from the delivery. Depending on the severity of the condition, the type of ventilation support required can range from an enclosed oxygenated cot to full artificial ventilation by machine.

Q MY BABY IS ON SPECIAL CARE BECAUSE SHE WAS "GRUNTING". WHAT IS THIS?

A Grunting implies that your baby's breathing is not as easy as it should be. This commonly improves within minutes or hours of delivery. Occasionally, though, the breathing may get worse, which means that your baby needs supplemental oxygen or even artificial ventilation. The causes of grunting include prematurity and infection.

Q WHY DOES MY BABY NEED VENTILATION? I HAD A CAESAREAN AT 37 WEEKS.

A A condition called transient tachypnoea of the newborn (TTN) is more common after Caesarean section, and especially so if a Caesarean is carried out before 39 weeks. This is probably because the baby's lungs are a little waterlogged immediately after delivery. Transient tachypnoea is not usually a dangerous condition, and improves within 24–48 hours, but your baby may need oxygen or ventilation for a short while. It is for this reason that planned Caesareans are now normally done after 39 weeks.

Q WHO CAN WE DISCUSS OUR CONCERNS AND WORRIES WITH?

A The paediatrician looking after your baby will be able to answer all your questions concerning the medical condition and the outlook for your baby. They may not always be available, but you can always voice your concerns to other members of staff. Do not be afraid to ask questions. Also, because no-one expects you to be able to cope all the time, specialist counsellors attached to the unit are available to listen and to help you through this difficult and distressing period.

Q CAN WE HELP TO CARE FOR OUR BABY IN SPECIAL CARE?

A Except in rare situations when your baby may be too ill or fragile to be touched, and there is a danger of infection, you and your partner will be encouraged to play a very important part in the well-being of your baby. Touching, cuddling, and talking to your baby can comfort and reassure him or her (see right). It may even be possible to help feed, clean, and change your baby.

Q CAN I BREASTFEED MY BABY WHILE HE OR SHE IS IN SPECIAL CARE?

A You can usually still breastfeed your baby. However, if your baby cannot suck properly because he or she is too small, a tube will be passed into your baby's stomach and your breast milk fed through this tube. To feed your baby this way, you will have to express your milk first, either manually or with a pump (see p. 218).

Q CAN I STAY IN HOSPITAL WHILE MY BABY IS IN SPECIAL CARE?

A You can spend as much time as you want with your baby in special care, although you will usually sleep on the post-natal ward. The midwives care for you there because you have just given birth. If your baby has to be in special care for some time, especially if born prematurely, you will be discharged from the post-natal ward but you can still visit your baby daily.

Q IF MY BABY NEEDS TO GO TO SPECIAL CARE, CAN I SEE HIM BEFORE HE GOES?

A This usually depends on the urgency with which he needs treatment or further observations. Ask your paediatrician if you can hold him for a few minutes before he is whisked away to the special care unit. In most circumstances, this will be possible.

Q HOW FAR WOULD DOCTORS GO TO SAVE MY BABY?

A Where there is any hope at all, your doctors will try to help your baby. Advances in fetal and neonatal medicine have been spectacular in the last ten years, and those caring for your baby will use every available option to help him or her survive. In some cases, this may mean transferring, with your agreement, you and your baby to a regional neonatal unit with more expertise and facilities.

CAN I TOUCH MY BABY?

Your baby may be put in an incubator to help maintain his or her body temperature and to monitor breathing. Some babies also need to be fed through a tube taped into their noses.

Physical contact

Although you may not be able to hold your baby, most incubators have special portholes in the side through which you can put your hands to touch or stroke your baby so that he or she knows you are close by. Tiny babies (especially premature ones) are much less able to cope with bacteria and viruses than adults and children and because there is a risk of infection, you will have to clean your hands with a special soap, and possibly wear a gown and gloves.

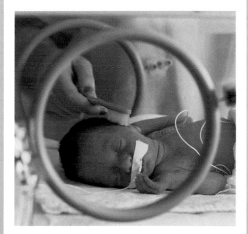

CARING FOR YOUR BABY
You can help look after your baby while in special care. Touching, stroking, and talking to your baby will also help him or her during this time.

IF YOUR BABY HAS A CONDITION AT BIRTH

Q WHAT IF MY BABY IS BORN WITH A MEDICAL CONDITION?

A There are medical conditions that result in a baby needing special attention and medical care after birth. A minor problem, such as jaundice, may only need short-term special care, or your baby may have a serious condition that requires surgery, such as a hole in the heart, or a long-term disabling condition, such as cerebral palsy or Down's syndrome (see opposite).

Q WHAT IS JAUNDICE?

A Jaundice is a blood condition that commonly affects newborn babies. It occurs for many reasons: usually, when red blood cells are broken down, the yellow pigment, bilirubin, is produced and is rapidly cleared by the kidneys and liver. If the bilirubin builds up, the body is unable to expel it and instead deposits it in the skin, causing the skin to develop a yellowish hue. Jaundice is more common in premature babies because their livers are not fully developed. It can also occur if your baby's head was bruised during a forceps or ventouse delivery. A mild form of jaundice is linked to breastfeeding.

Q IS JAUNDICE SERIOUS?

A Not usually. Mild jaundice, known as physiological jaundice, typically occurs about four days after birth, and commonly disappears without any treatment within ten days. More rarely, however, jaundice may be a sign of a more serious underlying condition such as a blood disorder, for example anaemia, or an infection, or a thyroid or liver problem. This type of jaundice is known as pathological jaundice.

Q WILL MY BABY NEED TREATMENT FOR JAUNDICE?

A This depends on how severe it is. Severe physiological jaundice is treated by photo-therapy: your baby is exposed to ultra-violet light for a few hours every day to break down the bilirubin beneath the baby's skin. Pathological jaundice requires further investigation (especially if anaemia is present) and your baby may need a blood transfusion. In certain situations drugs are given to stimulate the liver to get rid of excess bilirubin.

Q MY BABY HAS A GENETIC PROBLEM. I WAS TESTED FOR DOWN'S, SO WHAT'S WRONG?

A Down's is a condition in which there is an extra chromosome 21 in each cell of the baby's body. Most genetic conditions are more subtle than chromosomal syndromes, and affect the individual genes, of which there are many thousands making up each chromosome. Genetic conditions can affect any part of the body (see p. 39), are usually difficult to diagnose, even by specialists, and don't always have a specific diagnostic genetic test.

Q IF MY BABY NEEDS SURGERY, WHEN WILL IT TAKE PLACE?

A In many situations, surgery is most successful and least dangerous when the baby has matured a little and put on some weight, so surgery will only be carried out immediately if the situation is extremely serious or life-threatening (see p. 232). Minor abnormalities, such as club foot and extra fingers or toes, are not life-threatening and will normally be operated on within a few weeks or months of the birth (see p. 232). Hare lip, or a severe cleft palate may be dealt with sooner because they can cause feeding and, more rarely, breathing problems (see p. 233). A life-saving operation may be needed within a few days of birth if your baby has a hernia, either internal (affecting the lung) or external (around the umbilicus); hydrocephalus (water on the brain); heart problems; or, more rarely, problems of the bowel or windpipe.

Q DO I HAVE THE RIGHT TO SAY NO TO AN OPERATION ON MY BABY?

A Yes, it is your right to say no to any operation on your baby. If your baby has a very severe problem that is life-threatening, and an operation may well not be successful, you will have to make a decision (with the advice and guidance of the paediatric staff and the surgeon) whether or not to go ahead with the operation. In some situations, it may be more humane to hold off surgery and save your baby from further unnecessary pain. However, if the doctors feel that an operation has a high chance of success and you disagree, then they can make your baby a ward of court and act in his or her best interests. This only happens in extreme circumstances.

Q I'M DIABETIC, WILL MY BABY HAVE DIABETES?

A No, but your diabetes can cause a lot of blood sugar to cross the placenta to your baby while in your womb. In response to this, your baby's pancreas will have produced high levels of insulin to keep his or her own blood sugar levels under control in the womb. This supply of sugar stops at birth, but your baby's pancreas takes hours, or days, to adjust to the new, lower sugar levels. During this time, he or she will need to be closely monitored.

Q MY BABY WAS BORN WITH A HEART MURMUR, WILL THIS NEED TREATMENT?

A Most heart murmurs occur because of changes in the baby's circulation at or just after the birth. Usually, with this type of benign murmur, a baby is a healthy pink colour, feeds well, and the murmur disappears within a few days or weeks. Rarely, a murmur is present because of a structural problem in the heart, which causes a baby to turn blue and become ill. In this case, a heart scan is arranged and your baby will need surgery.

WHAT DOES HAVING A DISABILITY MEAN FOR MY BABY?

Disability is a term that covers everything from minor learning disorders to severe cerebral palsy. Your baby's disability may be mild, such as a degree of deafness or, more rarely, your baby's condition may be severe and include paralysis or mental disability. An increasing number of problems are detected before birth and successfully treated.

When will we know how severely our baby is affected?

Many disabilities can be detected at birth but it is often some time later before the extent of your baby's problem can be calculated. Once a problem is suspected, degrees of deafness or blindness can be picked up with tests and, if possible, treated immediately, whereas speech and learning difficulties will naturally take time to surface. If your baby is suffering from a condition such as cerebral palsy or Down's syndrome, he or she will have a more serious form of mental or physical disability and may need extensive help through childhood and in later life.

What is cerebral palsy?

Cerebral palsy is a rare disability that affects the baby's movements. It is caused by damage to the brain late in pregnancy, or during or after the birth, due to lack of oxygen or flow of blood to the brain. It usually affects the baby's muscle control, often causing a degree of paralysis of the limbs.

What is Down's syndrome?

A Down's syndrome baby suffers from an inherited chromosome defect causing some degree of mental disablement and physical abnormalities (see p. 144).

Will my baby get better?

With the recent advances in treatment, particularly of sight and hearing defects, a baby with an illness or a disability now has a better prospect of a more normal life. If your baby has a relatively minor problem, there is a good chance that he or she can be successfully treated. However, where the brain has been irreversibly damaged, the condition is essentially incurable, although much can be done to alleviate suffering and enhance quality of life. Surgery and physiotherapy can help physical problems, while sympathetic teaching can help those with mental disabilities.

How will we cope with a disabled baby?

Due to the extra needs involved, a disabled baby can be very hard and stressful work. He or she may take longer to feed, cry a lot, and show little or no response to you, or his or her surroundings. You will need to look into what professional care is available to help you and your baby, and plan ahead for any special schooling needs. Try not to blame yourself for your baby's condition because it is extremely unlikely that anything you did while pregnant could have affected your baby.

Where can we seek advice and support?

Talking to someone about how you feel can be a great comfort, and will help you and your partner to come to terms with what has happened. Friends and relatives may be your first thought, but it can also be helpful to talk to a community midwife, or health visitor, who can offer practical advice. There are also a number of help groups that offer information, advice and support; they may also put you in contact with other parents of disabled children (see p. 256).

SURGICAL PROCEDURES ON NEWBORNS

Q WHO WILL OPERATE ON MY BABY?

A Almost invariably (depending on the specific problem), a trained paediatric surgeon or an experienced surgeon with paediatric experience will do the operation. Operating on babies is completely different from on adults. This is why doctors dealing with babies are specially trained. The anaesthetist, who puts your baby to sleep, will also have special experience with small children and babies.

Q MY BABY HAS TALIPES (CLUB FOOT). WHEN WILL THE OPERATION BE?

A With talipes, depending on the severity of the condition, the first step is usually to arrange corrective physiotherapy (splinting/strapping legs); this may, on its own, cure the problem. If the talipes is more severe, however, an operation or a series of operations is needed, the first of which is usually before baby starts walking. An orthopaedic surgeon and physiotherapist will be able to give a plan of action. The good news is that your child should be able to run and walk, if not completely normally then almost normally, by the age of 6–8.

Q MY BABY'S INTESTINES ARE OUTSIDE HIS TUMMY. HOW CAN THIS BE FIXED?

A This condition is called either exomphalos (omphalocoele) or gastroschisis. These conditions are similar in some ways but have important differences: in gastroschisis, free loops of intestine float in the amniotic fluid; in exomphalos, the liver, and sometimes the stomach, finds its way outside the baby's tummy wall. As long as there are no other major conditions affecting the baby, and the baby's chromosome test is normal, an operation can be done that involves gently easing the baby's intestines back into the tummy. This cannot always be achieved at one operation, however.

Q HOW IS CLEFT LIP CORRECTED?

A There is a spectrum of severity, from cleft lip with an intact palate, to both baby's lip and palate being absent in the midline (under the nose). If only the lip needs to be repaired, this is a more straightforward operation, and usually gives a good cosmetic result. Opinions vary on when this operation is best done, but there is a strong move for it to be as soon as possible so that the baby goes home with the problem largely fixed.

COMMON REASONS WHY BABIES NEED OPERATIONS AFTER DELIVERY

The reasons why a baby needs surgery obviously vary considerably, but commonly include the following:

Within 48 hours

■ Gastroschisis: Intestinal loops that are lying in the amniotic fluid outside the baby's tummy.

■ Exomphalos (omphalocoele): Intestine, sometimes with baby's liver and/or stomach, lying in the amniotic fluid outside the baby's tummy.

■ Diaphragmatic hernia: A hernia allowing intestines, and/or stomach and liver to enter the baby's chest, potentially stopping the baby's lung development.

■ Certain heart conditions: For example, narrowing of the aorta, transposition of the vessels leaving the heart.

■ Hydrocephalus: Excess fluid in baby's brain.

■ Anal atresia: Blockage of the baby's bottom end caused by the intestine not linking up with the anus.

■ Intestinal blockages.

Within days to weeks

■ Cleft lip and/or palate.

■ Extra digits.

■ Kidney abnormalities/blockages.

■ Cystic adenomatoid lung malformation (CAM): Cysts in the baby's chest and lungs that show up as bright white areas on ultrasound scan.

Within weeks to months

■ Undescended testicles.

■ Talipes (club foot): Feet twisted either inwards or outwards at the ankle.

Q WHAT PROBLEMS CAN CLEFT PALATE CAUSE? HOW ARE THEY CORRECTED?

A If baby's lips and palate are affected, this means there are problems to be addressed beyond the cosmetic issues, and these can affect the eyes, nose, and lips. They include recurrent ear and throat infections, feeding, speech, hearing, and breathing problems, and the need for dental reconstruction. Several operations will be required, with surgery taking place well into childhood. Ideally, a baby born with cleft lip and palate should be fully assessed and a treatment plan made "under one roof". To facilitate this, many centres now offer a multi-disciplinary approach. This involves surgeons (plastic surgeons and ear, nose, and throat experts), speech therapists, and specialist nurses.

Q WHY WEREN'T MY BABY'S PROBLEMS DETECTED ON THE ULTRASOUND SCANS?

A Ultrasound scans are very good at identifying certain problems that your baby may have while in the womb, but other seemingly obvious conditions cannot be seen on the scan. These include oesophageal atresia (blockage in the food-pipe to the stomach), anal atresia (blockage in the back passage), dislocated hips, eye cataracts, and many facial abnormalities. Also, it is important to realize that some conditions may have developed since you had your last scan, which may have been at 18–22 weeks.

Q WILL MY BABY FEEL ANYTHING DURING THE OPERATION?

A No, nothing at all. Your baby will have an anaesthetic in just the same way as you would if you were undergoing an operation. Your baby's breathing, heart rate, and other vital functions will be monitored very closely, so that any minute changes are detected and adjustments can be made by the anaesthetist and theatre team.

Q WHY DO BABIES HAVE CHEST DRAINS?

A Babies' lungs, especially in a baby who is born prematurely or is being artificially ventilated, may blow a leak and collapse; this is called a pneumothorax. In such a situation, a small plastic tube is put into the baby's chest wall, and suction placed on it to re-inflate the lung. This is a very common procedure, and is usually performed by a doctor on the neonatal intensive care unit (NICU). Chest drains can normally be removed after a few days.

Q HOW CAN THE DOCTORS KNOW IF MY BABY'S IN PAIN AFTER THE OPERATION?

A There are specialized scoring systems that are based on the baby's heart rate, sweating, facial expressions, and other physiological responses. These allow the doctors and nurses to assess whether the baby is comfortable or whether the baby is in pain and needs more analgesic drugs.

Q CAN I GO INTO THE OPERATING THEATRE WITH MY BABY?

A Not normally, because operating theatres are often not especially large rooms, and are quite crowded with essential staff – doctors, nurses, and other theatre staff – all of whom are concentrating on your baby. You might feel quite uncomfortable in these surroundings, and may become distressed when you see your baby being operated on. There is usually a sitting room in, or just outside, the theatre suite where you can wait during the operation. The medical and nursing staff will keep you closely informed of what is going on.

Q WHERE WILL BABY GO AFTER THE OPERATION?

A After an operation and an anaesthetic, babies are normally looked after by specialist nurses and doctors on the neonatal intensive care unit (NICU). In this unit, they can be closely monitored and are sometimes ventilated. The babies are usually given fluids into a vein, and their temperature, heart rate, oxygen levels, blood tests, and urine output are checked frequently.

Q MY BABY NEEDS HEART SURGERY. WHERE WILL THE DELIVERY TAKE PLACE?

A In most cases, your baby can be delivered in your local large obstetric unit where there is a paediatric cardiologist, as opposed to a paediatric cardiac surgeon, on hand for advice. Your baby may be OK and "pink" (good levels of oxygen) rather than "blue" (poor levels of oxygen) after delivery, in which case the necessary arrangements can be made in good time for transfer to the surgical unit where cardiac operations are carried out. This may include an intravenous drip of prostaglandin to keep the baby's circulation from closing off. There are rare conditions such as hypoplastic left heart (HLH) or transposition of the great arteries (TGA), where delivery is best in the local paediatric cardiothoracic unit in case major surgery needs to be done shortly after delivery. This will be discussed with you once a diagnosis has been made.

PROBLEMS IN PREMATURE BABIES

Q WHAT DOES PREMATURE MEAN?

A Premature means that the baby is born early. Most women have their babies at 37–42 weeks. The due date (estimated date of delivery, EDD) is calculated to be 40 weeks. So, technically, any baby born before 37 weeks is premature. But in reality, prematurity is usually only a problem for babies born before 34 weeks. At less than 30 weeks, a baby will often need dedicated neonatal intensive care facilities and help with breathing and feeding. It is very rare for a baby born at less than 24 weeks to survive, even with the best facilities.

Q DO STEROID INJECTIONS BEFORE DELIVERY HELP A BABY TO BREATHE?

A Yes. If it is anticipated that your baby is going to deliver early (before 34 weeks), then giving you a course of two steroid injections (usually 12–24 hours apart) reduces the risk of your baby getting respiratory distress syndrome (RDS), which is the major problem for premature babies. The more preterm your baby, the more effect the steroid injection will have.

Q MY BABY WAS BORN AT 26 WEEKS. WHY CAN'T HE FEED?

A At 26 weeks, baby's intestines are still developing and are not capable of digesting fluids, milk, and foodstuffs as well as at term. Preterm babies are prone to a potentially serious condition called necrotising enterocolitis, in which the intestine develops a leak. The best way of reducing this risk is for the baby to be fed very small amounts of fluid and/or milk through a tube into his stomach until he is more mature and passes stool, and the doctors and nurses can be sure that his bowels are working.

Q HOW LONG WILL MY BABY STAY IN THE NEONATAL INTENSIVE CARE UNIT?

A Some babies spend only a few days on the NICU. Others spend weeks and weeks. It can be a roller coaster ride: one day things go well, the next day, badly. Any attempt to fix a date for your baby to be out is destined to be thwarted. A rule of thumb is that preterm babies are, on average, ready to be discharged around your original due date, but this is very variable!

WHY DO PREMATURE BABIES GET LUNG PROBLEMS?

Lung problems occur in preterm babies for several reasons. The lungs are not fully developed and coated with "surfactant", which allows them to function effectively,

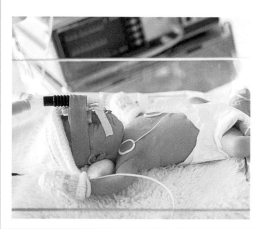

until after 36 weeks. Furthermore, premature babies are much more prone to respiratory infections than fully-grown babies. Finally, premature babies may need help breathing using mechanical ventilators (life-support machines), which, although life-saving, can themselves cause problems for the baby's lungs. Premature babies may develop a condition called respiratory distress syndrome (RDS), but this becomes progressively less likely as the weeks go by.

MECHANICAL VENTILATION
Babies can be ventilated through their noses, throats, or a tracheostomy (a surgically placed hole in baby's neck). Babies may need ventilating for several hours, days, or even weeks.

Q MY PREMATURE BABY HAD A FIT. IS THIS DANGEROUS?

A Fits can occur for many reasons – difficult deliveries, low blood sugar concentrations, infection, prolonged fetal distress in labour, bleeds into baby's brain and, very rarely, brain or genetic conditions. Usually, a fit is a one-off event and self limiting. Baby having a fit does not mean that she necessarily has a serious condition, nor does it mean as a result of the fit that her brain is damaged. The doctors will be doing tests and are the best people to advise you in this situation.

Q WHY DOES MY BABY NEED A BRAIN SCAN?

A Premature babies are at risk of small bleeds into the brain, especially if they have had fits, or have breathing and/or bleeding problems too. That is why an ultrasound scan of the brain is often done soon after baby has been delivered, and then some days or weeks later.

Q ARE PREMATURE BABIES ALWAYS HANDICAPPED?

A No, far from it. While in the best neonatal intensive care units the risk of handicap is highest at 23–24 weeks, and very low at 30 weeks, the risk for your baby depends on whether the baby has problems with liver, kidneys, or breathing, is underweight, or has other medical conditions. Problems with hearing, vision, or fine co-ordination skills are commonest in the more preterm babies. But many babies that survive after being born even at 24 weeks turn out to be absolutely fine.

Q DOES HAVING ONE PREM BABY MEAN MY NEXT ONE WILL BE PREMATURE TOO?

A This depends on the reason for your prem delivery. If it was because you went into premature labour, then there is a risk that it may happen again. However, if it was because of a condition affecting you or the baby that is highly unlikely to recur, then no.

Q MY BABY'S IN AN INCUBATOR AND I CAN'T BOND. WHAT EFFECT WILL THIS HAVE?

A There is no evidence that your baby being in an incubator reduces your ability to bond as parents later on, or to develop a loving relationship. Even very tiny babies in incubators can still be touched, and in some cases held, by their mums and dads. As your baby gets better, stronger and bigger, your contact can increase.

WHY ARE PRETERM BABIES MORE LIKELY TO HAVE JAUNDICE?

Preterm babies are more at risk of jaundice as they have an immature liver, which removes bilirubin from the body (see p.230). Bilirubin is the breakdown product of red blood cells. If it gets into the bloodstream, it colours skin yellow. Jaundice usually clears up without any problems in term babies, but high levels of bilirubin can, rarely, cause major damage to baby's brain, leading to a form of cerebral palsy. With good medical care, however, this is completely avoidable.

What can be done to help?

Ultraviolet (UV) light breaks down the bile pigments in the skin so that they can be safely excreted by the baby's kidneys. The ultraviolet light source may be a lamp in an incubator, with the baby wearing sunglasses or eye shields to prevent eye damage, or, as shown here, a UV light source wrapped around baby's trunk.

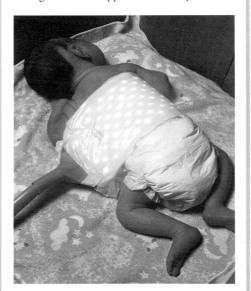

ULTRAVIOLET THERAPY
The baby shown here is wrapped in a UV light source blanket, so baby is not confined to an incubator and can move around at her leisure. The UV light breaks down bilirubin that is under the skin of the baby's trunk (chest and tummy).

LIFE AFTER BIRTH

Q HOW CAN I EXPECT TO FEEL IN THE FIRST FEW WEEKS AFTER THE BIRTH?

A In short, shell-shocked! Nothing can prepare you for the reality of having a baby, and the first few weeks will subject you to a barrage of new experiences and sensations. Powerful emotions will be evoked as you realize just how helpless and vulnerable your newborn is. The arrival of a new baby turns your whole world upside down, especially in the first few weeks, as you adjust to the demands of parenthood. Your baby will take up all your time and attention – for 24 hours a day – and you will feel tired and possibly tied down. Housework might pile up, social life and relationships could suffer, and your partner may feel neglected by your preoccupation with your baby.

Q MY BABY TAKES UP ALL MY TIME AND ENERGY. WILL IT ALWAYS BE LIKE THIS?

A Bringing up a new baby is hard work, especially in the early weeks. All the attention that was focused on you while you were pregnant is now being lavished on the baby – at a time when you could really do with being made a fuss of yourself. It is important to talk about your needs with your partner primarily, and also with your family and friends. This early phase of adjustment and chaos will not last too long. You will soon master the new skills of motherhood and, more importantly, how to juggle your needs, those of your partner and your baby all at the same time. In turn, you will gain in confidence and find the space to enjoy family life.

BONDING WITH YOUR BABY

Bonding is a term used to describe the initial building of a relationship between you and your new baby. Many people perceive it to be something that is instant and spontaneous. For some new parents it is, but for most, it will take time. You may feel that there is something wrong with you if it doesn't happen as soon as your baby is born. But having just survived the toughest physical and emotional challenge of your life, it is hardly surprising if you don't feel up to behaving how the books tell you to!

How should bonding happen?

There are no rules, procedures, or policies. You will eventually bond with your baby, whom you have cared for, nurtured from within, and longed for. It may take hours rather than minutes, weeks rather than days, but that doesn't mean that there is something wrong with you. Ask the staff caring for you to leave you and your partner alone with your new arrival as soon as possible. Remember you don't form "instant" relationships with people you love – it takes time for loving feelings to develop. Bonding describes the start of a long, lasting, and especially precious relationship.

What should I do if I don't feel that I'm bonding properly with my baby?

As we've already said, bonding won't necessarily happen instantly. If there were problems in your pregnancy, or with your baby and/or you after you have delivered, you may be confined to bed, on lots of medication, and feel in no mood to celebrate, despite your longed-for new arrival. Many mothers, and fathers too, secretly worry that they won't love their baby as much as they should, and fear that they might reject their baby. This only occurs, in our experience, extremely rarely. Take things as they come, relax, be comfortable, and a loving relationship will almost certainly develop as time goes by.

Is it possible to bond with my baby before he is born?

Many mothers do develop a close and intense feeling of bonding before the baby is even born. This is based on feeling the baby grow, kick, and move, and also from seeing him on the ultrasound scan monitor. Women who see their baby on ultrasound, or even real time 3-D ultrasound (which allows an almost life-like view of the baby), often say that this brings the experience of pregnancy to reality.

Q HOW CAN I MAKE SOME TIME FOR MYSELF?

A Try not to make the mistake of neglecting yourself at this time, or you'll soon feel as if you have reached the end of your tether. You need to be fit and rested to cope with a newborn baby, especially if you are breastfeeding, so make an effort to schedule some time for your own needs, perhaps by getting your partner to help out with some of the babycare chores. Your baby will probably sleep for an average of 16 hours a day, so try to rest when he or she is asleep; do not be tempted to use this time to catch up on housework or any other tasks that you feel you may have neglected. If you learnt any relaxation techniques in your antenatal classes, practise them now to help you relax, and to reduce stress. It is essential to have some time to yourself. As your baby gets older, perhaps you could have a reciprocal arrangement with a friend to look after each other's babies for a few hours each week.

Q I HAVE HAD TWINS – WILL I BE ABLE TO MANAGE ON MY OWN?

A Inevitably, looking after two babies is going to be hard work and is often more work than one pair of hands and one person's stamina can reasonably cope with. But don't panic. It is likely that you will stay in hospital for longer than usual, until you are quite happy that you can manage your babies' feeding, bathing, changing, and sleeping routines. Having someone to help you on a daily basis in the early days will make a big difference once you are back at home, so try to arrange this if you can. You should, as parents, plan ahead by making lists and writing things down. And learn to delegate – do not be afraid to ask friends and relatives to help with shopping and cleaning. If you have other children, ask someone to take them off your hands occasionally, to allow you to rest and recuperate. You and your partner will soon develop the routines that will allow you to cope sucessfully.

RESUMING SEX

Relationships change in many ways when you have a baby. Your partner is no longer just your lover – he is also your companion in parenthood. Sex can become a problem in the first few months after the birth, and this can make you both feel low.

When to begin?

The best time to start making love again is when you both feel ready. It's quite normal to experience a temporary lack of interest, or to feel too sore and tender to resume sex before your post-natal check. If you had an episiotomy, your partner should not attempt penetration until you are comfortable with this. Foreplay will be important because the glands that normally lubricate the vaginal area may not function as well for a short while after delivery, and you may need to use a lubricating cream or jelly.

Feeling unattractive

Many women feel unattractive after giving birth. Your body is probably still bloated or overweight, and it is difficult to feel sexually attractive if you are breastfeeding, have sore nipples, and leaking breasts. Starting post-natal exercises (see p. 240) to get back into shape will improve your self-esteem.

Partner's loss of interest

It is not uncommon for new fathers to lose their sex drive for several months after childbirth, especially if the baby is sleeping in their bedroom, and therefore a seemingly constant distraction. Your partner may also feel neglected because the baby takes up most of your time and energy. Both of you must be prepared for these distressing reactions, and try not to take them personally. Being open and talking about any problems is often the best solution but if, after several months, one of you is still feeling reluctant to resume your sexual relationship, seek professional advice. You'll be surprised how easy it is to talk about your problems with a third party. Consult your doctor about this; if necessary, you may be referred to a counsellor.

What about contraception?

Even if you are breastfeeding, or your periods have not begun again, you can still become pregnant again so you or your partner will need to use some form of contraception. Some contraceptive methods are recommended above others at this particular time, and your midwife or doctor will discuss these with you after the birth, and again at your six-week check (see p. 244).

PATERNAL CONCERNS

Q **WHAT DO I NEED TO DO BEFORE I BRING MY PARTNER AND BABY HOME?**

A Don't worry about trying to get everything perfect. Babies actually need very little, especially in the first few days. Just make sure that you have the basics, such as nappies, bottle-feeding equipment, milk, a well-stocked fridge, and a warm, dry, clean, and smoke free environment. Bring clothes for your partner and a warm shawl or blanket for the baby for the journey home.

Q **WHAT'S GOING TO HAPPEN TO MY SOCIAL LIFE?**

A You are about to discover the joys of the video store and the take-away. You will still be able to travel – but with an extra one, it takes longer and you'll need to take a lot more stuff with you. You will probably find that you'll spend more time with other parents who have young babies, rather than with your single friends.

Q **DO I HAVE TO BUY A SENSIBLE ESTATE CAR NOW?**

A Not necessarily. But on a practical level, to accommodate a growing family, baby, and all the equipment that goes with parenthood, the motor-bike or two-seater just isn't going to be the answer any more. So, your lifestyle may have to change, as well as your self-image and the belongings that defined you beforehand.

Q **I DON'T WANT OUR BABY SLEEPING WITH US IN CASE I SMOTHER HER. ANY ADVICE?**

A Yes, be reassured that's its virtually unheard of for a father (or a mother for that matter) to accidentally smother a baby in bed, so try to stop worrying.

Q **I CARE FOR MY BABY DURING THE NIGHTS, BUT I'M WORN OUT. ANY IDEAS?**

A If you're both doing a full-time job, share out the nights between you. During the week, it may be difficult, but at weekends try asking a friend to come round during the day and grab some sleep while you can. It's a tough physical, as well as emotional, time for dads, so eat regularly and well, have the odd night out with friends, and babysit while your partner does the same. Ask friends and family for help – they are usually delighted to be included in caring for the new baby.

Q **DO WE NEED TO USE CONTRACEPTION IF MY PARTNER IS BREASTFEEDING?**

A While breastfeeding, ovulation (release of eggs from the ovary) is suppressed. However, you shouldn't rely on it as a contraceptive method. Breakthrough periods can occur, especially if mixing breast- and bottle-feeding. Keep some condoms in the house so that you have something to use if the mood suddenly takes you both. Speak with your family doctor or family planning clinic when you both feel ready to consider alternative methods – coils (IUDs) and caps/diaphragms can be fitted after six weeks.

Q **I FEEL GUILTY TAKING PATERNITY LEAVE. SHOULD I?**

A Let's face it, things have changed during the last thirty or so years ago when the wife would obediently stay at home, cook, clean, and look after you and the baby. Also, family members, who might otherwise help, often live in another part of the country nowadays. Nor do many of us have nannies or domestic servants to help with the chores. Now, looking after a new baby is a time consuming, but very rewarding, job for two, and the greatest input is needed from you when and just after baby is born. So, in many countries, paternity leave is now a right, not a luxury, and let's hope it will make a difference to both of you in those first few critical weeks.

Q **WHAT IF SOMETHING HAPPENS WHEN I'M LEFT ALONE WITH THE BABY?**

A This is unlikely. Very little can happen in the hour or two that your partner is out. Dealing with babies is mostly a matter of common sense, so no need to panic. Make sure that you have her mobile number, or can contact friends or family for their advice

Q **SINCE SEEING THE DELIVERY, I'VE GONE OFF SEX. WILL THIS CHANGE?**

A Watching a partner deliver can be traumatic for some men, depending particularly on the type of delivery. If your partner feels ready, then it is unlikely you are going to hurt her in any way. You don't have to have full penetrative sex straight away, let her lead and see how you feel. Most importantly, tell her how you feel. After all, it's because you care about her that you feel this way.

Q WE HAVE A HOUSE FULL OF PETS. IS THIS BAD FOR MY BABY'S HEALTH?

A Pets can carry diseases that may affect the pregnancy. But to put things in perspective, many households have dogs and cats and it is very unusual for there to be a problem due to them. Do ensure, however, that you and your partner wash your hands any time you make contact with the pets, and that you are careful about disposing of pet waste. Your partner should wear gloves, especially when disposing of cat litter.

Q HOW CAN I KEEP IN TOUCH WITH MY FRIENDS WHO DON'T HAVE KIDS?

A It is a delicate balance between keeping up with them and not neglecting your time and "duties" as fatherhood approaches. You may not be able to enjoy carefree weekends and going out late with your friends at the moment, but you can still keep in touch – telephone, email, have a coffee after work, meet up at different times of day, and keep them up to date with what's happening to you and your family.

Q I NEED A HOLIDAY – HELP!

A When you feel up to travelling with your new baby, try sticking with a tried and tested holiday formula – start with a recommendation from someone who has done it before. Don't travel too far. Be realistic and try to stay in the same country or, failing that, go to somewhere you know well and where you know what to expect. It sounds obvious, but climate, safe water supplies, access to medical facilities, and clean accommodation are all important. You and your partner both need your holidays, but they should not end up becoming a major logistical nightmare that makes your work look like a walk in the park.

Q I FEEL AWKWARD WITH MY BABY. SHE'S GETTING ALL MY PARTNER'S ATTENTION.

A This is a very common feeling, that of being a little "left out" and even resenting the attention your partner gives to the baby. You should do two things. Firstly, explain to your partner what you are feeling. Secondly, banish these thoughts from your mind! Try not to focus so much on yourself, as it will prevent you from being constructive in the new and unfamiliar situation you find yourself in. You need to subjugate feelings of your own importance, and learn to move away from centre stage to accommodate someone else!

Q MY WIFE DOES EVERYTHING FOR THE BABY. WHAT CAN I DO TO HELP?

A Try getting more involved – ask your partner what she thinks you can do to help. Try to maintain contact with friends who have young children and help out with food when people visit. Parenting can and should be done together – it just takes time to work out a strategy.

Q MY WIFE SEEMS TO BE DEPRESSED SINCE THE BIRTH. WHAT CAN I DO?

A It is not unusual for a new mother to suffer with "baby blues", which lasts for a few days after the birth. However, if the depression lasts for weeks, and affects her eating and sleeping, then you should discuss this with your wife and encourage her to see her doctor or midwife to ensure that she is not suffering from post-natal depression. This is probably much more common than anyone realizes (see p. 249).

Q WE HAVEN'T HAD SEX FOR WEEKS. WHAT CAN I DO?

A Apart from feeling sore after the delivery, women often just don't feel very sexy, sometimes for weeks or months. Usually, they are simply exhausted and sex is low on the agenda. However, you can help and encourage your partner to get back in shape, to get plenty of rest, and to start feeling better. Reassure her that her body is still attractive and sexy. Try not to put pressure on her to feel or look a certain way – things will come naturally!

Q DOES QUALITY TIME WITH MY BABY CONSIST OF NAPPY CHANGING?

A If your baby is breastfeeding, then the answer is partly yes! You also get to bath the baby, soothe the baby, and babysit when your partner needs a break. Rest assured, it does get better very quickly, or perhaps you just get used to it!

Q I WORK WHILE MY PARTNER CARES FOR THE BABY. SHOULD I FEEL GUILTY?

A No! Unless you're extremely fortunate, one of you will need to be the breadwinner. If your partner is coping at home, you are supporting her practically and emotionally. It is normal and reasonable for you to get back to work, hopefully after a few weeks' leave during which you can be together and you can help for the first crucial weeks.

GETTING BACK INTO SHAPE

Q WHAT CAN I DO TO GET BACK INTO SHAPE?

A It is probably the last thing on your mind in the first few days after the birth, yet beginning gentle exercises for your pelvic floor and abdomen is important if you want to get back into shape as soon as possible. For a few weeks, while you are getting used to your new life, you will certainly feel and look very tired but if you make time for a regular exercise routine (see p. 242) you will find that it is doing far more for you than just reducing your waistline and rebuilding your muscle tone – it also increases your energy levels and enhances your emotional well-being.

Q HOW LONG WILL IT TAKE ME TO GET MY FIGURE BACK?

A Getting back into shape after having a baby doesn't happen overnight – you will have to work at it steadily and regularly. With daily exercises, your figure can return to normal in as little as three months after the birth, so begin exercising as soon as you can.

Q WHY ARE PELVIC FLOOR EXERCISES SO IMPORTANT AFTER BIRTH?

A As described in Chapter 5, the pelvic floor is the hammock of muscles that supports your bowel, bladder and womb. These muscles, which you tighten to help control your bladder and bowel when they are full, have been stretched and weakened by your pregnancy and labour, so you may find that you leak urine involuntarily when you cough, sneeze, or laugh. You may also experience decreased satisfaction during intercourse. Both these problems can be improved by toning your pelvic floor muscles with special exercises (see p. 111).

Q HOW LONG WILL IT TAKE TO STRENGTHEN MY PELVIC FLOOR?

A With regular exercise, the pelvic floor muscles should have regained their strength after a month or two. You can test this by jumping up and down with a fairly full bladder, and coughing. If you don't leak any urine while doing this, then your pelvic muscles are in good shape. Another good test is to grip your partner's penis with your vaginal muscles when you make love, and ask him if he can feel this.

Q I USED TO GO TO EXERCISE CLASSES, WHEN CAN I START AGAIN?

A Wait until you have stopped bleeding, your pelvic floor muscles have strengthened, and you have had your post-natal check at six weeks. Don't expect to be as energetic as you used to be at first. You'll have to start slowly again, perhaps in a beginners' class, to build up your fitness level.

Q HOW SOON CAN I EXERCISE AFTER A CAESAREAN?

A You can begin pelvic floor exercises immediately but should attempt nothing more until your post-natal check has given you the all-clear, and your wound has fully healed. You should avoid any exercise, such as sit-ups, that involves your abdominal muscles; also avoid any competitive sports for at least three months. Do not lift heavy weights, including shopping or even a toddler, for at least six weeks. When recovering from a Caesarean, listen to your body and stop if an exercise causes discomfort or you feel exhausted; and never exercise if you are feeling unwell.

Q CAN I START TO LOSE WEIGHT BY WATCHING MY CALORIE INTAKE?

A Much of the weight you gained during your pregnancy is nature's way of providing fat stores for you to draw on while breastfeeding, so it is not advisable to go on a diet until after you have stopped breastfeeding and even then you may not need to. Breastfeeding certainly helps you lose weight in the long run but you will also find that you need to eat more (about 2,500 calories a day) to maintain your energy levels as well as provide a good flow of milk.

Q IS MY DIET IMPORTANT EVEN IF I'M NOT BREASTFEEDING?

A Even if you are not breastfeeding it is essential that your diet is nutritious because you are recovering from the birth and now have a demanding baby to cope with. Try to start your day with a good breakfast; carbohydrates provide a good, steady supply of energy, and protein gives you a solid base (see p. 104), so choose wholewheat cereals, porridge, or eggs, bacon, and wholemeal toast. Later in the day, healthy sandwiches or snacks can keep you going; simple pasta or rice dishes are quick and easy to prepare in the evening.

IS THERE A SPECIAL DIET FOR BREASTFEEDING?

Most women find that they have a larger appetite when breastfeeding but to ensure that you are able to provide milk without taking from your own energy requirements you will need about an extra 500 calories per day. Eat nutritious food rather than sugary or salty snacks.

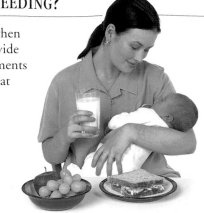

Eat more often

However tired or busy you are, it's important that you do not skimp on your meals. It may suit you to eat several lighter meals or snacks during the day, rather than one larger main meal that is harder to digest. Keep a stock of ingredients to make yourself quick and nutritious snacks.

Eat well

You need to eat plenty of protein and calcium, which are provided by eggs, dairy products, meat, or fish. (If you're a strict vegetarian, you will get your protein from wholegrains and pulses.) Be sure to include fresh fruit and vegetables to avoid constipation, carbohydrates such as rice, pasta, or potatoes for energy, and iron-rich foods such as sardines, green leafy vegetables, or dried fruit.

Take extra fluids

Always drink plenty of fluids when breastfeeding, preferably water, milk, fruit juices (except orange) or herbal teas instead of caffeinated drinks (see below).

FAST BUT NUTRITIOUS FOOD
You will need snacks and meals that require the minimum of preparation, for example, wholemeal bread sandwiches, fresh fruit, and a glass of milk.

QUICK HEALTHY SNACKS

- Baked potatoes with toppings such as cheese.
- Wholemeal sandwiches with healthy fillings.
- Hummus and pitta bread or toast.
- Pasta with melted butter or grated cheese.
- Milkshakes made with full-fat milk.
- Muesli with yogurt and fresh fruit.
- Soups and wholemeal bread.

WHAT SHOULD I AVOID?

Although you should avoid consuming any non-essential drugs, as well as alcohol while breastfeeding, many other ideas about what you can or can't eat are myths.

Drugs and alcohol

Drugs and alcohol enter the bloodstream and can be passed on to your baby through your milk, so it's vital that you tell your pharmacist or doctor that you are breastfeeding when prescribed any drugs; avoid alcohol, as your baby's system is unable to cope with it in the way that yours can.

Spicy foods, garlic, and caffeine

It is often said that certain foods such as oranges, onions, garlic, and spicy foods such as curries should be avoided because they can cause a baby to have loose stools or wind. This will not necessarily happen because the food you eat does not pass directly into the milk, but is first broken down by your digestive system. However, certain foods may change the acidity or taste of your milk and if you notice that a specific food upsets your baby, do not eat it. Try to avoid strong caffeinated drinks because caffeine could well affect your baby.

Empty calories

Even though you are short of time, try not to substitute fatty or sugary snacks – such as crisps, sweets, biscuits, and cakes – for proper meals. These snacks are usually high in calories but devoid of nutrients, and they can only give you a short burst of energy.

GETTING BACK YOUR FIGURE

With gentle daily exercise, your figure could return to normal within three months. You can begin to strengthen the pelvic floor and abdominal muscles straight after the birth, unless you had a Caesarean, in which case just practise the pelvic floor exercise until your doctor says you can be more active.

PELVIC FLOOR EXERCISE

Imagine that you are trying to stop yourself from passing wind, and at the same time trying to stop your flow of urine mid-stream. Squeeze and lift to close and draw up the back and front passages, hold for as long as you can, then rest for about four seconds. Don't tighten your stomach or buttocks, or hold your breath. Try to do about ten every hour.

BEFORE YOU EXERCISE

■ While you can begin these gentle exercises immediately, do not attempt any vigorous exercise until your bleeding has ceased, and your pelvic floor has strengthened (see p. 111).
■ If you have had a Caesarean, wait until you have had your six-week post-natal check-up before taking up any active exercise.
■ Never exercise if you feel exhausted or unwell.
■ If you have had back problems, consult your doctor about the suitability of these exercises.
■ Exercise little and often. Start with just one or two repetitions and build up to ten or more.
■ Do not attempt sit-ups or double-leg raises with your legs straight.
■ Remember to "exhale on the effort": breathe out when you tighten your stomach muscles.
■ Stop if an exercise hurts.

PELVIC TILT

Lie on the floor with your knees bent, feet flat on the floor, head and shoulders supported on a pillow. This is a good exercise for the first week after birth.

Tilt your pelvis as you draw your stomach in

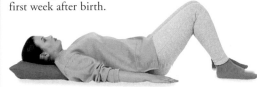

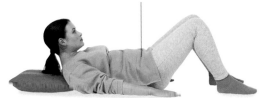

1 Draw in your stomach, pressing the small of your back into the floor. Hold for four seconds, but don't hold your breath, then gently let go.

2 As you get stronger, you can work your stomach muscles harder by holding the flattened position while you curl forward and lift your head.

CURL UPS

In the second or third week, you can try this more advanced position. Lie on the floor with your head on a pillow, knees bent, and feet slightly apart.

Always breathe out when you pull your stomach in

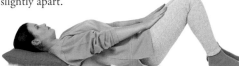

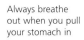

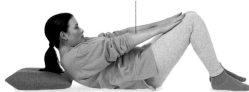

1 Breathe in, and begin the exercise by stretching out your arms and trying to reach your knees with your hands.

2 As you breathe out, pull in your stomach muscles and lift your head. Try to hold for a few seconds, and then rest.

DIAGONAL REACHES

Tighten your stomach muscles before you reach over, and relax them between reaches.

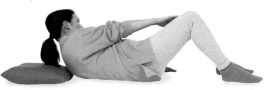

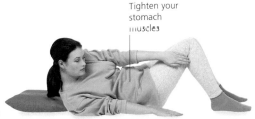

Tighten your stomach muscles

1 Lifting your head and right shoulder, reach the right arm across the body towards the left ankle.

2 Lie back and rest for a moment, then repeat the exercise on the other side.

LEG LIFTS

This exercise tones the hips and thighs. Use your hands and abdominal muscles for support and balance. Keep the leg straight but the knee soft.

1 Lie on your side, both legs directly in line with your hip and shoulder.

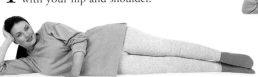

Foot faces forward

2 Keep the knees facing front, raise the upper leg more or less to shoulder height, and then lower the leg.

CAT STRETCHES

This is an excellent exercise for your back. Simply arch your spine towards the ceiling, like a cat having a good stretch.

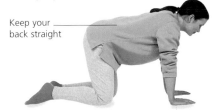

Keep your back straight

1 Get into position on all fours; make sure you start off with your back straight.

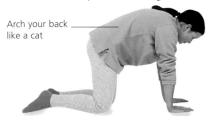

Arch your back like a cat

2 Slowly arch your back upwards without making yourself uncomfortable.

SIDE BENDS

Stand with your feet apart. Slowly and smoothly, bend sideways, keeping your hips steady and facing forwards, with your feet flat on the floor. Breathe out as you bend.

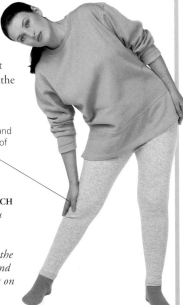

Rest your hand on the side of your knee

BEND AND STRETCH
Move as far as you comfortably can. Hold for a few seconds, return to the upright position and breathe in. Repeat on the other side.

YOUR POST-NATAL CHECK

Q WHY DO I NEED A CHECK-UP AFTER SIX WEEKS?

A Your recovery from pregnancy and labour should be almost complete six weeks after the birth, and your doctor will want to check that everything is returning to normal. By now, your stitches should have healed, your bleeding stopped, and your breasts adapted to feeding, or returned to normal if you are bottle-feeding. If you feel that anything is not quite right, this is an opportunity to get it checked by your doctor.

Q WHEN ARE MY PERIODS LIKELY TO START AGAIN?

A This date varies depending on individual circumstances. Your periods may begin before the post-natal check; if you are bottle-feeding (or you breastfeed only for a short time), your periods should return between two and four months after the birth but if you breastfeed for longer, your periods may not return until your baby starts to take solid food, or possibly even later.

Q WHEN DO I NEED TO START THINKING ABOUT CONTRACEPTION?

A Straight away, because even though your periods haven't started yet, it is important to realize that you could become pregnant again within a month or two of giving birth because ovulation can occur before your first period. Although breastfeeding reduces the likelihood of this, it is not a reliable form of contraception.

Q WHAT METHODS OF CONTRACEPTION CAN I USE?

A Condoms, diaphragms, and all barrier methods of contraception are safe to use at any time. You can take the Pill if you are bottle-feeding, but if you have chosen to breastfeed, your doctor will advise against hormonal contraception as oestrogen can inhibit milk production. The "Mini-pill" (containing only progesterone) is compatible with breastfeeding, but must be taken at the same time every day to be effective. There is also an electronic monitor available; this tests your urine for hormones, and shows the days when you are ovulating and those when you are safe. However, this system should not be used if you are breastfeeding.

WHAT HAPPENS AT THE POST-NATAL CHECK?

As well as a physical examination to check that you are fully recovered, the post-natal check is an ideal time to discuss any problems or incidents that occurred during your pregnancy or labour and why these occurred, and to express any other worries you may have (see opposite). It is normally carried out either at your doctor's surgery or at the hospital clinic; however, if you had a Caesarean, high blood pressure (pre-eclampsia), or any other complications, you will usually have to see the consultant at your hospital. Your doctor will also discuss your choice of birth control method.

Checks and advice

Any or all of the following checks will be carried out and appropriate advice given:
- Your urine is tested for protein, to check your kidney function and for urinary tract infection.
- Your weight is recorded.
- Your blood pressure noted.
- Your breasts and nipples are checked, especially if your are breastfeeding.
- Your abdomen is examined to check that your womb has shrunk back to its normal size.
- Any wounds (Caesarean or episiotomy) are examined.
- Your vagina and perineum are examined.
- You may be offered a cervical smear test if you have not had one recently, or if the last one gave an abnormal result.
- If there is any suspicion that you are anaemic, blood will be taken to test haemoglobin levels.
- If you are not immune to rubella (German measles), you will be offered a vaccination.
- You will be given advice about contraception: depending on your preference, you can have a new coil inserted or a new cap fitted; you can go on the "Mini-pill" (see left) or be given condoms.

I'M WORRIED ABOUT...

This is an excellent time to discuss with your doctor any health issues that you are concerned about, or any embarrassing problems that you are experiencing –

I am still sore in the perineal area

If you had an episiotomy (cut) or tear in the perineal area at the birth, the stitches should have dissolved, and the wound should have healed by now. If the area is still red or feels sore, there may be an infection present, and your doctor (or possibly an obstetrician) will check this now; you may need to take an antibiotic to help clear up the infection. Sometimes, if the stitches haven't dissolved properly, they have to be removed by the doctor.

My vagina feels different

It is common to feel that your vaginal area is "different" after having a baby and to some extent this is true: your pelvic floor muscles have been stretched and need to be exercised to regain their original elasticity (see p. 242). Some women fear that they have not been stitched back together properly. Although this is most unlikely, in extremely rare cases where the stitches have healed badly, the result can interfere with the ability to pass water and hold wind properly and even mar your sex life. In this case it may be necessary to have an operation, called a "refashioning of the perineum", to return things to normal.

I am leaking urine

Many women experience urine leakage (stress incontinence) after childbirth, so don't be embarrassed to talk about it. Most commonly it settles within a few weeks. The sooner you bring it to your doctor's attention the sooner you will be referred to a specialist unit if this is necessary. Usually it is the result of damaged or weak pelvic floor muscles.

A SYMPATHETIC EAR
Your doctor will be ready to discuss any problems you are experiencing during your recovery.

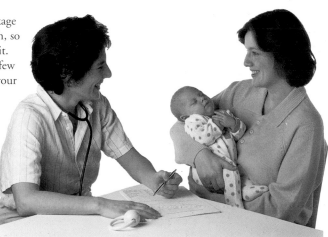

from soreness to your sex life. It will also put your mind at rest to discover that your fears and problems are very common and also easily remedied.

Sometimes exercises can help, or a simple treatment is all that is required. Infection can also make you leak, so a urine specimen is often asked for, or a course of antibiotics prescribed.

I feel weak after my Caesarean

If you had a Caesarean delivery, your stomach muscles can take some time to knit back together again and you will not have much strength in your abdominal area. You should avoid any lifting or driving for the first six weeks to give the wound time to heal properly; it will be at least three months before you can lift heavy objects, run, or take up sport again. Apart from the pelvic tilt (see p. 242), avoid any exercise until after six weeks.

I feel so tired

Many women feel exhausted in the weeks after the birth because of broken nights, but if your fatigue is accompanied by breathlessness and pallor, you may be anaemic. This can be caused by a lack of iron, or a loss of blood during labour. Normal blood loss does not cause a problem because your body rapidly makes up the oxygen-carrying blood cells. If you had a Caesarean, you may have lost twice as much blood as after a vaginal delivery, so you may need to take iron tablets to replenish your body's stores.

POST-NATAL ISSUES

Q I HAVE NO ENERGY SINCE THE BIRTH. WILL I EVER FEEL NORMAL AGAIN?

A Yes, of course you will. However, you will feel better now if you are able to get as much sleep and rest as possible. Make sure that you are resting whenever your baby is asleep, and don't take on any other major projects until the most demanding weeks of your baby's life have passed. Even if you don't sleep, try the relaxation techniques you learned to use during labour.

Q MY BABY WAS BORN THREE WEEKS AGO. I FEEL OVERWHELMED. WHAT CAN I DO?

A This is an exhausting, though exhilarating, time in your life. Take a little time every day for yourself – plan little treats that will make you feel pampered. Ask your partner, family, or friends for support during these special times so that you have a little uninterrupted space just for you!

Q I WANT TO SEE MY FRIENDS BUT IT ALL SEEMS TOO DIFFICULT. ANY IDEAS?

A Start with having your friends around to you, then go out for an hour without the baby. Leave her with your partner or a friend. As you grow in confidence, be more adventurous – gradually you'll find you are coping with getting out and about.

Q I FEEL ENGULFED BY BREAST MILK AND NAPPIES. AM I DEPRESSED?

A Probably not. It's more likely that you are suffering from an identity crisis as motherhood puts everything else in the shade. This is common in the early weeks after giving birth as everyone's attention focuses on the new arrival, but this will improve as your baby gets older. Spare a thought for your partner too. He's probably feeling the same!

Q WHO SHOULD I GET TO LOOK AFTER MY BABY WHEN I RETURN TO WORK?

A That depends on what is right for your family and lifestyle. Cost is a consideration, as is your child's welfare. You need to sit down and work out the practicalities. For example, if you are expected to work late or at little notice, a crèche that closes at 5pm will be of little use to you. Work out what is essential and desirable to your childcare situation, and you will be able to answer your own question.

Q I'M WORRIED ABOUT LEAVING MY BABY IN THE CRÈCHE. IS THIS NORMAL?

A Of course it is. You have no proof yet that the crèche and your child are right for each other. But as time goes by, this will be evident, so try not to worry for now. Most mothers feel guilty about going back to work and question whether the crèche, nanny, or au pair is a good enough substitute for a parent. However, it is neither wise nor practical for your baby to live in your pocket. Try to think of the crèche not as somewhere you dump your baby so you can go to work, but rather as a place you provide for your child to learn social skills, widen vocabulary, and make friends, all under the supervision of trained professionals.

Q I'M DREADING GOING BACK TO WORK. WHAT CAN I DO?

A Well, to start with, look at why you are dreading going back to work. If it is because you don't want to leave your baby, then you need to put this in perspective. There are times when you have to be apart and you need to be with adults some of the time. If you have sorted out childcare and love your work, try to focus on the positive and start looking forward to getting back. After all, if it doesn't work out, you can change it. Women sometimes worry that things will have changed whilst they have been away and that they will be unable to cope with the work. However, once you get back into the swing of work, you will feel differently.

Q I FEEL CUT OFF FROM THE REAL WORLD. I LOVE MY BABY, BUT WHAT ABOUT ME?

A This is a very common feeling in new mums. If you think about it, you are encouraged to mix with others in pregnancy, herded together in the antenatal clinic and post-natal ward, to share stories and experiences. Then, when you have had the baby, you go home behind closed doors never to be seen again! It can be lonely – you are cut off from most adult company, and feel at your most social during unsocial hours. Try to get out with a friend, preferably one with no children, where you can just talk about you and what interests you both. Get someone else to keep an eye on your baby and have some time off for good behaviour!

Q I'M AFRAID TO LEAVE MY BABY WITH ANYONE. WHAT IF SHE NEEDS ME?

A Plan for this eventuality. Get a mobile phone and write down the number on which you can be called. In other words, do something about it if you can and if it is something you can't do anything about, stop worrying. This is for the rest of your life, so start small. Maybe just go to a friend's house in the same street for an hour. Then go shopping (with your mobile), or go out with your partner for the evening. Gradually, as you have proof that you can safely leave your baby, your confidence will increase and the world will be your oyster!

Q I HEAR ROUTINE IS A GOOD IDEA. IS IT TOO EARLY TO START YET?

A Routine is vital for family life but a newborn cannot adapt immediately and so needs to dictate the routine for a while, which means there is no routine! Clearly though, a routine gradually evolves over the first few weeks and then months, and involves more than just eating and sleeping. This is the stage where your baby is awake for much longer periods. You must then determine bedtimes and rest times, rather than waiting for your baby to decide when he is tired. By the time your baby has worked out he needs to sleep, he is actually over-tired and probably difficult to settle.

Q WHAT SHOULD I DO TO GET MY BABY INTO A SLEEP ROUTINE?

A When your baby is a few months old (not just weeks), you can try to put her down to sleep at a regular time. As you do this, give your baby something to keep her entertained, such as music, stories on a tape, or a colourful mobile above the cot. This way, she'll have her playtime without you having to be there to entertain her. Once you have established a sleeping pattern, you will be able to claim your evenings back, and may even start socializing again.

Q I NEED TO LOSE WEIGHT, BUT I JUST GRAZE ON LEFTOVERS. ANY IDEAS?

A Firstly, stop grazing. If your partner is not at home for a meal and you find that you do not have the motivation to cook just for yourself, buy a healthy ready-prepared dinner for one from the supermarket. Stop eating your child's or partner's leftovers. It may sound wasteful, but cover the food with washing up liquid as soon as you clear away the dishes. The leftovers aren't doing you any good, so it's preferable to waste the food. Even better still, think about getting a dog – not only would you have a ready recipient for any leftovers, but walking the dog would give you a form of healthy extra exercise.

POST-NATAL PHYSICAL ACTIVITY

Exercising may be the last thing on your mind after you've just had your baby! But seriously, the routines you establish now will see you through the next few months while your body regains its normal shape.

A physical regime made up of many different "mini-routines" (for example, morning stretching exercises, two walks a day, a swim twice a week) will help you to regain your figure that much more quickly.

How do I lose the weight that I put on during my pregnancy?

Try to maintain the healthy eating habits that you developed during your pregnancy, but remember that you need less food now than you did in the last few weeks before the birth. Start an exercise routine that fits in with your life. If this is not producing results by the time you go for your post-natal check, try joining a reputable local slimming group or club that can give you advice and support – your midwife can provide help, too, especially if you are breastfeeding.

I have always been fit. How do I get back into shape after my baby is born?

Looking after a newborn baby is a full-time job so, to begin with, do your exercises with your baby. Start by going for a short walk as soon as possible after the birth. Make the walk a little longer each day, and get extra exercise by pushing the pram. Take a few moments each day to do pelvic floor and abdominal exercises, too, even if you have to do them with your baby lying beside you. You will soon find that your body regains its natural fitness.

POST-NATAL HEALTH

Q I WAS ANAEMIC IN PREGNANCY AND NOW I FEEL COMPLETELY DRAINED. WHY?

A It takes quite a long time for your iron stores to build up again, and red blood cells to come back to their pre-pregnancy level. Therefore, you don't just recover from anaemia after you have had your baby. In fact, it may get worse if you are breastfeeding and/or if you have some vaginal bleeding. Although a balanced diet will help, it is wise in this situation to take iron supplements as prescribed by your doctor.

Q I WAS DUE A SMEAR TEST BEFORE I WAS PREGNANT. WHEN SHOULD I HAVE IT?

A The best time to have a smear is when you've stopped having any bleeding or discharge, at or after the six week post-natal check-up. Any earlier, and the results of the test may be difficult to interpret. But if you were due one, remember to mention it to your doctor, nurse, or health visitor.

Q I HAD AN EPISIOTOMY THREE WEEKS AGO AND IT'S STILL SORE. WHAT'S WRONG?

A If you had stitches, these normally dissolve in 10–14 days and therefore don't need to be taken out. Sometimes, however, little bits of stitch can hang around for weeks, causing vaginal soreness. It is rare for an infection to develop at the stitch site, but if it's very tender, swollen, and you have a yellow-coloured discharge, see your doctor, who may give you antibiotics.

Q MY LEG IS RED, TENDER, AND PAINFUL TO WALK ON. IS THIS SERIOUS?

A Probably not. It may well be phlebitis, inflammation of the small vessels in the skin. However, if you have these symptoms, it is very important that you see a doctor. Sometimes, these symptoms indicate a clot in the deep veins of the leg (deep venous thrombosis, or DVT). This is a potentially serious complication, and may need immediate treatment.

Q MY CAESAREAN SCAR FEELS NUMB. IS THIS NORMAL?

A Yes. When you have a Caesarean, the incision on your tummy cuts through some of the nerve fibres supplying your skin. It takes some time for these to reconnect, but they will. Your scar may feel numb for some months yet.

Q I'VE HAD A CAESAREAN SECTION. CAN I STILL LIFT MY CHILDREN?

A You shouldn't do this for some weeks, as your muscles and tummy wall have been weakened by the Caesarean. This will not only make it very painful to lift, but may strain the scar, which is trying hard to heal. Wait six to eight weeks before returning to full lifting duties.

Q MY CAESAREAN SCAR FEELS REALLY LUMPY AND HARD. WHAT CAN I DO?

A After a Caesarean, there is invariably some bruising and a little bleeding in the layer under the skin (the subcutaneous tissue). Don't worry, as this will improve over several weeks as the blood clot dissolves and becomes soft. Also, don't be concerned if after a few days a little old dark blood seeps out through the skin – better out than in! If your scar is infected, it will be tender and swollen, and discharging blood mixed with pus.

Q CAN MY NORMAL ACTIVITIES CAUSE MY CAESAREAN SCAR TO BURST?

A Any surgical scar may rupture, but this is very rare indeed. It would only happen if the scar were weakened already, so doing normal activities won't cause it to burst on its own. It can occur a few days after the operation and is highly traumatic, especially if your intestines come through the scar. This may happen if the internal stitches break or pull through. Luckily, this is not normally as dangerous as it seems: lie flat, get someone to put a warm, clean, damp sheet over your tummy and get an ambulance to take you to hospital. Don't walk around, eat, or drink.

Q IT'S A MONTH AFTER THE BIRTH. WHY DO I LEAK URINE WHEN I COUGH OR SNEEZE?

A After a vaginal birth, your tissues (including the bladder, vagina, and the skin and muscles of your perineum), which have all been stretched, need to get back in shape. This can take months, so it is very common to leak a bit in the first few weeks. A physiotherapist or health visitor can show you pelvic floor exercises to tone up your vaginal muscles. However, if you have a burning sensation when you pass urine, or if you are peeing very often, you must tell your doctor, as you may have an infection.

POST-NATAL DEPRESSION

Q WHAT ARE THE SYMPTOMS OF POST-NATAL DEPRESSION?

A Classical symptoms include waking early in the morning, poor concentration, and a feeling of "slowing down" mentally. Also, you may feel guilty about yourself, worthless, and lacking in confidence – sometimes this is so bad you cannot face meeting friends. Other features include insomnia, eating very poorly, and worrying about even minor things.

Q WHY CAN'T MY DEPRESSION BE TREATED WITH HORMONES?

A There have been several studies using high dose oestrogens or progesterone, to treat post-natal depression, with varying degrees of success. Neither has become a standard treatment, however, and it is not at all clear how they might work, as oestrogen and progesterone have opposite effects.

Q MY HEAD'S WHIRRING AND I'M WORRIED ALL THE TIME. AM I DEPRESSED?

A It is much more likely that you are just worn down by having too much to do and too little sleep. Mild post-natal depression, sometimes known as "baby blues", makes you feel anxious and tearful within days of having your baby. It affects up to 10 per cent of women and usually gets better within weeks. However, if you are finding it difficult to cope, speak to your doctor about your feelings. Visiting a trained counsellor may also help.

Q THERE IS DEPRESSION IN MY FAMILY. WILL I GET POST-NATAL DEPRESSION?

A No. Although there is a weak family link in depressive illnesses, there are many different types of depression, and these are caused by different circumstances.

WHY AM I DEPRESSED?

Most women expect to feel euphoric once their baby is here, but many feel low for several days after giving birth; this is known as "baby blues". Doctors are not entirely clear why this happens, but it is probably due to the adjustments that your body undergoes after the birth, and the sudden change in hormone levels, which can deeply affect your emotions. You are more likely to get the blues if you usually suffer with premenstrual depression, if you were depressed during the pregnancy, and/or if you have just had your first baby.

How will the blues affect me?
You may feel miserable and tearful and you may even feel strangely distant from your baby. This can happen when your milk first comes in, or because your sleeping and eating routines are disturbed. At times your spirits will lift – only to plummet again rapidly. These emotional highs and lows usually last for a day or two and you will be more able to cope if you understand what is causing this. You will need plenty of support from your partner and family. The midwife can also be a source of advice.

What is post-natal depression?
About one in ten women suffers from post-natal depression. This is a more prolonged bout of "baby blues" and usually starts a week or two after the baby is born – often when you get home from hospital. You may feel weepy, irritable, confused, and tired, have difficulty concentrating, and may even doubt your ability to look after your baby.

Why does it happen?
However much you longed for the event, the reality of having a baby can take some getting used to. Depression can result from the difficulty of adjusting to motherhood, or be the expression of a grieving process for the loss of your previous lifestyle. In your new, changed life you still need to feel that you are a person in your own right, and not merely an appendage to your baby.

How long does post-natal depression last?
The symptoms of post-natal depression usually diminish within a few weeks, but if they persist you may be suffering from severe depression and should see your doctor; you may benefit from anti-depressant drugs and further specialist medical care. There may be a counsellor to whom you could talk, or you could join a support group.

YOUR BABY'S SIX-WEEK CHECK

Q HOW HAS MY BABY DEVELOPED OVER THE FIRST SIX WEEKS?

A You will find that your baby has become a more responsive individual, and less of a noisy, demanding bundle. You may also find that he or she does not cry as much as before, and that there is a longer wakeful period during the day. Control over the limbs has increased and the fists have unclenched, enabling objects to be grasped more easily. You will notice how your baby enjoys kicking his or her legs in the air. When lying face down, your baby may be able to lift his or her head momentarily, but will remain unable to do this when sitting.

WHICH IMMUNIZATIONS AND CHECKS WILL MY BABY NEED?

The six-week check is the first part of your baby's medical programme and is followed by check-ups and vaccinations up to four years old. Some vaccines are long-lasting, others need to be boosted at regular intervals. Call the Department of Health for a schedule (see p. 256).

Immunizations

AGE	IMMUNIZATION
2, 3, 4 months	DTP – Diphtheria, tetanus, polio, pertussis (whooping cough)
12 – 15 months	MMR – Measles, mumps, rubella
3 – 4 years	Pre-school booster of MMR, plus polio, diphtheria, and tetanus

Check-ups

■ At eight months, your baby's hearing, growth, and development are tested.
■ At two years, your baby's walking, talking, comprehension, and co-ordination (fine motor skills) are assessed.
■ At three-and-a-half years, the physical development, speech, and hearing are checked.

Q CAN MY BABY RECOGNIZE ME OR MY PARTNER YET?

A Yes, one of the biggest thrills for you and your partner is that your baby now has a range of facial expressions and can respond to you both. Your baby's head turns upon hearing your voice, and he or she will stare at your face when you are talking, meeting your eyes and smiling at you.

Q IS IT NORMAL FOR A PREMATURE BABY TO BE REALLY DIFFICULT AT FIRST?

A Premature babies can be especially difficult during the first six weeks, crying incessantly and refusing to be comforted, no matter how hard you try, or be very sleepy and reluctant to feed. He or she needs extra care, more frequent feeding, and lots of warmth – but because there is less response you may feel rejected. As he or she matures, you will see a reaction to your care. The check-up is a good time to ask about any problems that are worrying you.

Q CAN IMMUNIZATIONS REALLY CAUSE BRAIN DAMAGE?

A There have been alarming stories about the side-effects of vaccinations, but these cases are rare. There is no firm evidence that immunizations cause brain inflammation (encephalitis) and brain damage. Some babies and children have developed fits and subsequent brain damage shortly after being immunized, but as these problems afflict some babies anyway – even if they are not immunized – it may well be a matter of chance that some of them had received immunizations only a few days earlier.

Q IS THE COMBINED MEASLES, MUMPS, AND RUBELLA (MMR) VACCINATION SAFE?

A There is a balance between the real risks to your child of measles, mumps, and rubella, against a hypothetical and unproven risk of inflammatory bowel disease or autism. There is no evidence that giving separate doses of MMR reduces the risk of adverse effects. In fact, with single doses, your child may miss an injection or it may be delayed, and complete immunity will not occur for many more months compared to the combined MMR. However, single doses are preferable to nothing at all. Ask your doctor, midwife, and health visitor for the most current information.

WHAT IS THE DOCTOR LOOKING FOR?

The six week check is the first of the major developmental assessments for a new baby. Your doctor or local baby clinic will carry out the check in relaxed surroundings. This is a good time to raise any queries you may have about the daily care of your baby.

ROUTINE CHECKS

Your baby is undressed so that the doctor can observe how he or she moves her limbs. Your baby will be examined in detail from head to foot to ensure that physical progress is normal, and you will be asked questions about your baby's feeding and toilet habits, as well as general well-being.

General assessment

The head circumference is measured to check for normal growth, and the fontanelles (soft parts of your baby's head at the front and back where the skull bones meet) are checked for abnormalities. His or her eyes, ears, and mouth are examined; the chest and breathing are checked, and the genitals inspected. The doctor will also feel your baby's abdomen to ensure that the liver, stomach, and spleen are all dpeveloping normally; by manipulating your baby's legs, the hips are checked for possible dislocation.

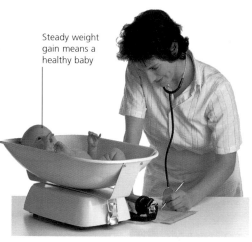

Steady weight gain means a healthy baby

WEIGHING
Your baby will be weighed regularly and the weight gain compared with the birth weight. Normal weight gain usually means a healthy baby; the weight chart will be an important record for months to come.

TONE AND GRASP
The doctor will observe your baby's muscle tone and how the limbs are working. She will also check the "grasp reflex", which demonstrates that your baby can now grasp a finger and hold on.

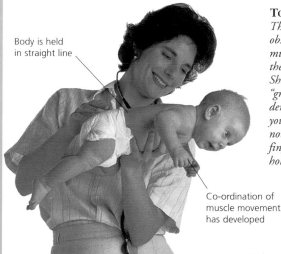

Body is held in straight line

Co-ordination of muscle movement has developed

CONTROL OF HEAD
Now that your baby has some control over the neck muscles, the doctor will see if he or she holds the head in line with the body while being held in the air, and even when moved into a sitting position.

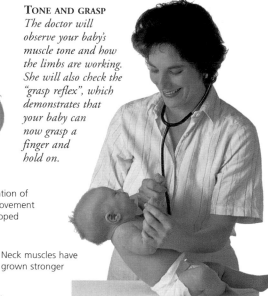

Neck muscles have grown stronger

ENJOYING LIFE WITH YOUR BABY

Q I'M FINDING IT HARD TO ESTABLISH A ROUTINE, WHEN WILL THIS GET EASIER?

A The first weeks following the birth of your baby will have been a period of great upheaval as you juggle the needs of the new baby and those of your partner. So much has had to be learned in a short time, and all your time and energy have been focused on the new arrival. Rest assured that whatever your experience, or lack of it, you will eventually establish a way of life that suits your family and gives you more breathing space. Nights of broken sleep will become easier to cope with or become less frequent. Your baby will soon begin to know the difference between night and day, and become more responsive to you and your partner, making babycare easier and more fun.

Q AM I RIGHT TO WANT TO SPEND ALL MY TIME WITH MY BABY?

A You will automatically feel that the helpless little bundle that you have brought into the world demands all of your time – time you will naturally want to give. What you should do, however, is to try to give your own well-being a high priority; being fit and rested is particularly important if you are breastfeeding. Remember to keep things in perspective. Spend as much time as you want with your baby, but don't forget about yourself and your partner. When you feel ready, ask a family member, friend, or neighbour to mind your baby for an hour or so, so that you can spend time on your own or with your partner.

Q HOW CAN I KEEP IN CONTACT WITH FRIENDS AND FAMILY?

A Once your baby has arrived, it is important to keep in touch with your friends and family for adult conversation, support, and advice, because the constant care of a baby can be quite a burden to shoulder without company, especially if your partner has returned to work. There are usually local "mother and baby groups", which you may already know about through your antenatal classes. If not, your local baby clinic should be able to give you information and addresses. If your antenatal group has a reunion at about six weeks after the birth, this is a good time to find out how everyone else is coping with parenthood.

Q WHEN CAN WE HAVE A NIGHT OUT AND LEAVE THE BABY WITH SOMEBODY ELSE?

A It depends on your confidence. It may be a few weeks or months before you feel relaxed enough to allow others to look after your baby. An evening out with your partner is a major step, but the break from the constant caring for your baby and the return to normality will probably be greatly appreciated by you both. If you are breastfeeding, expressing your milk allows you to leave your baby for a few hours knowing that he or she can be fed.

Q WHAT DO I NEED TO THINK ABOUT BEFORE GOING OUT WITH MY BABY?

A If you use public transport, you will need something lightweight, portable, and easy to assemble and collapse; a pushchair that adapts into a fully reclined position can be ideal (see opposite). A traditional pram is sturdy and excellent for walks, but it is difficult to manage on buses or trains. If you use a car, your pram or pushchair will have to fit into the boot when folded. Also consider whether you and your partner are very different heights; if so, an adjustable pushchair is probably more practical. If you have twins, you can choose either a side by side or back-and-front pushchair; a side-by-side is wider and therefore more difficult to manoeuvre; both have advantages and disadvantages.

Q WHAT CAN I LOOK FORWARD TO IN THE COMING MONTHS?

A Babies are hard work but they are also enormous fun. Watching your baby grow, develop, and discover the world around him or her, makes parenthood a journey of learning that is probably one of the most satisfying experiences that life can offer you and your partner. Your baby will also be learning from you and can detect your moods; the more confident and relaxed you become, the happier he or she will be. As a parent you will have a major influence on the life and personality of your child. The year ahead will be one of unequalled development for your baby and, looking back at the end of the year, it will be difficult to imagine that the laughing boisterous one-year-old toddler was ever a helpless little infant.

GETTING OUT

There is no need to feel marooned at home with your young baby because there is a wide range of prams, buggies, and car seats available. Before buying any equipment, check that it is safe and comfortable for your baby, as well as easy to use and store.

CONVERTIBLE PRAM

This is ideal for a newborn because your baby can lie flat. The carrycot can be removed from the chassis and used as a bed. At six months, a pushchair seat fits on instead.

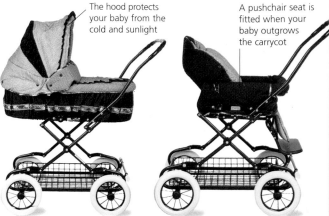

The hood protects your baby from the cold and sunlight

A pushchair seat is fitted when your baby outgrows the carrycot

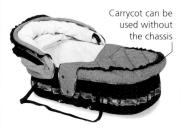

Carrycot can be used without the chassis

CARRYING YOUR BABY

Instead of a pram or a pushchair, you could use a front-carrying sling or a car seat to carry your baby around, giving yourself more freedom of movement.

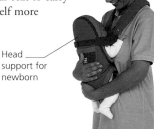

Head support for newborn

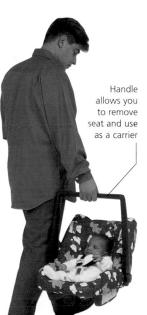

Handle allows you to remove seat and use as a carrier

FRONT-CARRYING SLING
This convenient sling leaves your hands free.

Always strap your baby in

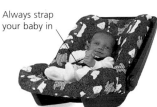

REMOVABLE CAR SEAT
Most car seats can be used as a carrier or low seat. Check that it is the right size for your baby's weight.

THE CHANGING BAG

This is invaluable when you are out and about because it contains everything you need to change and, if necessary, feed your baby.

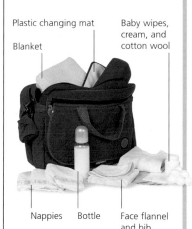

Plastic changing mat

Blanket

Baby wipes, cream, and cotton wool

Nappies   Bottle   Face flannel and bib

WHAT TO PACK
You need the essentials for feeding and changing your baby's nappy (see p. 211), a blanket, a change of clothes for your baby, and later, a favourite toy.

YOUR RIGHTS AND BENEFITS

As soon as you become pregnant you are eligible for certain rights and benefits (see below). To claim these, you should get the appropriate forms from your midwife, doctor's surgery, or local Social Security office. There are deadlines by which you should apply for your benefits, so check the Rights and Benefits Summary (see below, opposite) to ensure that you do not miss out. Soon after the birth, you must register your baby's name and birth at a register office (see opposite). Your rights concerning maternity leave are outlined below.

BENEFITS

■ While pregnant and for a year after the birth, you are entitled to free NHS dental care and prescriptions.
■ If you're a single parent, you may be entitled to one-parent benefit, but not if you co-habit.
■ If you are on a low income, enquire about the possibility of Income Support, Family Credit, Maternity Payments, Housing and Council Tax Benefits, and Health Benefits.

■ If you or your partner is on Income Support, unemployed, or disabled, you may be entitled to a Maternity Payment. This is a single payment to help buy necessities for your baby.
■ Child benefit is a tax-free weekly benefit given irrespective of National Insurance contributions or income. You must register for it within six months of your baby's birth; it will be backdated to the birth date.

IF YOU WORK

If you work for an employer, talk to your employer as soon as possible about your maternity leave and pay. At least 21 days before you intend to stop work, you should confirm in writing to your employer the date you intend to leave, when your baby is due, and when you are planning to return to work. This will protect your right to Statutory Maternity Pay (SMP). If you are self-employed, you are not entitled to SMP, but you may be entitled to a Maternity Allowance. These are both payable for up to 18 weeks.

Maternity leave
■ You are entitled by law to at least 14 weeks' maternity leave, as long as you notify your employer in writing at least 21 days before your maternity leave starts, and your job must be kept open for your return.
■ The earliest date that maternity leave can start is 11 weeks before the week your baby is due.
■ If, by the eleventh week before the expected week of confinement, you have worked for your employer continuously for two years, you're entitled to extended maternity leave of 40 weeks in total.
■ You are entitled to take paid time off work to attend your antenatal clinics and classes.
■ When you are pregnant, you are also protected under the Employment Protection Act against unfair dismissal for maternity-related reasons. If you are suspended from your job for health or safety reasons, your employer is legally obliged to offer you another suitable position or to give you full pay during the period of suspension.
■ To protect your right to return to work, write to your employer at least 21 days before you intend to return.
■ By law, if you have still not returned to work 29 weeks after the birth of your baby, you may lose your right to return to your previous job.

Statutory Maternity Pay
You are entitled to SMP if you have been working for the same company for 26 weeks by the fifteenth week before the week your baby is due, and have earned enough to pay class 1 National Insurance. You will receive 90 per cent of your average weekly earnings for the first six weeks and a flat rate for the next 12 weeks.

Maternity Allowance
If you're not entitled to SMP, perhaps because you have recently given up your job, changed jobs, or you are self-employed, but have paid National Insurance contributions for at least 26 of the 66 weeks before your baby's due date, you can get Maternity Allowance. This is paid for up to 18 weeks, starting any time from 11 weeks before your baby is due. If you don't qualify for SMP or Maternity Allowance, but have paid some National Insurance contributions over the previous three years, you may be entitled to Incapacity Benefit, a weekly benefit paid from six weeks before the birth until two weeks after.

REGISTERING YOUR BABY'S BIRTH

You must register your baby's birth with the Registrar of Births, Deaths, and Marriages within six weeks in England, Northern Ireland, and Wales, and within three weeks in Scotland. Go to the register office local to the hospital where your baby was born because the hospital will have sent details of your baby there. You will be given a birth certificate and a form that will enable you to get a medical card with a National Health Service number so that you can register your baby with your doctor, and a child benefit claim form.

What you need to know

If you are married, only one of you needs to see the registrar. If you are not married to the baby's father and you want his details on the birth certificate, the father must be with you. You must be absolutely clear about your baby's name; if you wish to change even minor details, like the spelling, after the certificate has been issued, you will have to pay for a new certificate, and you can do this only once. A basic certificate is free but there is a more elaborate version for a small fee.

A father's rights

If you are married to the mother of your child, you will have a right to be registered as the father on your child's birth certificate. If you are not married to the mother but you wish to be registered as the father, you must both attend at the registering of the birth.

Registering a stillbirth or a baby who has died

If your baby was stillborn after 24 weeks or died after the birth (regardless of how premature he or she was) your baby should still be registered so that you can get a certificate of burial. You are also still entitled to all benefits, including free prescriptions, dental treatment, Maternity Allowance, and SMP if your baby dies.

RIGHTS AND BENEFITS SUMMARY

WHEN	WHAT TO DO	WHY
As soon as you know you are pregnant	■ If you are working, inform your employer ■ If you're not entitled to SMP, find out about Maternity Allowance (MA)	■ To establish eligibility for SMP and so that you can organize paid time off for antenatal visits
3 weeks before intending to stop work	■ Confirm to your employer in writing when you will stop work, and your return date	■ To protect your right to return to work; and to get SMP
14 weeks before the week your baby is due	■ Ask your doctor/midwife for a maternity certificate (MAT B1; in Northern Ireland, MB1)	■ Your employer needs this
11 weeks before the week your baby is due	■ You can leave work from this date	■ SMP and Maternity Allowance are paid if you have stopped work
As soon after the birth as possible	■ Register the baby's birth ■ Apply for Child Benefit	■ To get a birth certificate, form for an NHS card, and child benefit form
By 6 weeks after the birth (3 weeks in Scotland)	■ You should have registered the baby's birth	■ This is the latest date
7 weeks after the baby was due	■ Write to your employer to confirm that you are returning to work	■ To protect your right to return to work
3 weeks before returning to work	■ Write to your employer with date of return to work	■ To protect your right to return to work
6 months after the birth	■ The latest date to claim Child Benefit and get it backdated to the birth	■ You cannot backdate this more than 6 months
29 weeks after the birth	■ The latest date to return to work	■ You may lose your right to return

USEFUL CONTACTS

LABOUR AND BIRTH

The Active Birth Centre
020 7482 5554
www.activebirth.com

APEC (Action on Pre-eclampsia)
020 8863 3271
www.apec.org.uk

Caesarean Support Network
01624 661269 (after 6 pm)

National Childbirth Trust (NCT)
0870 444 8707
www.nct-online.org

RCOG (Royal College of Obstetricians and Gynaecologists)
020 7772 6200
www.rcog.org.uk
Helpline and leaflets

Splashdown Waterbirth Services
020 8422 9308
www.splashdown.org.uk

TENS Hire
0800 371614

COMPLEMENTARY MEDICINES

British Acupuncture Council
020 8735 0400
www.acupuncture.org.uk

British Homeopathic Association
020 7566 7800
www.trusthomeopathy.org

British Hypnotherapy Association
020 7723 4443

National Institute of Medical Herbalists
01392 426022
www.btinternet.com/~nimh

PARENT GROUPS

Cry-sis Helpline
020 7404 5011
Advice on babies with sleep problems

Gingerbread National Office
020 7488 9300
www.gingerbread.org.uk
Support for one-parent families

National Childminding Association
020 8464 6164
www.ncma.org.uk

National Council for One-Parent Families
0800 018 5026
www.oneparentfamilies.org.uk
Support for those raising a family on their own

The National Meet-a-Mum Association (MAMA)
020 8771 5595
www.mama.org.uk
Help for new mothers, especially those with post-natal depression

TAMBA (Twins and Multiple Birth Association)
0151 348 0020
www.tamba.org.uk
Support for families with twins or higher multiples

Well-being
020 7262 5337
www.wellbeing.org.uk
Women's and babies' health; problems during and after birth

SUPPORT GROUPS

Association for Spina Bifida and Hydrocephalus
01733 555988
www.asbah.org

BLISS
020 7831 9393
www.bobsh.demon.co.uk/bliss
Advice and support for parents with special-care babies

British Diabetic Association
020 7323 1531
www.diabetes.org.uk

British Epilepsy Association
Freephone 0808 800 5050
www.epilepsy.org.uk

Council for Disabled Children
020 78431900
www.ncb.org.uk

Down's Syndrome Association
020 8682 4001
www.dsa-uk.com

MENCAP (Royal Society for Mentally Handicapped Children & Adults)
0207 454 0454
www.mencap.org.uk
For people with learning difficulties

Scope (formerly the Spastics Society)
Helpline 0808 800 3333
www.scope.org.uk

Sickle Cell Society
020 8961 7795
www.sicklecellsociety.org

BREASTFEEDING

Association of Breastfeeding Mothers
020 7813 1481
http://home.clara.net/abm/

La Leche League (Great Britain)
020 7242 1278
www.laleche.org.uk

MATERNITY RIGHTS

AIMS (Association for Improvement in Maternity Services)
01753 652781
www.aims.org.uk

The Maternity Alliance
020 7588 8582
www.maternityalliance.org.uk

MIDWIVES

Association of Radical Midwives
01695 572776
www.radmid.demon.co.uk

Independent Midwives Association
01483 821104
www.independentmidwives.org.uk

Royal College of Midwives
020 7312 3535
www.rcm.org.uk

BEREAVEMENT

ARC (Antenatal Results and Choices)
020 7631 0285

The Foundation for the Study of Infant Deaths
Helpline: 020 7233 2090
General enquiries: 020 7222 8001

The Miscarriage Association
01924 200799
www.miscarriageassociation.org.uk
For advice, information, and support

SANDS (Stillbirth and Neonatal Death Society)
020 7436 7940
www.uk-sands.org

FAMILY PLANNING

British Pregnancy Advisory Service (BPAS)
08457 30 40 30
www.bpas.org

Brooke Advisory Centre
0800 0185023
www.brooke.org.uk

FPA (formerly The Family Planning Association)
020 7837 5432
www.fpa.org.uk

Issue (The National Fertility Association)
01922 722 888
www.issue.co.uk

GENERAL

Association for Post-natal Illness
020 7386 0868
www.apni.org

Department of Health
020 7210 4850
www.doh.gov.uk
www.nhs.uk

Genetic Interest Group
020 7704 3141
www.gig.org.uk

Health Education Agency
020 7222 5300
www.hea.org.uk

UK National AIDS Trust (NAT)
020 7814 6767
www.nat.org.uk

Royal Society for the Prevention of Accidents (RoSPA)
0121 248 2000
www.rospa.co.uk

A GUIDE TO DRUGS IN PREGNANCY

The list below can give only an overview of the most important categories of drugs. For specific requests, you should contact your doctor, pharmacist, or drug manufacturer. Be aware that sometimes not taking a drug means that you are at risk (for example, failing to take anti-malarial or anti-epileptic drugs), and this must be balanced against the negligible risk to the baby's health.

The advice we give is general, and is split into the following categories:

◆ Drugs commonly used in pregnancy and not considered to be associated with serious risk to the baby.

● Drugs that may be used in pregnancy under careful medical supervision. However, they may be associated with fetal side effects.

■ Drugs that would not normally be prescribed in pregnancy.

Analgesics (pain-killers)
◆ Low dose aspirin: (<150mg/day) used to reduce the risk of pre-eclampsia and growth restriction.
● Aspirin in higher doses, and aspirin-like drugs to treat acute or chronic pain: these are best avoided because of their effect on bleeding and fetal kidney function.
◆ Paracetamol: regarded as very safe in the correct dosages.
◆ ● Opiates (pethidine, morphine, heroin): for acute severe pain or in labour: pass to the baby, but safe in short courses.

Anti-acne drugs
■ Oxytetracycline: affects baby's bones and teeth.
■ Retinoic acid-based drugs: these can cause birth defects. Should be avoided for at least three months before becoming pregnant.

Antacids
● Most antacid syrups (used to treat heartburn) are safe, but check instruction/data sheet.

Anti-asthma drugs
◆ Inhaled steroids: these are safe – very little of the dose reaches your own circulation.
◆ Inhaled beta-agonists: these are considered safe.

Antibiotics
◆ Penicillins, erythromycin, and cephalosporins are safe.
■ Tetracycline can affect the baby's bones and teeth.
● Chloramphenicol can affect the baby's bone marrow.
● Co-trimoxazole: these should not be used in the first trimester.

Anti-cancer drugs
● ■ Anti-cancer drugs should be avoided except in rare circumstances. When they are considered essential for the health of the mother, they should be administered after the first trimester, where a small risk to the baby may be weighed against the risk of not treating the mother.

Anti-coagulants
◆ Heparin and other injectable preparations: do not cross the placenta.
● ■ Warfarin: best avoided in first and third trimesters because of the risk of birth defects (first trimester) and fetal bleeding (third trimester).

Anti-depressants
● Lithium is best avoided, but may be used if no alternative available.
◆ Newer generation antidepressant drugs (SSRIs) are probably safe, and haven't been linked to birth defects.

Anti-emetic (sickness) drugs
◆ ● Most are safe but check with your doctor or pharmacist first.

Anti-epileptic treatments
● Carbamazepine, valproate, and phenytoin increase the risk of birth defects slightly if taken in the first trimester, but should not be discontinued in pregnancy, except under expert medical advice.
◆ Newer anti-epileptic drugs may not have this effect.

Anti-hypertensives (high blood pressure drugs)
◆ Methyldopa, labetalol, and nifedipine are considered very safe.
◆ ● Beta blockers may be used in certain circumstances.
■ ACE inhibitors may cause birth defects and fetal kidney damage, and should be avoided.

Anti-malarial drugs
● ■ Best avoided, especially in the first trimester, unless travelling to a malaria endemic zone.

Anti-thyroid drugs
◆ ● May be taken, but may affect baby's thyroid function depending on the dosage used.

Diabetes drugs
◆ Insulin is safe in normal doses.
● ■ Anti-diabetes tablets are not recommended in pregnancy.

Herbal remedies
● Depends on which one. Quality control and analysis of contents is often uncertain. Not recommended unless clearly safe.

Homeopathc remedies
◆ ● Usually safe, but check with prescriber/seller.

Steroids (oral)
◆ ● Unlikely to cause fetal problems; theoretical but very rare risk of fetal cleft palate if taken in large doses early in pregnancy.

Thyroid hormone (thyroxine)
◆ Completely safe, as it doesn't cross the placenta.

GLOSSARY

Abruption Premature separation of the placenta from the wall of the womb.

Amniocentesis A procedure in which a small sample of amniotic fluid is removed from around the baby.

Amniotic fluid The fluid surrounding your baby (known as the waters)

Amniotomy (artificial rupture of membranes ARM) Breaking the membranes using a special plastic hook.

Anaemia Lack of haemoglobin in red blood cells, due to iron deficiency or disease.

Antenatal Before birth.

Antepartum haemorrhage (APH) Vaginal bleeding that happens after 24 weeks of pregnancy and before delivery.

Anti-D An injection of antibodies given to women whose blood group is Rhesus negative, if there is a chance that they have been exposed to fetal blood cells.

Breech The baby is lying bottom down in the womb.

Cardiotocograph (CTG) An electronic monitor used to record the baby's heartbeat and the mother's contractions.

Cephalic The baby is lying head down in the womb.

Chorion villus sampling (CVS) A method for sampling placental tissue for genetic or chromosome studies.

Cilia The fine hairs that line the Fallopian tubes.

Cordocentesis The procedure for taking blood from the baby's umbilical cord via a needle through the abdomen.

Cystitis Infection of the bladder.

Dizygous Non-identical (fraternal) twins.

Doppler A form of ultrasound used specifically to investigate blood flow in the placenta or in the baby.

Down's syndrome (trisomy 21) A disorder caused by the presence of an extra chromosome (21) in the cells.

Ectopic pregnancy A pregnancy that develops outside of the womb.

Embryo The medical term for the baby from conception to about six weeks.

Epidural anaesthesia A method of numbing the nerves of the lower spinal cord to ensure a pain-free labour.

Episiotomy A cut of the perineum and vagina performed by a midwife or doctor to make the delivery easier.

Fallopian tubes Two tubular structures (one on each side of the womb) leading from the ovaries to the womb.

Fetus Medical term for the baby from six weeks after conception until birth.

Fibroid A benign (non-cancerous) growth of muscle of the womb, usually spherically shaped.

Forceps Metal instruments that fit on either side of the baby's head and are used to help deliver the baby.

Fundus The top of the womb.

Haemoglobin (Hb) The oxygen-carrying constituent of red blood cells.

Hepatitis Viruses (named A, B, C, E, and others) that infect the liver, causing jaundice and generalized illness.

Hypertension High blood pressure.

Induction of labour (IOL) The procedure for starting off labour artificially.

In utero death (IUD) The death of the unborn baby after 24 weeks.

In vitro fertilization (IVF) A method of assisted conception in which fertilization occurs in a "test tube" and the embryo is replaced in the womb.

Lanugo The fine hair that covers the fetus in the womb.

Liquor See amniotic fluid.

Lochia Blood loss after the birth.

Membranes Two sets of protective sacs enclosing the baby, called the amnion and the chorion.

Miscarriage The loss of a baby before 24 weeks of pregnancy.

Monozygous Identical twins.

Neonatel A baby less than 28 days old.

Nuchal scan A special ultrasound scan that can check for Down's syndrome.

Oedema Swelling of the fingers, legs, toes, and face.

Oocyte One egg that is released from the ovary at each ovulation.

Placenta A flat, thick disc-shaped organ that supplies the fetus with oxygen and nutrients.

Placenta praevia A placenta situated over, or near to, the cervix which makes a vaginal delivery unlikely.

Post-natal After birth.

Post partum haemorrhage (PPH) Excessive bleeding following delivery.

Pre-eclampsia A condition that features high blood pressure, oedema, and proteinuria. May be mild or serious.

Presentation Describes the way the baby is lying in the womb.

Preterm (premature) labour Labour before 37 weeks of pregnancy.

Puerperium Just after and up to six weeks after delivery.

Rhesus(Rh) factor Blood is either Rhesus positive or Rhesus negative.

Spinal anaesthesia An injection of anaesthetic into the spine for pain relief in labour (similar to an epidural).

Stillbirth Birth of a baby after 24 weeks of pregnancy who shows no signs of life.

Sutures Stitches.

Thrombosis A blood clot, commonly occurring in the calf; most dangerous if in the lungs (pulmonary embolus).

Toxoplasmosis A parasite infection that can be caught from cats or other pets.

Transverse The baby is lying sideways in the womb.

Urinary tract infection (UTI) Infection affecting the kidneys and/or bladder.

Uterus Womb.

Vernix Thick, greasy substance covering the baby's skin in the womb.

INDEX

MEDICAL REFERENCES

The papers listed below will give you an opportunity to read for yourself the original papers that help to shape current practice.

Breastfeeding, worldwide and historical perspectives
Gdalevich M, Mimouni D, Mimouni M. Breast-feeding and the risk of bronchial asthma in childhood: a systematic review with meta-analysis of prospective studies. *Journal of Pediatrics*, 2001; vol. 139(2): pp. 261–6.
Lupton D, Fenwick J. "They've forgotten that I'm the mum": constructing and practising motherhood in special care nurseries. *Social Science Medicine*, 2001; vol. 53(8): pp. 1011–21.

Caesarean section
Graham W J, Hundley V, McCheyne A L, Hall M H, Gurney E, Milne J. An investigation of women's involvement in the decision to deliver by caesarean section. *British Journal of Obstetrics and Gynaecology*, 1999; vol. 106(3): pp. 213–20.
McGurgan P, Coulter-Smith S, O'Donovan P J. A national confidential survey of obstetrician's personal preferences regarding mode of delivery. *European Journal of Obstetrics, Gynecology and Reproductive Biology*, 2001; vol. 97(1): pp. 17–9.

Morning sickness (hyperemesis) and eating disorders
Franko D L, Spurrell E B. Detection and management of eating disorders during pregnancy. *Obstetrics and Gynecology*, 2000; vol. 95(6 Pt 1): pp. 942–6.
Knight B, Mudge C, Openshaw S, White A, Hart A. Effect of acupuncture on nausea of pregnancy: a randomized, controlled trial. *Obstetrics and Gynecology*, 2001; vol. 97(2): pp. 184–8.

Pelvic pain in pregnancy
Albert H, Godskesen M, Westergaard J. Prognosis in four syndromes of pregnancy-related pelvic pain. *Acta Obstetrica Gynecologia Scandinavica*, 2001; vol. 80(6): pp. 505–10.

Prediction of pre-eclampsia
Aquilina J, Thompson O, Thilaganathan B, Harrington K. Improved early prediction of pre-eclampsia by combining second-trimester maternal serum inhibin-A and uterine artery Doppler. *Ultrasound in Obstetrics and Gynecology*, 2001; vol. 17(6): pp. 477–84.
Lees C, Parra M, Missfelder-Lobos H, Morgans A, Fletcher O, Nicolaides K H. Individualized risk assessment for adverse pregnancy outcome by uterine artery Doppler at 23 weeks. *Obstetrics and Gynecology*, 2001; vol. 98(3): pp. 369–73.

Pregnancy, mood changes and depression
Evans J, Heron J, Francomb H, Oke S, Golding J. Cohort study of depressed mood during pregnancy and after childbirth. *British Medical Journal*, 2001; vol. 323(7307): pp. 257–60.
Hayes B A, Muller R, Bradley B S. Perinatal depression: a randomized controlled trial of an antenatal education intervention for primiparas. *Birth*, 2001; vol. 8(1): pp. 28–35.

Screening for Down's syndrome
Cuckle H. Biochemical screening for Down syndrome. *European Journal of Obstetrics, Gynecology and Reproductive Biology*, 2000; vol. 92(1): pp. 97–101.
Nicolaides K H, Heath V, Liao A W. The 11–14 week scan. *Baillieres Best Practice and Research in Clinical Obstetrics and Gynaecology*, 2000; vol. 14(4): pp. 581–94.
Spencer K, Souter V, Tul N, Snijders R, Nicolaides K H. A screening program for trisomy 21 at 10–14 weeks using fetal nuchal translucency, maternal serum free beta-human chorionic gonadotropin and pregnancy-associated plasma protein-A. *Ultrasound in Obstetrics and Gynecology*, 1999; vol. 13(4): pp. 231–7.

Water birth
Eckert K, Turnbull D, MacLennan A. Immersion in water in the first stage of labor: a randomized controlled trial. *Birth*, 2001; vol. 28(2): pp. 84-93.
Ohlsson G, Buchhave P, Leandersson U, Nordstrom L, Rydhstrom H, Sjolin I. Warm tub bathing during labour: maternal and neonatal effects. *Acta Obstetrica Gynecologia Scandinavica*, 2001; vol, 80(4):pp. 311–4.

ACKNOWLEDGMENTS

The authors would like to thank:
Christoph Lees would like to thank Deb and Patrick Conner, Hugh and Patricia Sergeant for their helpful comments and input; to Trish Chudleigh; Dr Edward Petch for advice on mental illness in pregnancy; Dr Lesley Roberts for scouring the text and posing for photographs. Finally, thanks to the staff in the obstetric units at Greenwich and King's Hospitals who, although they may not realize it, inspired this book. Grainne McCartan would like to thank her parents Marion and Xavier; also Gretta Duffy, Xavier McCartan, Sen, Brian, Kim, Patsy, Jenny, Juliet, Peter, Sandra, Linda, Briege, Shirley, Alicia, and Jack for all their help and support.

Dorling Kindersley would like to thank the following:
DESIGN AND EDITORIAL ASSISTANCE Jennifer Bayliss, Sue Callister, Evan Jones, Claudine Meissner, Kylie Mulquin, Fergus Collins, Maureen Rissik, Katherine Robinson, Debbie Voller, Pippa Ward.
DTP ASSISTANCE Ian Merrill, Rachel Symons.
ILLUSTRATORS Joanna Cameron, Karen Cochrane, Sandie Hill, Paul Richardson, Gill Tomblin, Halli Verrinder.

PICTURE CREDITS Chelsea and Westminster Hospital/Dr Paula Ameida 17tl, 17tr; Collections/Anthea Sieveking 159br, 180cl, c, cr, 181l, r, 186br, 202br; Sally Greenhill: 341l, 168bl; Oxford Scientific Film: /Derek Bromhall 61tr; Science Photo Library: /BSIP VEM 59tr; /Dr. Jeremy Burgess 65tr; /J. Croyle/Custom Medical Stock 92; Aaron Haupt 235br; /Joseph Nettis 229br; /Petit Format/Nestle 8tl, 46, 53tr, 63tr; /Row Sutherland 197br; Toshiba Medical Systems:/ Dr Schwerdtfeger 38bl;The Wellcome Institute Library: /Fiona Pragoff 234bl. Every effort has been made to trace the copyright holders and we apologize in advance for any unintentional omissions. We would be pleased to insert the appropriate acknowledgment in any subsequent edition of this publication.

ADDITIONAL PHOTOGRAPHY Eddie Lawrence.
MODELS Sue Berry, Amber Bezer, Ellie Blancke, Tracey Blancke, Emma Burt, Angie Callan, Sue Callister, Louise Clairmont, Roberto Costa, Felicity Crowe, Duane Duncan, Jo Evans, Yvette Fernandez, Lee Goodger, Joany Haig, Toby Judge, Leesa Kotting, Silvia Lagreca, Andrew Lecoyte, Shahida Majeed, Ian Merrill, Mutsumi Niwa, Kelly Priestly, Eleanor Roberts, Leslie Roberts, Katherine Robinson, Charlie Rutherford, Derek Rutherford, Ellena Rutherford, Faye Rutherford, Jo-anne Skinner, Shannon Skinner, Emily Wood.

MAKE-UP Karen Fundell, Lynn Percival.
HOME ECONOMIST Alison Austin.
PROPS, CLOTHES AND EQUIPMENT John Bell & Croydon, Kings Health Care NHS Trust, Mothercare, Blooming Marvellous, Bumpsadaisy, Early Learning Centre.

INDEXER Indexing Specialists, Hove